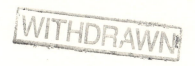

LIVER TRANSPLANTATION: PRACTICE AND MANAGEMENT

LIVER TRANSPLANTATION: PRACTICE AND MANAGEMENT

Edited by

James Neuberger

Consultant Physician
Queen Elizabeth Hospital, Birmingham, UK

Michael R Lucey

Associate Professor of Internal Medicine
Medical Director, Liver Transplant Program
University of Michigan Medical School
Ann Arbor, Michigan, USA

Published by the BMJ Publishing Group
Tavistock Square, London WC1H 9JR

© BMJ Publishing Group 1994

British Library Cataloguing in Publication Data
A catalogue record for this book is available from the British
Library

ISBN 0 7279 0787 5

Typeset, printed and bound in Great Britain by
Latimer Trend & Company Ltd, Plymouth

Contents

IV Management in the transplant unit

V After discharge

VI   Public health issues

List of Contributors

William F Balistreri
Professor of Paediatrics
Department of Paediatric Medicine and Nutrition
Children's Hospital Medical Center
Cincinnati, Ohio, USA

Janet Bellamy
Hospital Chaplain
Queen Elizabeth Hospital
Birmingham, UK

Martin Benjamin
Professor
Department of Philosophy
Michigan State University
East Lansing, Michigan, USA

Thomas Beresford
Professor of Psychiatry
University of Colorado
Psychiatry Service (116A)
Veterans' Administration Medical Center
Denver, Colorado, USA

Mary Beth Becht
Dietitian Specialist
Department of Liver Transplantation
Children's Hospital Medical Center
Cincinnati, Ohio, USA

Daniel K Braun
Assistant Professor of Internal Medicine
Division of Infectious Diseases
Department of Internal Medicine
University of Michigan Medical School
Ann Arbor, Michigan, USA

Christoph Broelsch
Professor of Surgery
University of Hamburg
Universitäts Krankenhause Eppendorf
Hamburg, Germany

Kimberley Ann Brown
Lecturer in Medicine
Division of Gastroenterology
Department of Internal Medicine
University of Michigan Medical School
Ann Arbor, Michigan, USA

Stirling Bryan
Research Fellow
Health Economics Research Group
Brunel University,
Uxbridge, Middlesex, UK

John A C Buckels
Consultant Surgeon
Liver Unit
Queen Elizabeth Hospital
Birmingham, UK

Martin J Buxton
Professorial Research Fellow
Director
Health Economics Research Group
Brunel University
Uxbridge, Middlesex, UK

Mervyn Davies
Research Fellow
Liver Unit
Queen Elizabeth Hospital
Birmingham, UK

Elwyn Elias
Consultant Physician
Liver Unit
Queen Elizabeth Hospital
Birmingham, UK

Robert House
Associate Professor
Department of Psychiatry
University of Colorado School of Medicine
Denver, Colorado, USA

S G Hubscher
Senior Lecturer in Pathology
Department of Pathology
University of Birmingham Medical School
Birmingham, UK

Deidre A Kelly
Consultant Paediatric Hepatologist
Liver Unit
Children's Hospital
Birmingham, UK

John R Lowes
Senior Registrar
Liver Unit
Queen Elizabeth Hospital
Birmingham, UK

Michael R Lucey
Associate Professor of Internal Medicine
Medical Director, Liver Transplant Program
University of Michigan Medical School
Ann Arbor, Michigan, USA

David Mayer
Consultant Surgeon
Liver Unit
Queen Elizabeth Hospital
Birmingham, UK

Geoff McCaughan
Professor
AW Morrow Gastroenterology and Liver Center
Royal Prince Alfred Hospital
Camperdown
New South Wales, Australia

Paul McMaster
Consultant Surgeon
Liver Hepatobiliary Unit
Queen Elizabeth Hospital
Birmingham, UK

Robert M Merion
Associate Professor of Surgery
Chief, Division of Transplantation
Department of Surgery
University of Michigan Medical School
Ann Arbor, Michigan, USA

David Mutimer
Research Fellow
Liver Unit
Queen Elizabeth Hospital
Birmingham, UK

Miquel Navasa
MD
Liver Unit
Hospital Clinic i Provincial
Barcelona, Spain

James Neuberger
Consultant Physician
Liver Unit
Queen Elizabeth Hospital
Birmingham, UK

Michael J Nowicki
Senior Fellow
Department of Paediatric Gastroenterology and Nutrition
Children's Hospital Medical Center
Cincinnati, Ohio, USA

Suzanna I Park
Assistant Professor of Medicine
Lexington Clinic
Gastroenterology Division
Lexington, Kentucky, USA

Antoni Rimola
Associate Professor of Medicine
Liver Unit
Hospital Clinic i Provincial
Barcelona, Spain

Joan Rodés
Professor of Medicine
Liver Unit
Hospital Clinic i Provincial de Barcelona
Barcelona, Spain

Xavier Rogiers
Department of General Surgery
University Hospital
Hamburg, Germany

Frederick C Ryckman
Associate Professor of Surgery
Division of Paediatric Surgery
University of Cincinnati
Cincinnati, Ohio, USA

Susan Pederson Ryckman
Manager
Department of Liver Transplantation
Children's Hospital Medical Center
Cincinnati, Ohio, USA

Christopher S Shorrock
Lecturer
Department of Medicine
Queen Elizabeth Hospital
Birmingham, UK

Jeremiah G Turcotte
Professor of Surgery
Director of Organ Transplantation Center and Liver Transplant
  Program
University of Michigan Medical Center
Ann Arbor, Michigan, USA

Preface

The last decade has seen a dramatic increase both in the numbers of patients receiving a liver transplant, and in the length and quality of survival after transplantation. Because of this, an increasing number of primary care physicians are looking after patients who either are potential liver allograft recipients or have received a liver allograft. Our own experience suggests that there is little readily accessible information to assist primary care physicians with the practical aspects of management of such patients. Therefore, we felt that there was the need for a book aimed primarily at experienced physicians who see patients both pre- and post-transplantation, but whose practice is not based in liver units. It is for these doctors that this book is designed. We hope that this book will prove a valuable guide also to medical students and physicians in training, as a brief but comprehensive handbook for their time passing through a liver transplant service.

Although this book has been written primarily by members of the liver units in Ann Arbor and in Birmingham, we have drawn on the experience of experts in a number of other centres around the world. We appreciate that every liver transplant unit has its own management protocol, and so have tried to illustrate the general principles and give specific details as appropriate. We realise that there are some duplication and divergence of views. We have not edited these to produce uniformity because they serve to illustrate areas of uncertainty.

Finally, we would like to thank all those who have made this book possible – the contributing authors; our secretaries, Miss Michelle Calcutt and Mrs Evonne Levigne; Dr Belinda Keogh and Dr Patricia Hughes; finally we would like to thank Dr Robert Allan, Editor of *Gut* for the idea for the book, and Mary Banks at the BMJ and Jane Sugarman for their editorial skills and assistance.

James Neuberger, Michael Lucey
November 1993

I: Introduction

1: The development of liver transplantation

PAUL McMASTER

Few undertakings in clinical surgical practice can have presented quite the challenges involved in the development of liver transplantation. Not only were the complexities of the surgical technique involved formidable, but all too often the organs implanted were of poor quality. Patients often succumbed to technical complications or graft failure, and those who survived were exposed to the ravages of graft destruction from rejection. Understandably, therefore, the risks of the procedure were such that few patients would be grafted unless in a late phase of liver decompensation often with multiorgan failure, gross clotting derangement, and usually sepsis. Many patients died while waiting for organs to become available, and before the concept of brain stem death and the retrieval of organs from heart-beating cadavers, the potential donor grafts experienced significant deterioration just before harvesting. Liver grafting was little more than a high risk, complex, emergency procedure in the critically ill.

It is therefore perhaps inevitable that few patients survived these early efforts at transplantation; there were those who called for a moratorium until many of the principal difficulties could be overcome. Slowly, the initial pioneering programmes became established, with early clinical attempts in 1963 by Starzl,[1] building on the 1950s laboratory work of Welch[2] and others. In Europe, Calne[3] (Cambridge, 1968) instituted a major programme in conjunction with King's College Hospital which was to contribute so much to our understanding of liver transplantation. An operation with such a pernicious reputation for massive haemorrhage and with consumption of blood products often running to hundreds of units was to come slowly under control as more effective monitoring of intra-operative coagulopathy, using thromboelastographs, and blood saving autotransfusion and bypass, was developed. Soon, blood product needs were little more than those used for other complex major surgery; currently, it is not uncommon for transplantation to be undertaken without the use of blood at all.

In part, this more effective control of bleeding was related to a marked improvement in quality of donor organs. Those clinicians who have not lived through the experience of organ retrieval from non-heart-beating cadavers will rarely appreciate the anguish of waiting until there is no clinical sign of cardiac activity. The liver often became irreparably damaged in the 20–30 minutes it took for cardiac function to cease, although this fact only became clear after implantation, when primary graft failure occurred with death of the recipient. The concept of brain stem death, and its much wider recognition and support in the late 1970s and 1980s, led to fewer poor quality organs being harvested and more liver grafts becoming available for transplantation. Although, in the early stages, as many as half the patients would die while waiting for a transplant, a progressive reduction in deaths on waiting lists occurred as better quality organs increasingly became available. Even so, such operations were for the most part undertaken in haste, with teams rushing to potential donor hospitals and long operations being undertaken through the night. The introduction of improved organ perfusion with the solution developed at the University of Wisconsin was an important practical and logistical step forward; this solution extended the time that the organ could be stored with excellent function. Suddenly liver transplantation could become a semi-elective procedure with grafts being stored for 10–14 hours.

Although initially the operation itself had presented major clinical challenges in some respects, the postoperative period represented an even greater challenge. Patients returning after such major surgery, who had been critically ill at the time of liver grafting, had poor tolerance of the high steroid schedule so often used, in the early years, to prevent rejection. Biliary complications frequently led to sepsis and the "lethal triangle" of sepsis, rejection, and technical complication often led to failure. All too often it was necessary to stop immunosuppression to prevent patients dying from sepsis, only to result in rejection of the liver. Re-transplantation became increasingly accepted as a means of salvaging such patients, and some teams had re-transplantation rates approaching 20%. Nowadays many groups have re-graft rates of less than 5%, and chronic rejection is infrequently seen.

As, slowly, the risks of transplantation decreased, so the spectrum of patients accepted was extended. Emergency liver grafting for fulminant hepatic failure had long been felt to be inappropriate both because of the difficulty in categorising the nature of fulminant hepatic failure and its prognosis, and because a successful outcome to liver grafting was rarely possible as a result of the instability of the patient; nowadays, liver transplant operations for fulminant hepatic failure represent nearly a third of clinical programmes. The young infant of less than 10 kg weight and the "old" of over 60 years, who were initially excluded, can now expect excellent rehabilitation. Currently, more than 80% of patients will be active and well at 1 year post-transplantation. In 1980 the figure was a mere 30%.

Improved survival has been associated with improved quality of life. The introduction of cyclosporin A (cyclosporine) was a seminal event, leading not just to improved liver graft survival but to a reduction in the steroid complication previously seen so frequently and which had increased risk of infection. Children now grow normally; none of the cushingoid facies resulting from high dose steroids and complications associated with diabetes or bone necrosis has been seen. Patients can now truly be considered to follow a normal life pattern; indeed, for the majority, studies show that self-esteem and personal fulfilment are often higher than in the "normal" population!

Barely a decade ago, liver transplantation was still considered by many gastroenterologists to be a dangerous and almost experimental undertaking. Very few patients were referred and transplant numbers were small. In 1980 fewer than 50 grafts were performed across Europe, whereas in 1990 more than 2000 patients were transplanted by more than 60 clinical groups. In North America, a new stimulus for the growth of liver transplantation was the National Institutes of Health's Consensus Development Conference on Liver Transplantation in 1983, which declared that liver transplantation was a "therapeutic modality for end-stage liver disease that deserves broader application". This indicated that liver transplantation had advanced from being an experimental procedure to becoming a legitimate form of therapy. The expansion of liver transplantation in North America has mirrored that in Europe; in

5

1990 more than 2600 liver transplantation procedures were performed in more than 85 centres.

From an infrequent, hazardous emergency and an often heroic endeavour, which usually followed a dramatic dash across the countryside with police escort, liver grafting can now usually be considered as almost a semi-elective undertaking. Although organ shortage remains a problem, particularly in children, harvesting can frequently take place early in the evening with organ preparation and recipient counselling, and surgery can be commenced semi-electively the next morning. Procedures are usually completed within 4 or 5 hours with minimal blood loss, and patients returned to the general ward after less than 48 hours of intensive care. Our increased immunosuppressive armamentarium, combined with greater histological monitoring for early signs of graft damage or rejection, mean that for many the postoperative period can be relatively straightforward provided that the hazards of infection and rejection can be successfully avoided.

Liver transplantation is thus a treatment that should be constantly borne in mind by clinicians caring for patients with advancing liver disease. The care of such patients – from the very first recognition of hepatic problems to the eventual successful long-term outcome after grafting – requires careful monitoring and review. Through the recognition of the gravity of the hepatic problem, a clear plan of appropriate care is instituted. The avoidance of inappropriate procedures, which may be of little benefit, is also important and surgical portal shunting has become a less frequent procedure. Thereafter, the successful evaluation and undertaking of transplantation will require teams working closely together, supported by high quality laboratory services, physiotherapists, social workers, transplant organisations, and coordinators. The combined care of these patients, in the long term, requires careful monitoring of the immunosuppressive agents to avoid complications.

In many ways, the final phase in the development of liver transplantation will be total incorporation of all those patients with additional complex problems, such as intestinal failure, those who require composite multi-organ grafts, such as liver and small bowel, and others who require liver and kidney, liver and heart/lungs transplantations. Attempts at xenografting humans are already under way, and perhaps the use of temporary auxiliary grafts will find an appropriate place in the support of patients with potentially reversible liver conditions. Many major challenges remain for the future: the need to contain the cost of transplantation; the need to increase organ availability; the search for alternatives to orthotopic human grafts, such as using xenografts or isolated hepatocytes; alternative strategies for immunosuppression by, for example, making the recipient more tolerant; and more successful methods to prevent or control disease recurrence.

There could be no better reward than the current clinical successes, now seen almost routinely in major transplant programmes, for those who struggled for years to develop liver transplantation in order to support patients with critically injured livers.

There are few endeavours in clinical/surgical practice at this time that can transform such critically ill patients to normal rehabilitation.

References

1 Starzl TE. *Experiences in Hepatic Transplantation*. Philadelphia: WB Saunders, 1969.
2 Welch CS. A note on transplantation of the whole liver in dogs. *Transplant Proc* 1955; **2**: 54–8.
3 National Institutes of Health Consensus Conference. *Hepatology* 1984; **4**(suppl 1).

II: When to refer for transplantation

2: General considerations

JAMES NEUBERGER, CHRISTOPHER S SHORROCK

The current results of liver transplantation are such that no patient should die from liver disease without liver transplantation having been considered by his or her physician. In some patients clearly this may be no more than a passing thought to be rapidly dismissed, although current evidence and experience suggest that many people who are potential transplant recipients are dying without transplantation having been considered as a therapeutic option.[1] In the early days of liver transplantation, patients were often referred in a terminally ill state, and surgeons were expected to perform miracles, resuscitating dying patients. As confidence in liver transplantation has grown among members of the medical profession, patients are being referred at a more appropriate stage. If the patient is referred too late then the chances of a successful outcome after transplantation are severely limited. Conversely, because of the short and long term risks of the procedure, if a patient is referred and transplanted too early in the course of the illness, then there is a significant risk that the patient's life will be prematurely shortened. Thus, appropriate timing of referral and transplantation is all important for the optimal management of the patient. The best way to ensure this is close liaison between referring physicians and transplant centres to facilitate mutual appreciation of one another's problems: timely referral of the patient will allow the patient time to consider all options; and appropriate timing of listing will allow for the inevitable and increasing delay in finding an organ, before progression of the disease reduces the patient's chances of surviving the procedure or else precludes transplantation altogether.

In general terms, orthotopic liver transplantation is considered for one of two indications:

- Anticipated length of life of less than one year resulting from liver disease.

● Quality of life is intolerable for the patient as a result of liver disease.

These two principles, which are relatively easy to define in theory, are often very difficult to extrapolate to the individual patient. As discussed later, when different diseases are considered, those factors that predict reduced survival can be relatively well defined for a population, and yet extrapolation to the individual, because of the uncertainties of unpredictable events such as sepsis or variceal haemorrhage, makes accurate prediction difficult. Although the development of prognostic models has been of great help, the wide confidence limits when applied to an individual pose severe limitations on their over-zealous application.

Equally, quality of life is difficult to define for the individual. A quality of life that is acceptable to one patient may be intolerable to another. Although the physician is usually able to make a reasonable assessment of the patient's prognosis, assessment of the patient's quality of life is very subjective. As discussed elsewhere, chronic illness has a major effect on both the patient and his or her family: coping mechanisms include the development of a sick role. Correction of the liver disease is not necessarily associated with an alteration in the sick role.

There are a few circumstances when it may be appropriate to offer a transplant to a patient who has a normal liver; such indications are rare and may include, for example, those metabolic diseases where a consequence of any liver abnormality results in the likelihood of early death. One example is familial hypercholesterolaemia where the child may die at a young age from coronary artery disease. Liver transplantation will correct the metabolic defect and some centres are now using liver transplantation before the development of significant coronary atheroma.

It is important to consider the patient's age; initial studies confined transplantation to patients aged below 55 years, but as results improved and indications widened, the age limit increased. Few centres now have an upper age limit on potential candidates, and consider biological age rather than chronological age. This has the advantage of being less readily definable. As most series suggest that survival in the highly selected patients aged over 60 years is at least as good as in those who are younger, it seems sensible to consider each patient on his or her own merit; the decision to offer transplantation will depend on the extent of restriction and the expectation of life in the absence of liver disease. Such babies and neonates are considered in the paediatric section (p 84–87).

There are six factors that should be considered in any patient who is a potential candidate for transplantation, and these relate to the following questions:

- Are the patient's symptoms due to liver disease?
- Have less aggressive treatments been tried?
- Will transplantation "cure" the patient?
- Are there technical problems precluding a successful outcome?
- When is the optimum time to offer transplantation?
- Does the patient want a liver transplant?

Are the patient's symptoms due to liver disease?

Although for many patients the answer to this question is straightforward, in some instances it may be less difficult to answer. For example, lethargy may be difficult to define and to disentangle the lethargy associated with chronic cholestatic liver disease from an associated depression is often difficult. It is important to exclude other treatable causes such as myxoedema, Addison's disease, or nutritional deficiency which may be responsible for the patient's symptoms.

Are there other treatments available?

As a result of the associated morbidity and mortality of liver transplantation, it is important to consider all other medical therapies before transplantation is indicated.

In some instances, surgical intervention may be indicated. For example, in a patient with recurrent, life threatening, variceal haemorrhage, but good liver function, it may be worth doing a transjugular intrahepatic portosystemic shunt (TIPS) or a surgical shunt. If encephalopathy develops, then transplantation is indicated.

Will liver transplantation "cure" the patient?

There seems little point in asking a patient to go through a transplant procedure unless the patient is likely to be cured or have his or her symptoms alleviated for a reasonable period of time. Thus, in patients with hepatic malignancy, if there is evidence of extrahepatic spread, it is extremely unlikely that the patient will live long enough to derive the benefits of the procedure and, therefore, transplantation is inappropriate. Nevertheless, the effect of recurrence and the associated morbidity need to be considered.

Some metabolic diseases may recur or persist. However, clinically significant recurrence of disease may be delayed so that it becomes appropriate to transplant patients even if a cure is not possible. Such instances include transplantation for carcinoid type tumours and for those metabolic diseases, such as haemochromatosis, where the disease is likely to recur, and in autoimmune diseases, such as primary biliary cirrhosis, where recurrence of disease has been suggested despite remaining controversial. There is more uncertainty about the role of transplantation in those diseases where recurrence is likely to recur in a shorter period of time, e.g. the rare metabolic disease sea blue histiocyte disease or protoporphyria.

As discussed elsewhere, transplantation for primary hepatic malignancy remains controversial. The major risk is that of disease recurrence which may occur 3–5 years after transplantation. Nevertheless, in the absence of transplantation, the prognosis of a patient with primary hepatic malignancy is very bleak, and so the patient and his or her medical advisers may feel that transplantation is appropriate even though the chances of long term success (i.e. greater than 10 years) may be limited.

Transplantation for infective hepatitis may be associated with disease recurrence. Where graft infection is likely to be associated with clinically significant disease and poor survival, such as hepatitis B virus (HBV) DNA positive patients, transplantation may not be indicated. In contrast, with hepatitis C virus (HCV) infection, graft infection is not associated with any reduction in quality of life in the medium term, and, therefore, the possibility of disease recurrence is not a contraindication to grafting.

Are there technical reasons precluding a successful outcome?

As the experience of both surgeons and anaesthetists has increased, and newer techniques have been introduced, the contraindications to transplantation have decreased. Considerations apply broadly in two areas: vascular and extrahepatic disease. In the early years a thrombosed portal vein was considered an absolute contraindication to transplantation, but in recent years it has become appreciated that portal blood can be provided to a graft from either the superior mesenteric vein or the splenic vein. In the presence of thrombosis of both these veins, then it may not be feasible to perform at transplantation. Equally, thrombosis of the inferior vena cava may preclude successful transplantation.

The presence of previous upper abdominal surgery, although it may considerably increase the technical problems associated with the procedure, does not pose an absolute contraindication to a procedure. Previous gastric surgery, in particular in patients with established portal hypertension, presents major technical challenges.

Extrahepatic considerations include those conditions that will result in the patient being unable to survive the surgery or the perioperative period. Thus, advanced cardiac or pulmonary disease (discussed below) will prevent successful transplantation. Attention must also be paid to extrahepatic disease that may affect patient rehabilitation after successful surgery, e.g. those with progressive neurological disease may survive the early operative period, but are not restored to a satisfactory level of health.

Does the patient want a liver transplantation?

In patients with fulminant hepatic failure, the patient may be encephalopathic on arrival at hospital; clearly he or she will be in no position to make his or her wishes known. In such cases the decision has to be made by the relatives. The inherent problems associated with the patient unable to give consent are linked to significant problems of rehabilitation in the short term. Thus, patients who, prior to the recent onset of the illness, will have been in perfectly normal health will require medical supervision and medication, with all its consequences, for the rest of their lives. Despite the excellent quality of life that may be achieved after transplantation, it is unrealistic to claim that this is completely normal.

In contrast, patients with chronic liver disease are accustomed to suboptimal health and, therefore, any improvement is usually greatly appreciated. It is usually extremely valuable for the patient to come to the transplant centre well before the time of transplantation, so that the patient can meet not only the transplant team but also other patients and their relatives. Only in this way can the patient fully appreciate all the inherent stresses associated with the procedure and also the stresses and traumas of being on the waiting list; it is also then possible to assess the complications and problems after the transplantation. In order for the patient to form a balanced view of the risks and benefits of liver transplantation and to make an informed decision, the patient must be in possession of all the facts.

When is the optimum time to offer the patient for transplantation?

This is perhaps the most difficult area to define. For those receiving a transplant for intolerable quality of life, transplantation is indicated as soon as it becomes clear that the patient's quality of life is unacceptable and there is no chance of improvement either because of disease progression or from therapeutic intervention.

Timing of transplantation for patients with chronic disease is far more difficult to define and involves assessment of the risk factors both of surviving in the absence of transplantation and of dying from the procedure. Until such time that these can be accurately quantified for any individual patient, assessment of timing is largely a matter of clinical experience and judgement. Because of the inherent difficulties of such an approach, such considerations are discussed in much greater detail later in the book.

Unsuitability for transplantation

Having decided that the patient's condition is severe enough to warrant liver transplantation, it is necessary to consider those factors that would seriously impair or prevent survival during the first 2 years following transplantation. Because of the need to undergo prolonged general anaesthesia and major abdominal surgery, general principles regarding fitness for surgery apply. Also patients will need to take life-long immunosuppressive treatment, and will need to be suitably motivated, and capable of taking potentially complicated and changing drug regimens.

There are no absolute rules about coexisting extrahepatic disease, but a number of significant specific conditions need mentioning, and these are dealt with below, and in the boxes.

16

BOX A   Absolute contraindications to transplantation

AIDS
Active sepsis
Metastatic cancer
Extrahepatic cancer (other than local skin cancer)
Severe pulmonary hypertension
Advanced cardiac disease
Advanced pulmonary disease

BOX B   Relative contraindications to liver transplantation

Age >65 years
Diabetes mellitus
Previous malignancy
Past psychiatric illness
Active alcohol abuse
Cardiac disease
HIV infection
Hepatitis B virus DNA positivity
Previous biliary surgery

Diabetes mellitus

Well controlled non-insulin and insulin-dependent diabetes, without evidence of end organ damage, produce few additional management problems during transplantation and are, in general, not a contraindication. FK506 and, to a lesser degree, cyclosporin A (cyclosporine) have a tendency to induce diabetes; thus, following transplantation hypoglycaemic requirements may increase and blood sugar is more difficult to control. Corticosteroids will also exacerbate the tendency to diabetes and increased insulin requirements. Hyperglycaemia before transplantation may, in part, be due to end organ resistance resulting from the liver disease and as such reverses following surgery.

Diabetic patients with liver disease have a greater incidence of autonomic neuropathy, which may significantly increase the risk of intraoperative death. The presence of a diabetic retinopathy is often associated with nephropathy and peripheral neuropathy. As with any patient with liver disease, there are multiple potential causes of renal impairment and in those with significant nephropathy (proteinuria, miscroscopic haematuria, or creatinine clearance of less than 60 ml/min), a renal biopsy often gives useful information. In the presence of a diabetic nephropathy, liver transplantation alone is considered inappropriate in many centres.

Cardiac disease

The purpose of cardiac screening is to identify ischaemic heart disease and cardiomyopathy which would increase the risk of death. Initial screening will include history taking and a clinical examination. Investigations at this stage include chest radiograph and ECG in all potential candidates. Additional investigations are routinely performed in some centres. Further evaluation is recommended in patients who are at greater risk of heart disease, such as those aged over 45 years and smokers, those with a history of ischaemic heart disease, peripheral vascular disease, hypertension, or hyperlipidaemia, and those with alcoholic liver disease and haemochromatosis. The available additional tests include exercise ECG, multigated acquisition (MUGA) or thallium scanning, echocardiography, or coronary angiography. The relative value of these tests as predictors of outcome after liver transplantation has not been studied prospectively.

Significant and surgically correctable cardiac lesions should be treated before liver transplantation. This should be considered after discussion with the transplant team. In those with a left ventricular ejection fraction of below 40%, transplantation is inappropriate.

Peripheral vascular disease

Due to the generalised nature of the disease, clinical evidence of significant peripheral vascular disease usually precludes transplantation as an option for liver disease.

Pulmonary disease

Patients can only be considered for liver transplantation if they have sufficiently good pulmonary function to survive prolonged periods of ventilation; standard lung function tests and blood gases should be measured. Patients with irreversible airway disease and lung function tests less than 65% of predicted values are, in general, not suitable for liver transplantation. However, lung function tests must be assessed with regard to the patient's clinical condition; the presence of ascites or massive hepatomegaly may be associated with restrictive lung function tests. These abnormalities will be corrected when the ascites is removed or the liver size returned to normal. The presence of a pleural effusion, which may be associated with ascites, may also give misleading lung function tests. Pulmonary hypertension may be associated with liver disease, especially primary biliary cirrhosis, or portacaval shunting. Significant pulmonary hypertension greatly increases the risks of using an anaesthetic. Such patients may require combined heart/lung and liver transplantation.

The presence of arterial hypoxia (arterial oxygen partial pressure or Pao_2 of < 6.65 kPa or 50 mmHg) is reported to be an absolute contraindication to transplantation. Although some patients may have intrinsic lung disease, the presence of the hepatopulmonary syndrome must be considered. Intrapulmonary shunts are associated with chronic liver disease and these may improve with time following successful transplantation.

Reversible airway obstruction (asthma)

In well controlled patients this usually produces few additional problems but severe asthmatic individuals may not be appropriate candidates.

Renal disease

Of all the risk factors suggesting a poor outcome after surgery, most series have shown that impaired renal function is one of the best prognostic indicators of poor outcome. Renal disease may be due to intrinsic renal disease or hepatorenal syndrome. In the latter case, successful transplantation will be associated with a return to normal of renal function. However, in the presence of other causes of chronic renal disease, the nephrotoxic effect of cyclosporin A or FK506 may lead to progressive renal damage such that dialysis is required. Alternatively, it may be appropriate to do a combined liver and kidney transplantation.

Psychiatric disease

It is clear that patients with long-standing major psychoses are inappropriate candidates for transplantation either if they would not benefit from the procedure or if they would find the stresses of the follow up unacceptable. Nevertheless, psychiatric assessment and evaluation of a patient with liver disease are often very difficult: the mental state may be affected by subclinical hepatic encephalopathy or there may well be a depression that is consequent upon the chronic state of ill health. In general, the patient is well able to make decisions and commonsense usually dictates the appropriate course of action.

Drug dependence

For patients with a drug dependence, the decision to offer patients transplantation may be difficult. Problems associated with dependence on alcohol and/or other drugs are discussed elsewhere (p 27–32); however, previous use of "recreational" drugs is not a contraindication to grafting, although continued and active use of such drugs does pose a bar to grafting because of the risks of non-compliance and of acquiring infections.

Previous abdominal surgery

Previous operations such as portosystemic shunt, cholecystectomy, or biliary tract surgery do not preclude transplantation but make the operation technically more difficult and carry a higher risk of perioperative problems. With the exception of biliary tract surgery in patients with primary sclerosing cholangitis, the presence of right upper quadrant surgery has not been shown to affect the outcome significantly.

Infection

As a result of the effects of surgery and the subsequent immunosuppression, patients with active sepsis should not be considered until the sepsis has been treated. Dental sepsis is not uncommon in patients with chronic liver disease. In all cases, the teeth should be assessed and any infection treated aggressively before listing.

Most centres will exclude those who are HIV positive. Current

---

BOX C Effect of immunosuppression on pre-existing cancers (from Penn[2])

Tumours with low recurrence rate (0–10%)
    Incidental renal neoplasm
    Testicular tumours
    Thyroid carcinoma
    Lymphoma
Tumours with intermediate recurrence rate (11–25%)
    Carcinoma of the body of the uterus
    Wilms' tumour
    Colon carcinoma
    Prostate adenocarcinoma
    Breast cancer
Tumours with high recurrence rate (>26%)
    Bladder carcinoma
    Sarcoma
    Melanoma
    Myeloma

---

evidence suggests that patients who are HIV positive, but do not have any AIDS related symptoms, do reasonably well after surgery although those who have either AIDS related complex (ARC) or AIDS will have their condition exacerbated by the immunosuppression.

Previous malignancy

This is a difficult area. Our view is that recurrent malignancy is an absolute contraindication to transplantation; the presence of previous malignancy will depend on the nature of the cancer, its probability of cure, and the time that has elapsed since the cancer was diagnosed. Although there is an increased risk of de novo malignancy after transplantation, the question of whether immunosuppressive therapy will affect the rate of growth of pre-existing malignancy remains uncertain. In general, patients with a history of malignancy should be considered as suitable candidates when all indications suggest that the tumour has been successfully removed. Penn[2] has identified those tumours with low, intermediate, and high risk of recurrence (Box C).

Electrolyte disturbance

In patients with no intrinsic renal disease, such abnormalities are usually the result of hepatorenal failure, inappropriate use of diuretics, and other measures. Correction of electrolytes is important before transplantation and this can be done either by medical means or by use of dialysis.

If the serum sodium is below 125 mmol/l, there is a significant risk that replacement of body fluids will be associated with a rapid change in serum sodium leading to central pontine myelinolysis. So, where possible, serum sodium should be gradually corrected before surgery, by discontinuing diuretics, by water restriction, or even by dialysis, as appropriate.

Variceal haemorrhage

It is preferable for variceal haemorrhage to be controlled before transplantation. Although injection sclerotherapy is highly effective in controlling variceal haemorrhage, the high incidence of oesophageal ulcers consequent upon sclerotherapy puts the patient at risk of developing empyema in the post-transplantation period. However, the advent of banding techniques and percutaneous portosystemic shunts may allow more rapid control of variceal bleeding tendencies without risk of inducing other complications.

Nutrition

Many patients with end stage liver disease are malnourished; the reasons are multifactorial, including poor intake, malabsorption, and poor hepatic function. Although there is increasing evidence that those who are malnourished fare worse after grafting, there is little evidence in adults that preoperative feeding alters the outcome. It is clearly sensible to correct any vitamin deficiency and encourage patients to take a high protein diet; advantages of correcting protein deficiency outweigh the potential disadvantages of precipitating encephalopathy.[3]

Logistical considerations

The patient must be made aware of the other, non-medical implications of transplantation. Financial implications must be carefully considered. Even when the cost of the actual procedure is borne by the state or an insurance company, there are the additional costs incurred for the patient or members of his or her family through time off work, the additional costs of travel to and from hospital, and, depending on the situation, costs of drugs and tests. All these factors need to be considered before embarking on transplantation.

Psychological support also needs to be assessed. Most patients will need strong psychological support at all stages. In many cases, this support will be provided by the patient's family, but, in some, this may not be possible or appropriate. Before a patient goes on the transplant list, the need for, and provision of support before, during, and after, must be discussed. Although the decision to accept transplantation must be made by the patient, we believe that it is very important to discuss the full implications and to gain the support of the patient's partner or family.

Alternatives to orthotopic liver transplantation

The vast majority of organ transplantations are performed using orthotopic liver transplantation, ie, the diseased liver is removed and the donor liver (or part of the donor liver) is grafted in that site. Thus, orthotopic liver transplantation corrects not only the metabolic abnormalities, but also the associated portal hypertension. There are alternatives to orthotopic liver transplantation. Auxiliary transplantation has also been advocated; the donor liver can be located either in the right iliac fossa or in the space provided by resection of the recipient left lobe. This approach has several theoretical advantages, particularly in those where there is the possibility that the host liver may recover (as may occur in some instances of fulminant hepatic failure) and allow removal of the graft or where the donor liver can correct metabolic abnormalities (as may occur in primary hypercholesterolaemia).[4-6] Auxiliary liver transplantation was introduced when the recipient hepatectomy was a major problem, often needing 100 or more units of blood; now blood use is much less and the median blood usage in adults in our centre is 5 units.

Initial results of auxiliary grafts were poor, resulting from a combination of factors, including lack of space in the abdomen and vascular problems. These technical problems have been largely overcome. The role of auxiliary liver transplantation remains uncertain. In those with pre-existing cirrhosis, there is the proven possibility of hepatocellular carcinoma developing in the host liver. There are studies currently under way to compare orthotopic and auxiliary liver transplantation in different clinical settings.

Because of the scarcity of donor organs and because of the many problems still outstanding with liver transplantation, alternative approaches are being assessed. These alternatives include the use of hepatocyte transplantation and of xenografts. At present, these remain largely experimental but are likely to reach clinical practice in the future.

Conclusions

The decisions about who to refer and when to refer must be based on individual considerations of both indications and contraindications. The absolute contraindications are relatively few. Optimal management of any patient who is a potential candidate for transplantation is dependent on close liaison and mutual confidence between the attending physician and the transplant unit. The development and maintenance of close communication should allow for optimum management of such patients.

References

1 Davies MH, Langman MJS, Elias E, Neuberger J. Liver disease in a district hospital remote from a transplant centre: a study of admissions and deaths. *Gut* 1992; **33**: 1397–9.
2 Penn I. Effect of immunosuppression on pre-existing cancers. *Transplant Proc* 1993; **25**: 1380–2.
3 Kearns PJ, Young H, Garcia G, *et al*. Accelerated improvement of alcoholic liver disease with enteral nutrition. *Gastroenterology* 1992; **102**: 200–5.
4 Terpstra OT. Auxiliary liver grafting: a new concept in liver transplantation. *Lancet* 1993; **342**: 758.
5 Boudjema K, Jaeck D, Simeoni U, Bientz J, Chenard MP, Brunot P. Temporary auxiliary liver transplantation for subacute liver failure in a child. *Lancet* 1993; **342**: 778–9.
6 Whitington P, Emond JC, Heffron T, Thistlethwaite JR. Orthotopic auxiliary liver transplantation for Crigler–Najjar syndrome type 1. *Lancet* 1993; **342**: 779–80.

3: Psychiatric evaluation of liver transplant candidates

ROBERT HOUSE, THOMAS BERESFORD

In this section psychiatric factors impinging on selection of suitable candidates for liver transplantation are reviewed, together with those factors that clinical experience has noted as salient in preoperative care of such patients. The reader is referred to Craven and Rodin[1] and Vaillant[2] for further specific in-depth information.

Psychiatric symptoms

With the diagnosis of advanced liver failure patients often pass through a series of psychological stages: denial, anger, accentuation of personality characteristics, magical expectations, idealisation, and acceptance.[3] Denial often takes the form of disbelief that a transplant is needed. Without resolution the patient may reject the recommendation of transplantation or be non-compliant with treatment. Anger, depression, and grief may follow. Progressive, physically restrictive symptoms may serve as a reminder of the patient's illness and mortality. Personality traits may be accentuated during this time. Patients with significant maladaptive traits may develop behavioural disturbances; such behavioural problems may provide clues to patients' abilities to cope in the future. During the phase of "magical expectations" patients may minimise risks and complications of transplantation. Idealisation of the treatment team may occur during this time. The final stage is one of acceptance.

As patients' end stage liver disease progresses, frequent hospitalisations and a worsening quality of life may led to depression, anxiety, and organic mental disorders. Some degree of anxiety and depression is to be expected as patients' physical health fluctuates.

Adjustment disorders are common and occur in 20–25% of patients.[4,5] Major depression is hard to assess in the presence of end stage liver disease. Watts[6] suggested that suicidal thinking, feelings of worthlessness, and constricted affect were indicative of a major depression; it is well known that patients with depression are at risk for surgical morbidity.[7]

Anxiety is common and often relates to the patient's state of health. Somatic symptoms of anxiety may include: shortness of breath, hyperventilation, diaphoresis, palpitations, chest pains, nausea, and vomiting. However, such symptoms may also be due to the patient's liver decompensation making diagnosis difficult.

Organic mental disorder is a frequent problem.[8] Patients with liver failure are particularly susceptible to delirium. Classic signs include a decreased level of consciousness and liver flap on physical examination. Confusion, memory impairment, and lability of affect may be seen on examination for mental status. Such symptoms can be documented by family, friends, and other physicians.[5] Concentration problems may be indicated by decreased ability to read, to carry out tasks of daily living, to manage finances, and so on. Prolonged delay before assessment may result in further deterioration. Therefore, evaluation for transplantation should be done as early in the clinical course as possible, so as to provide education and obtain informed consent.

Medications for most psychiatric disorders are broken down in the liver, so minimal use is recommended. If indicated, tricyclic antidepressants such as desipramine and nortriptyline may be initiated at 25 mg daily and increased in 25 mg increments until a satisfactory clinical response is obtained. Blood levels should be followed closely for toxicity. Some of the newer antidepressants, e.g. fluoxetine, must be followed closely because of their long half-life. For anxiety, oxazepam and lorazepam are recommended because of their short half-lives and because their metabolism only requires glucuronide conjugation before excretion in the urine. Both may also be useful for insomnia; in addition diphenhydramine may also be used for this purpose. Patients with organic mental disorders may benefit from low dose neuroleptics, e.g. 0·5 mg haloperidol daily. These may be particularly helpful for agitation and psychotic disorders of thought or perception.

Two disorders that can be considered under psychiatric evaluation are those of alcohol use and polydrug dependence. These are discussed below, although alcohol use disorder is also considered later in the section on alcoholic liver disease (p 56–9).

Alcohol use disorders

The most frequent and most worrisome of the psychiatric disorders seen in the setting of liver transplantation include those relating to the heavy or uncontrolled and frequent use of alcohol over a long period of time. Several diagnostic schemata are available to assist the clinician, both in evaluation and in diagnosis of these disorders. Two schemes currently in use, the *Diagnostic and Statistical Manual of Mental Disorders*, 3rd edn – revised (DSM-III-R)[9] and the *International Classification of Disease*, 10th revision (ICD-10)[10] are contrasted in Table I. The DSM-III-R and its subsequent version (DSM-IV) constitute the diagnostic standard in North America whereas the ICD-10 serves a cognate function in most European countries. The reader will note that there is overlap in both instruments but there are also some criteria that might qualify a patient as alcoholic on one side of the Atlantic but not on the other.

Practically, it may be preferable to consider alcohol use disorders

TABLE I—*Comparison of two alcohol dependence criteria**

DSM-III-R criteria	ICD-10 criteria
1 Drinking > intent	2 Awareness of impaired control
2 Unable to cut down/stop use	2 Awareness of impaired control
3 Much time used to get/use/recover	No counterpart
4 Use despite obligations or hazards	No counterpart
5 Activities given up due to drinking	7 Neglect of alternative pleasures
6 Continued use despite problems	8 Persistent use despite harm
7 Marked tolerance	5 Evidence of tolerance
8 Characteristic withdrawal symptoms	4 Physiological withdrawal state
9 Alcohol use to treat withdrawal	3 Alcohol effective for withdrawal
No counterpart	1 Desire/compulsion to drink
No counterpart	6 Narrowing drinking pattern
No counterpart	9 Relapse leads to rapid return of symptoms

*Adapted from Atkinson.[11]

from the perspective of three general phenomenological domains: physical dependence, lost or impaired control of drinking, and social or physical deterioration. The first of these, physical dependence, rests on the development of tolerance to alcohol, and on the subsequent occurrence of characteristic alcohol withdrawal symptoms. Tolerance may be assessed by contrasting the patient's alcohol use at a point early in the drinking history with the point at which the patient reports the quantity and frequency of his or her drinking to have been at a maximum. For example, a patient may relate feeling lightheaded or sick after two 12 ounce cans of beer drunk at age 18 as compared to the same sense of lightheadedness or vague sense of nausea occurring after drinking 12 cans of beer at age 35. In some standardised definitions, a 50% increase in alcohol intake to reach the same subjective end point is viewed as evidence of tolerance. Clinically, this must be judged in the individual case based on the total amount of alcohol drunk in one day on a regular basis.

The classic withdrawal symptoms are shown in Table II. A history of encountering such symptoms regularly indicates an irritable response in a nervous system that has become used to large doses of this depressant drug. Many patients will say that they do not encounter withdrawal symptoms despite evidence of a large tolerance to alcohol. In such cases it is important to enquire whether or not the patient is regularly taking benzodiazepines or other sedative medications – these could mask withdrawal symptoms – and whether the patient is drinking regularly in the morning to calm the withdrawal syndrome with more alcohol.

TABLE II—*Alcohol withdrawal symptoms*

Symptom experienced after cessation of drinking for		
6–12 hours	24–36 hours	72 + hours
Tremor	Ankle clonus	Delirium tremens
Nausea, vomiting	Seizure(s)	
Anxiety		
Diaphoresis		
Hyperreflexia		
Tachycardia		
Tachypnoea		
Hypertension		
Fever		

The phenomenon of loss of control or impaired control is at the centre of a diagnosis of alcohol dependence. It refers to an inability to drink in a regular and predictable fashion. At interview, alcohol dependent patients frequently describe having a very difficult time stopping drinking once they have begun a drinking bout. Because of this patients or corroborating family members will often report such phenomena as making rules about drinking – for example, only drinking certain beverages or not beginning drinking until a certain time each day – many attempts at quitting or cutting down alcohol use followed by resumption of drinking leading to the previous high levels of use, or drinking until reaching an externally controlled end point, such as exhausting the supply of alcohol, drinking until passing out, or reaching an alcoholic blackout. The dependent drinker is generally unable to drink in regular and predictable fashion – for example, no more than two standard drinks daily – over a significant period of time; either alcohol use increases beyond this amount or the drinker must cease use altogether.

When drinking has become uncontrolled, when tolerance dictates more and more alcohol to reach a desired effect, and when withdrawal symptoms intervene if the alcohol supply is foreshortened, alcohol dependent persons characteristically spend more and more time and energy in efforts to perpetuate their drinking in socially acceptable forms. As this occurs they characteristically spend less time and energy in other areas of their life resulting in a number of social sequelae. These may include lost time or frequent tardiness at work, difficulty with the legal system, particularly drunken driving charges, and, most frequently, strained family relationships with spouse and children. Family members are often the most knowledgeable on this score and, in the case of alcoholic transplant candidates, they *must* be interviewed at least to corroborate the dependent patient's own version of the clinical history.

In most diagnostic approaches, alcohol dependence is present when there is a history of physiological dependence, on the one hand, and of either the loss of control phenomena or social problems due to drinking, on the other. Once made, to the best of present knowledge the diagnosis of alcohol dependence in most patients carries with it a very high risk for resumption of uncontrolled drinking for the indefinite future.[2, 12, 13]

This may be contrasted to a lesser form of alcohol abuse which is shown when a patient has developed a tolerance to alcohol but has no other symptoms of alcohol dependence. This would suggest a much more optimistic prognosis for sustained abstinence and a much lower risk of progression to uncontrolled drinking. It is important for the clinician to recall that as many as 10% of patients with a history of alcohol abuse who request liver transplantation will fall into this more ameliorative category, whereas approximately a further 10% will fail to meet any diagnosis of alcohol abuse or dependence. As a result of this, proper attention to diagnostic concerns is crucial.

For the busy internist (houseman) or general practitioner, the time required to make a diagnosis of alcohol dependence and to corroborate this with a family member may not allow for evaluation in a large number of cases. At Colorado the use of screening examinations for alcoholism is recommended in this instance, particularly the four CAGE questions (see Chapter 4, Box A), which appear to be very useful in medical populations. In hospital or clinic settings, patients answering in the affirmative to two or more of the CAGE questions appear to have a 90% probability of qualifying for the more stringent alcohol dependent diagnosis.[14]

Prognosis

Assessing the prognosis for long term abstinence among alcohol dependent patients is often a difficult clinical task.[15] Current knowledge suggests that the patients who are likely to maintain long term abstinence are the following:

- Those who recognise their alcohol dependence and accept it as a condition to be dealt with
- Those who present a socially stable living environment
- Those who are free of intercurrent psychiatric disorders, such as schizophrenia, affective disorders, or severe anxiety disorders
- Those who have resources that can be used to help in the service of continued abstinence.

Vaillant's work in the last category is particularly pertinent.[2] In an 8-year prospective study of alcohol dependent persons, he noted that those who remained abstinent for 3 years or more had two of four prognostic indicators. First, they were able to structure their time with the use of substitute activities, thereby limiting free time that could be spent drinking. Second, they could identify an important relationship in their life with a person who was committed to their well-being but who also set clear limits on tolerance of any further drinking episodes. This could include any of a number of people: a knowledgeable spouse, a physician, a clergyman, a sponsor in Alcoholic's Anonymous (AA), or a number of others. Third, long term abstinent individuals often possessed a sense of hope or of improved self-esteem with which to counteract the intense guilt that resulted from uncontrolled drinking and its consequences. Fourth, and finally, the presence of a noxious and certain result of drinking was significant; this included phenomena such as abdominal pain from pancreatitis, the ethanol–disulfiram reaction, or a return to incarceration or some other punishment directly related to alcohol use. Liver failure and other more subtle forms of alcohol related injury did not qualify because of their subtlety.

The assessment of all these factors has become a necessity in conducting a careful selection of transplantation candidates for alcohol related liver disease. This is an exercise that requires that time be spent by one or more clinicians knowledgeable about alcoholism. Many, if not all, of the prognostic factors are present in the natural course of postoperative care of transplant recipients during the first 6–12 months. Prognostic assessment seeks to identify those who have the resources to maintain abstinence beyond that period, inevitably requiring that transplant teams continue to work with alcohol dependent graft recipients in assuring that abstinence factors are kept in good repair. This may include referral to alcoholism treatment as needed, continued follow up with the transplant team itself, or a combination of both.

Polydrug dependence

The foregoing discussions are germane for the vast majority of persons who suffer from alcohol dependence in the absence of other forms of drug addiction. There is a much smaller but more seriously ill population for whom polydrug addiction is a prime characteristic, which may include dependence on alcohol. Broadly speaking, this subgroup usually presents a history of psychiatric disorders before the age of 15 years and of multiple drug use starting in adolescence and often lasting through the third and fourth decades of life. There

31

may also be a history of legal involvement and of long standing difficulties in work and interpersonal relationships. Studies of the natural history of this population suggest that the drug use behaviour often wanes by the late thirties or early forties. Patients with this disorder are, generally, more likely to remain alcohol and drug free if by this age they have shown a significant period of drug and alcohol free living in addition to Vaillant's prognostic factors.

Present data suggest that for most non-polydrug abusing alcoholics the length of abstinence prior to acceptance for transplantation has little to do with the prediction of abstinence post-transplantation. The opposite may be true for patients presenting a polydrug addiction history along with liver failure due to alcohol use. Studies of sufficient numbers of such patients to allow generalisation do not exist. Clinical evaluation of polydrug patients should include corroborated histories of abstinence and prognostic resources. Current knowledge suggests wisdom in approaching this problem of candidacy in a conservative manner.

References

1 Craven J, Rodin GM. Liver transplantation. In: *Psychiatric Aspects of Organ Transplantation*. New York: Oxford Medical Publications, 1992.
2 Vaillant GE. *The Natural History Of Alcoholism*. Cambridge, MA: Harvard University Press, 1983.
3 Reither AM, Libb JW. Heart and liver transplantation. In: Soudemire A, Fogel BS, eds. *Medical Psychiatric Practice*. Washington, DC: American Psychiatric Press, 1991: 309–46.
4 Trzepacz PT, Brenner R, Van Thiel DH. A psychiatric study of 247 liver transplantation candidates. *Psychosomatics* 1989; **30**: 147–53.
5 Surman O. Liver transplantation. In: Craven J, Rodin GM, eds. *Psychiatric Aspects of Organ Transplantation*, New York: Oxford Medical Publications, 1992: 177–88.
6 Watts D, Freeman AM, McGriffin DG, *et al.* Psychiatric aspects of cardiac transplantation. *Heart Transplant* 1984; **3**: 243–7.
7 Surman O. The surgical patient. In: Hackett TP, Cassem NH, eds. *Massachusetts General Hospital Handbook of General Hospital Psychiatry*, 1st Ed. St Louis, MO: CV Mosby, 1978: 64–92.
8 Tarter RE, Van Thiel DH, Hegedus AM, Schade RR, Gavaler JS. Neuropsychiatric status after liver transplantation. *J Lab Clin Med* 1984; **103**: 776–782.
9 American Psychiatric Association. *Diagnostic and Statistical Manual of Mental Disorders* 3rd edn, revised. Washington, DC: American Psychiatric Association, 1987.
10 World Health Organization. *International Classification of Diseases*, 10th revision. Geneva: WHO, 1988.
11 Atkinson RM. Aging and alcohol use disorders: diagnostic issues in the elderly. *Int Psychogeriatr* 1990; **2**: 55–72.
12 Schuckit MA. *Drug and Alcohol Abuse. A Clinical Guide to Diagnosis and Treatment*. New York: Plenum, 1991.
13 Polich JM, Armor DJ, Braker HB. *The Course of Alcoholism: Four Years After Treatment*. New York: Wiley, 1981.
14 Beresford TP, Blow FC, Hill E, Singer K, Lucey MR. Comparison of CAGE question-

naire and computer-assisted laboratory profiles in screening for covert alcoholism. *Lancet* 1990; **336**(8713): 482–5.

15 Beresford TP, Turcotte JG, Merion R, *et al.* A rational approach to live transplantation for the alcoholic patient. *Psychosomatics* 1990; **31**: 241–54.

4: Specific indications

CHRONIC PARENCHYMAL LIVER DISEASE

ANTONI RIMOLA, MIQUEL NAVASA,
JOAN RODÉS, ELWYN ELIAS, JAMES NEUBERGER,
MICHAEL R LUCEY, CHRISTOPHER SHORROCK

General

The main objective of liver transplantation is to improve the survival and quality of life of patients. Therefore, this therapy should be indicated when the probability of patient survival after liver transplantation is significantly greater than the survival expected with conventional treatment, or when the patient's quality of life is unacceptable as a result of liver disease.

According to the European Registry of Liver Transplantation, the cumulative survival reported in transplant recipients since 1988 is 71% at 12 months, 66% at 24 months, and 63% at 36 months after the procedure.[1] It seems reasonable therefore to indicate liver transplantation in those patients whose survival probability when receiving standard therapy is lower than these figures. As the estimation of the probability of survival is therefore crucial for selecting the adequate timing for liver transplantation, the natural history and prognostic factors in patients with chronic liver diseases most frequently treated with liver transplantation are discussed. It is also important to identify those patients in whom transplantation is contraindicated because of technical reasons, poor prognosis, or early death from recurrent disease.

Evaluation of patients with chronic liver disease as candidates for liver transplantation

The evaluation of potential candidates for liver transplantation can be divided into three main areas:

● To confirm the necessity of indicating liver transplantation.

- To investigate the possible existence of contraindications to the procedure.
- To identify those pre-transplantation data that may be important for the peri- and postoperative periods.

The evaluation work up of liver transplant candidates followed in the authors' hospital in Barcelona is summarized in Table I.

After the evaluation, the final decision to accept or reject candidates for liver transplantation is usually made by a multidisciplinary team formed by members of the different departments involved in the liver transplant programme. Around 60% of the patients evaluated as candidates for liver transplantation are finally accepted for the therapeutic procedure,[2-5] thus indicating that a high proportion of patients initially considered as adequate candidates are rejected for liver transplantation after careful evaluation.

Contraindications for liver transplantation

Liver transplant candidates must be evaluated for contraindications in order to reject those patients in whom the risk of postoperative death (and, consequently, the risk of graft loss) is unacceptably high despite theoretical indications for liver transplantation. The reasons for this are to ensure the best and most profitable use of every liver transplant in the present climate of donor liver shortage. The circumstances currently considered to be general contraindications for liver transplantation in patients with chronic liver diseases are listed in Table II.[6-8]

Liver transplantation is also contraindicated in patients with active alcoholism.[9] As almost all patients receiving liver transplantation for hepatitis B virus (HBV) related cirrhosis and high viral replicative state (hepatitis B antigen (HBeAg) and/or HBV DNA positive) develop recurrence of the HBV infection in the transplanted liver, which is usually followed by rapidly progressive liver disease and loss of the graft,[10] most authors consider liver transplantation to be contraindicated in these patients, outside the context of specific trials.

Prognosis

In cirrhotic patients with ascites

The development of ascites carries a poor prognosis. However, as patients with ascites represent a mixed group with regard to clinical

TABLE I—*Evaluation work up of liver transplant candidates with chronic liver disease in the Hospital Clinic i Provincial of Barcelona*

History of hepatic and possible extrahepatic diseases
Complete physical examination
Study of the liver disease:
  Standard liver function tests
  Viral hepatitis markers:
    HBsAg; if positive: HBeAg, anti-HBe, and HBV DNA
    Anti-HCV
  Upper gastrointestinal fibreoptic examination
  Other biochemical, immunological, radiological, and histological examinations
  necessary to confirm diagnosis and assess current status of liver disease
Study of hepatic vessel patency:
  Abdominal ultrasonography using a Doppler technique
  Celiac axis and superior mesenteric arteriography with portal vein system
  phlebography (optional in patients with severe coagulopathy or renal failure)
Respiratory function evaluation:
  Chest radiograph
  Arterial blood gas determination
  Pulmonary ventilation tests
Cardiocirculatory system evaluation:
  ECG
  Echocardiography in alcoholic patients, patients older than 55 years, and
  patients with suspicion of valvular heart disease
  Ophthalmoscopic examination
  Plain abdominal radiograph (searching for arterial calcification)
Haematological evaluation:
  Red blood cell, white blood cell and platelet counts
  ABO and Rh group determination
  Serum anti-erythrocyte antibodies
  Serum anti-HLA antibodies
Metabolic evaluation:
  Blood glucose level
  Standard renal function tests
Baseline status of infectious disease processes:
  Antibodies to HIV, cytomegalovirus, Epstein–Barr virus, herpes virus,
  syphilis, and *Toxoplasma* sp.
  Tuberculin skin test
  Dental examination (searching for inapparent infectious foci)
In alcoholic patients:
  Psychological assessment to estimate prognosis of alcohol re-intake after
  transplantation
  Brain computed tomography scan in patients with apparent neurological or
  intellectual function disturbances

and laboratory parameters, the identification of subgroups of ascitic patients with different survival probability is of importance for selecting the best time for liver transplantation in these patients.

TABLE II—*General contraindications to liver transplantation in patients with chronic liver diseases*

Advanced age*
Complete portal vein thrombosis
Serious extrahepatic infection, including HIV infection
Severe extrahepatic problems (mainly cardiocirculatory, respiratory, renal, or
  neurological) unrelated to the liver disease
Low probability of complying with the necessary postoperative follow up and
  treatment

---

*Limit is not well established. At the hospital in Barcelona the limit is 65 years.

Different authors have identified several clinical and laboratory data, particularly those relating to renal function and haemodynamics, as prognostic factors in cirrhotic individuals with ascites. In the centre at Barcelona, criteria for liver transplantation in cirrhotic patients having ascites are based on prognostic factors that are easily available and associated with a survival probability of less than 50% at 2 years of follow up in conventionally treated patients;[11, 12] these include:

- Mean arterial pressure < 85 mmHg
- Poor nutritional status
- Past history of spontaneous bacterial peritonitis
- Absence of hepatomegaly
- Functional renal failure
- Urinary sodium excretion < 1·5 mmol/day
- Serum sodium concentration < 133 mmol/l
- Serum albumin < 28 g/l.

For cirrhotic patients with ascites meeting these criteria and who underwent liver transplantation in hospital at Barcelona, the cumulative survival is 75% at 1 year, 67% at 2 years, and 67% at 3 years after surgery (Figure 1), which is much higher than that expected theoretically using standard management.

Recently, a prognostic index for predicting survial in cirrhotic patients with ascites has been developed.[13] This prognostic index is calculated from the following variables: hepatomegaly, serum albumin, nutritional status, mean arterial pressure, serum urea, serum sodium concentration, and urinary sodium excretion. Based on this index, patients can be classified into three groups:

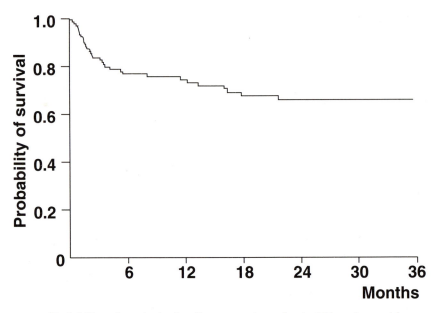

FIG 1—*Probability of survival after liver transplantation in 121 patients with non-biliary cirrhosis and ascites.*

1 Group I – patients with good survival probability (approximately 80% at 1 year of follow up).
2 Group II – patients with medium survival probability (around 60% at 1 year).
3 Group III – patients with poor survival probability (lower than 20% at 1 year).

Using the cumulative survival shown in Figure 1 as a reference survival probability for cirrhotic patients with ascites, this therapeutic procedure would be indicated in patients from groups II and III but not from group I. This index must, however, be adequately validated in prospective studies and should therefore be used cautiously in the decision making process taken for liver transplantation in these patients.

In cirrhotic patients with variceal haemorrhage

As actively bleeding patients are not generally considered as liver transplant candidates until haemorrhage has ceased, prognosis is only considered in the posthaemostasis period. After cessation of

TABLE III—*Child–Pugh classification*

Points scored	Encephalopathy grade	Bilirubin		Albumin (g/l)	Prolongation of prothrombin time (seconds)
		µmol/l	mg/dl		
1	–	<25	<1·5	>35	1–4
2	I, II	25–40	1·5–2·3	28–35	4–6
3	III, IV	>40	>2·3	<28	>6

Grade A = 5–6.
Grade B = 7–9.
Grade C = 10–15.

haemorrhage the natural history and prognostic factors can be extrapolated from studies used to investigate rebleeding and survival rates in relation to different therapeutic modalities, such as surgery, sclerotherapy, and β-blocker administration. From most of these studies, parameters that estimate hepatic function reserve are the best factors for predicting patient survival after an episode of variceal haemorrhage whatever the type of therapy. By using the Child–Pugh score to classify cirrhotic patients recovering from an episode of gastrointestinal haemorrhage (Table III), the survival rate of class A patients treated by any of the currently available therapies for preventing new haemorrhagic episodes is consistently good (approximately 75–100% at three years of follow up), and the expectancy of survival for class C patients is generally poor (around 20–45% at three years). In contrast, survival in Child–Pugh class B patients largely varies among series, ranging from 40% to 85% at three years.[15–23]

The probability of survival in patients with non-biliary cirrhosis receiving liver transplantation is usually greater than 60% three years after the procedure.[24] As post-transplantation survival of these patients is not influenced by the presence or absence of a past history of gastrointestinal haemorrhage,[25] survival after liver transplantation in cirrhotic patients who had presented with variceal haemorrhage can reasonably be assumed to be more than 60% at three years. As an example, the cumulative survival in a series of patients, with non-biliary cirrhosis and a history of variceal bleeding, who had undergone liver transplantation in the hospital at Barcelona was 79% at one year and 65% at three years after the procedure (Figure

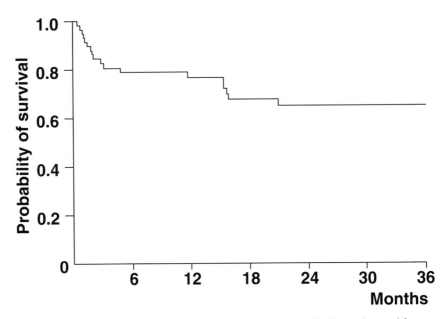

FIG 2—*Probabiliity of survival after liver transplantation in 62 patients with non-biliary cirrhosis and past history of variceal haemorrhage.*

2). By comparing survival obtained with liver transplantation to that without in this type of patient, it can be concluded that liver transplantation is indicated in Child–Pugh class C patients and not in Child–Pugh class A patients; however, the decision to perform liver transplantation in Child–Pugh class B patients is unclear. Further studies are needed to ascertain whether other clinical and laboratory parameters that have prognostic significance in cirrhotic patients, such as age, hepatic encephalopathy, alcohol intake in alcoholic patients, very sensitive liver function tests, or haemo-dynamic data, could be useful in the decision of whether to transplant the liver in patients from Child–Pugh class B. The possibility of improving survival in bleeding cirrhotic patients by recently introduced therapies, such as transjugular intrahepatic portosys-temic shunting, is still unknown.

In other patients

The natural history and prognostic factors in patients with non-biliary cirrhosis, and with other conditions that are less frequent

40

than ascites or gastrointestinal haemorrhage (for example, patients with marked changes in liver function tests but without overt clinical decompensation of the liver disease, or patients in whom hepatic encephalopathy is the only clinical manifestation), have not been investigated adequately. Liver transplantation in these patients is usually indicated after careful individual evaluation. Similarly, as prognosis in cirrhosis has mainly been studied in patients with alcoholic, post-hepatitis, and cryptogenic cirrhosis, indication for liver transplantation in patients with cirrhosis of uncommon aetiologies, such as haemochromatosis or Wilson's disease, is also based on individual selection.

Cryptogenic cirrhosis and chronic active hepatitis

The major indications for transplantation for both these conditions are discussed later in this chapter. The most common features indicating the time for transplantation are:

- Diuretic resistant ascites
- Spontaneous bacterial peritonitis
- Grossly disabling lethargy
- Low serum albumin ($<26\,g/l$)
- Progressive jaundice
- Muscle wasting
- Encephalopathy (either spontaneous or following a bleed or sepsis).

These patients are the most difficult to judge for the optimal timing of grafting. Patients often remain stable for many months and deterioration is gradual until a major life threatening event occurs.

In patients with autoimmune chronic active hepatitis, corticosteroids should be reduced as far as possible once the decision has been made for transplantation, not only to reduce the susceptibility to infection, but also to reduce the effect of osteoporosis.

Primary biliary cirrhosis

PBC is associated with many extrahepatic diseases: sicca syndrome and thyroid disorders; less common diseases that are

41

associated are: pernicious anaemia, coeliac disease, arthralgia, and an increased tendency to extrahepatic malignancy (especially breast).

The disease is associated with a widespread disturbance of the immune system, but the presence of elevated serum IgM and anti-mitochondrial antibodies is the most specific. There is no form of therapy (other than transplantation) that has been shown to be associated with a clinically significant improvement in survival, although some authors have claimed that benefit is achieved with ursodeoxycholic acid.

Recently it has been recognised that those patients with a biochemical and histological picture of PBC, but who are anti-mito-chondrial antibody negative and anti-nuclear antibody positive, may have a different condition – an immune cholangitis. Recognition of this condition is important because there is a significant biochemical and histological response to corticosteroids. Whether the use of corticosteroids alters the prognosis is, as yet, uncertain.

Indications for transplantation may be for either symptomatic disease or end stage disease.

Symptomatic disease

The two most common symptoms for which patients with PBC may be considered for transplantation are lethargy and pruritus. Less commonly, transplantation may be considered for osteoporosis.

Lethargy, as a consequence of liver disase, may be overwhelming and the patient's quality of life severely reduced as a result. Care must be taken in excluding any treatable causes of lethargy:

- Depression
- Thyroid disease
- Addison's disease
- Medication induced lethargy (especially sleeping tablets and antihistamines).

Pruritus may also be intractable and severe enough to warrant consideration of grafting. It is important to try all potential therapies for relief of itching. Cholestyramine is the mainstay of therapy, but many patients find the powders difficult to take or the side effects intolerable. Cholestyramine (Questran preparations) is best taken just before and just after breakfast, with additional doses before other meals. Alternative approaches include the following:

- Questran A contains aspartame in place of sorbitol – the major factor causing nausea, bloating, and diarrhoea associated with standard Questran. Many patients unable to tolerate Questran can control itching with Questran A.
- Colestipol is rarely effective when cholestyramine fails to control itching.
- Antihistamines are usually disappointing in treating pruritus in PBC; the major consequence is sedation rather than relief of itching.
- Plasmapheresis is effective in controlling itching, but the medical side effects and need for repeat hospital attendances may outweigh any benefits.
- Ursodeoxycholic acid is reported in most trials to reduce the severity of itching, but, at least in our experience, this agent has not proven effective in otherwise intractable itching.
- Surgical biliary diversion via a fistula has been shown to be effective, but the need for surgery in patients who may require surgery makes the approach less than ideal.
- Use of oil of evening primrose, simple emollient creams, rifampicin, phenobarbitone (phenobarbital), and exposure to ultraviolet light has been reported to be effective, but, in our experience, results have been disappointing for most patients. Intravenous infusion of naloxone or propofol may relieve itching but cannot readily be given long term.

Bone disease is a common associated feature of PBC. Although vitamin D-responsive osteomalacia is uncommon, it should always be considered in any patient with PBC, especially if the patient is of Asian origin, cholestatic, or taking cholestyramine. Osteoporosis or, more accurately, hepatic osteopenia is much more common and less readily treated. The presence of bone pain or the occurrence of fractures is a strong indication for consideration of early transplantation. It must be remembered that the inevitable bed-rest and use of corticosteroids following surgery may, in the short term, exacerbate osteoporosis, but once the patient is ambulant and steroids reduced, then bone mass often increases, although rarely to more than that observed before transplantation. In patients with osteoporosis, transplantation should be considered early because limb fractures may immobilise the patient and rib fractures will increase the tendency to chest infections.

End stage disease

Most patients with PBC are grafted for end stage disease and, as with other parenchymal diseases, indications are relatively simple to define:

- Bilirubin >180 µmol/l (10 mg/dl) (should suffice even in the absence of any of the following)
- Diuretic resistant ascites
- Spontaneous bacterial peritonitis
- Hepatic encephalopathy
- Progressive muscle wasting
- Recurrent variceal bleeding.

Patients often undergo transplantation with several of the above features in combination.

Of the various serological markers, the serum bilirubin remains the best single guide to prognosis; a serum bilirubin greater than 180 µmol/l (10 mg/dl) suggests a prognosis of less than 18 months. Because hepatoctye function is well preserved, serum albumin and the prothrombin time are often within normal limits until very late stages of the disease. In contrast, because of a pre-sinusoidal element of portal hypertension, features such as bleeding varices and ascites may present before the patient develops a true cirrhosis; hence, histological staging should not be considered as a major factor in the timing of transplantation.

In recent years, a number of prognostic models have been developed and validated. The initial model[26] was derived from an international, multicentre study of the effects of azathioprine in PBC.[27] The prognosis for an individual patient can be calculated from the formula:

$2{\cdot}51 \times$ log serum bilirubin (µmol/l)

$+$ age $\times e^{(\text{age in years} - 20)/10}$

$+ 0{\cdot}88$ (if cirrhosis present)

$- 0{\cdot}05 \times$ serum albumin (g/l)

$+ 0{\cdot}68$ (if central cholestasis present)

$+ 0{\cdot}52$ (if treated with azathioprine)

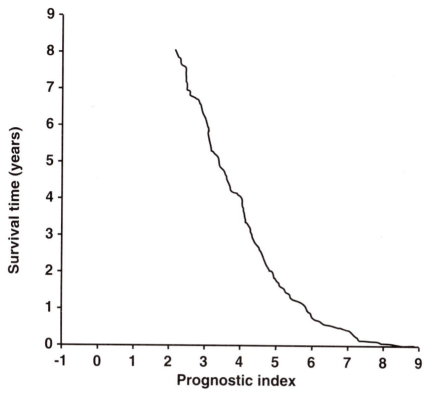

FIG 3—*Estimated median survival time by the prognostic index. (Reproduced with permission from Christensen et al.[26])*

The product of the above formula is calculated to give a score (the prognostic index, PI). This figure can be translated into an estimate of the median expected survival time or the probability of surviving a given number of years (Figures 3 and 4).

The Mayo Clinic[28] used a similar approach to develop a prognostic model, which did not contain any histological data. The R value is calculated as:

$0.871 \times \log_e$ bilirubin (mg/dl)
$-2.53 \times \log_e$ albumin (g/dl)
$+0.039 \times$ age in years
$+2.38 \times \log_e$ prothrombin time (seconds)
$+0.859$ if oedema present

Both these models have been validated and compare well with

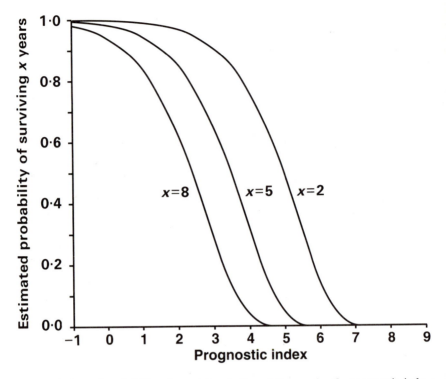

FIG 4—*Estimated probability of surviving 2, 5, and 8 years by the prognostic index;* x = *no. of years. (Reproduced with permission from Christensen* et al.[26])

each other. However, as indicated earlier, these models are only valid when used at presentation and cannot be used repeatedly. Just as life expectancy changes with age, so do the prognostic models. Indeed, a recent study from New York, applying the Mayo Clinic model to a group of patients followed over many years, indicated that the model lost accuracy in patients who survived for less than 2 years.[29] Thus, these models may be helpful in selecting patients for therapeutic trials, but should not be used for determining when to refer a patient for transplantation, and do not replace clinical judgement.

In order to overcome these problems, time dependent models have been developed. Hughes and colleagues[30] have developed one time dependent model in which the patient's estimated probability of survival includes serum bilirubin and serum albumin, age, and history of ascites and variceal haemorrhage. The time dependent model proposed by Christensen is the following:

$2.53 \times \log$ serum bilirubin $(\mu\text{mol/l}) - 1.53$
$+ 1.39$ if ascites present
$- 0.085 \times$ serum albumin $(\text{g/l}) - 34.3$
$+ 0.4 \times$ age (years) $- 55$
$+ 0.65$ if gastrointestinal bleeding present

Again, as with the earlier models, the prognostic indicator can be translated into a survival probability.

Although the models do have many advantages in identifying the important prognostic factors and in evaluating the effect of transplantation in populations, it is unlikely that these models will achieve widespread use and should not be used in isolation.

Other markers have been proposed as having value in assessing prognosis in PBC, particularly: type III procollagen aminopropeptide; serum hyaluronic acid; and functional tests such as aminopyrine clearance and galactosamine elimination clearance. None has achieved widespread support, and serial estimations of serum bilirubin remain the most practical and useful test to help decide the timing of transplantation in patients with PBC.

Primary sclerosing cholangitis

In contrast to PBC, the clinical course of PSC is more variable and less predictable. Episodes of jaundice may be transient, often associated with biliary sepsis. Overall, however, there is a relentless progression, for which there is no definitive therapy.

PSC is associated with inflammatory bowel disease, especially ulcerative colitis. The severities of the two conditions do not parallel each other; most patients with PSC have a quiescent pancolitis, although the entire spectrum of the disease may be seen. Removal of the colon does not affect the progression of the liver disease.

In PSC, there is evidence of immunological abnormality; a characteristic marker of the disease is the presence of anti-neutrophil cytoplasmic antibodies, which have a perinuclear distribution.

The disease must be considered as a premalignant condition, because many patients develop cholangiocarcinoma.

The usual indications for transplantation are:

• Deepening jaundice, which is progressive, not fluctuating
• Intractable pruritus

- Weight loss and muscle wasting
- Decompensated cirrhosis.

Other, less drastic, procedures for relief of cholestasis have to be approached with extreme caution. Death has followed directly or indirectly from intrahepatic biliary sepsis induced by endoscopic retrograde cholangiopancreatography (ERCP) in patients who are cirrhotic from PSC. Similarly, introduction of contrast above biliary strictures should be limited to strict clinical indications and not purely for visualisation. In our view, the risks of introducing biliary stents to deal with anything other than a single, well-defined, extrahepatic stricture outweigh any benefit. Thus, once the diagnosis of PSC has been confirmed, repeat examination should be for defined indications only and these are very few.

The presence of colitis is not in itself a contraindication to grafting, although there is a reluctance to graft in the presence of an active colitis. In those with long standing colitis, a colonoscopy has been carried out to exclude the presence of a colonic tumour. Caution should be used in the presence of ascites, because bacterial peritonitis may be induced, even if prophylactic antibiotics are given. In our view, the presence of low grade dysplasia is not a contraindication, but high grade dysplasia is of concern, because of the effects of the immunosuppressive drugs.

As with PBC, prognostic models have been developed but the most recent one, developed from a multicentre study, is not time dependent.[31] The prognostic factor, R, can be calculated as:

$0.535 \times \log_e$ serum bilirubin
$+ 0.486 \times$ histological stage
$+ 0.041 \times$ age (years)
$+ 0.705$ if splenomegaly present.

The risk score, R, is calculated and, from Table IV, $So(t)$ is derived. The probability of surviving t more years ($S(t)$) is calculated from the equation: $S(t) = So(t)e^{R-3.326}$.

As before, the format of the model makes it unlikely that it will achieve widespread use in clinical practice.

The major difficulty in timing of transplantation for PSC is the anticipation of complicating carcinoma which will occur in about 20% of cases. Any sudden deterioration (jaundice and weight loss) suggests this diagnosis. Dilatation of intrahepatic ducts on ultrasonography is another sign suggesting the development of cholangiocarcinoma. In such a patient, exclusion of a neoplasm involves a careful work up including:

- Serum carcinoembryonic antigen
- Biliary cytology
- Biopsy of the stricture where possible
- Imaging for a mass, enlarged nodes, vascular invasion, or distant spread. Ultrasonography, scanning, and angiography computed tomography (CT) and magnetic resonance imaging (MRI) should all be considered.

In the absence of proven malignancy the patient proceeds to transplantation aware that a cholangiocarcinoma could be discovered during the operation, or subsequently on histological examination of the hepatectomy specimen. Frozen section histological examination of enlarged hilar and peribiliary nodes may be performed at the onset of laparotomy to exclude metastatic disease. Because aggressive recurrence of disease is usual when cholangiocarcinoma has metastasised, the transplantation is stopped under such circumstances so that the donor liver can be given to another patient.

Viral disease

Viral hepatitis

A comprehensive review of viral hepatitis will not be attempted here. Aspects of viral hepatitis that particularly impact on liver

TABLE IV—*Survival probability in primary sclerosing cholangitis*

Time (years)	So(t)
1	0·951
2	0·951
3	0·871
4	0·844
5	0·799
6	0·752
7	0·741

From Dickson *et al.*[31]

49

TABLE V—*Major viral causes of liver failure*

Disease	Virus	Genome	Genome length (kb)	Mode of transmission	Incubation* (days) Mean	Range
Hepatitis A	Picornavirus	RNA	7·5	Faecal–oral Parenteral	28	15–50
Hepatitis B	Hepadnavirus	DNA	3·2	Parenteral Sexually transmitted ?Faecal–oral	84	28–160
Hepatitis C	Flavivirus	RNA	10·2	Parenteral ?Sexually transmitted ?Faecal–oral	56	14–160
Hepatitis D	Viroid	RNA	1·67	Parenteral	–	–
Hepatitis E	?Calicivirus	RNA	7.6	Faecal–oral	40	22–60

*Time from exposure to clinical hepatitis.
†Especially in pregnant women in the third trimester.

transplantation will be emphasised. Table V lists the viruses that cause liver failure to the extent that liver transplantation is required.[32]

Hepatitis A

Hepatitis A virus (HAV) is an enteric virus which, on rare occasions, causes fulminant hepatic failure. HAV is implicated as an aetiological factor on the basis of serum antibody tests. Table VI shows the interpretation of anti-HAV serology. The natural history of fulminant hepatitis due to HAV is often benign and in some series up to 50% of patients who progress to grade III encephalopathy recover fully without transplantation. Nevertheless, occasionally HAV infection may progress to a stage that requires liver transplantation. Inactivated HAV vaccines have now been developed which are highly efficacious in healthy persons. Their suitability for use in immunocompromised hosts has not been studied.

TABLE V—*contd*

		Consequence of infection		Infection post-transplantation	
Acute hepatitis	Fulminant hepatic failure	Chronic hepatitis	Hepatoma	Recipient to allograft	New acquisition
Yes	Yes	No	No	No*	No
Yes	Yes	Yes	Yes	Yes	Yes
Yes	Uncertain	Yes	Yes	Yes	Yes
Yes	Yes	Yes	No	Yes	Uncertain
Yes	Yes†	No	No	Uncertain	No

*Occurs rarely.

Hepatitis B

The presence of positive hepatitis B virus (HBV) related serological tests in a patient with liver failure often poses a clinical challenge. Table VII summarises the interpretation of HBV serological tests. When presented with a patient with liver failure and positive HBV serologies, the physician should try to ascertain the following: categorise the infection as acute or chronic; determine whether HBV is in a replicative state; and determine whether other viruses such as hepatitis C virus (HCV) or hepatitis D virus (HDV) are present. Recently, attention has been drawn to genetic variations

TABLE VI—*Hepatitis A*

Anti-HAV IgG	Anti-HAV IgM	Interpretation
+	+	Acute HAV infection occasionally may persist up to 6 months
+	−	Previous exposure to HAV, now immune

51

TABLE VII—*Serological patterns of HBV infection and their implications*

HBsAg	HBeAg	HBV DNA	Anti-HBs	Anti-HBc (IgG)	Anti-HBc (IgM)	Anti-HBe	Transaminases	Interpretation
+	+	+	-	+/-	+	+/-	↑	Stereotypical acute acquisition with active viral replication
+	+	+	-	+	+/-	-	Usually↑	Chronic HBV infection with active viral replication. Low level anti-HBc (IgM) may be positive particularly after recent reactivation from chronic carrier state
+	-	-	-	+	-	+	Normal	Chronic carrier. Typically no or low grade viral replication only (ie, HBeAg−, HBV DNA−) and no ongoing liver injury
+	-	+	-	-	-	+	↑	Viral replication (HBV DNA+) plus HBeAg−, anti-HBe+, suggests presence of HBV pre-core mutant
+	-	-	+/-	+	-	+	↑	Elevated transaminases in absence of active replication suggests (a) presence of other viruses – ie, HCV, HDV; (b) other toxins; (c) recent seroconversion to non-replicative state; (d) hepatoma; (e) incorrect data
-	-	-	+	-	-	-		Stereotypical pattern for a person who has received HBV immunisation
-	-	-	+	+	-	+/-		Prior exposure to HBV wild type, now immune

52

in HBV which may influence its clinical characteristics. The "pre-core mutant" variant, which may be associated with fulminant or aggressive hepatitis, is characterised by positive results for serum HBV DNA and anti-HBe antibody, and by the absence of HBe antigen (HBeAg).

A careful search for hepatoma should be made in all HBV chronically infected persons undergoing evaluation for liver transplantation. Abdominal ultrasonography or CT scan, and serum α-fetoprotein measurement are reasonable screening tests in this population.

The major impediment to successful liver transplantation in HBV infected persons has been recurrence of HBV in the allograft[33, 34] (see p 81-2, 269-72, 304). This risk appears to be greatest in patients with evidence of active viral replication (ie, serum HBV DNA + or HBeAg +). The source of the HBV that infects the allograft is unknown, but may include extrahepatic loci such as spleen and peripheral blood mononuclear cells. Attempts have been made to ameliorate the risk of transmission to the graft by administration of interferon in the pre-transplantation period and by hepatitis B immunoglobulin and interferon in the post-transplantation period. Immune responses, which are a major mechanism of injury to the HBV infected hepatocytes, may be increased by exogenous interferon. Thus, treating HBV infected patients, who had poorly compensated liver function, with interferon runs the risk of precipitating further liver injury.[35] For this reason, interferon has been used in these patients in defined study protocols, usually at much reduced doses compared with that used in patients with intact liver function.[35]

Furthermore, some authors have noted loss of serum HBV DNA after low dose interferon has been given to serum HBV DNA positive patients awaiting liver transplantation. As the risk of transmission of HBV seems greatest in HBV DNA positive hosts, it might be anticipated that loss of HBV DNA would portend a reduction in HBV transmission. Unfortunately, no such reduction has been recorded. This may be because small amounts of intact virus remain which are sufficient to infect the allograft. Other antiviral agents are currently being studied in this context, but no results are available. The efficacy of post-transplant HBV treatment is reviewed later in the book (p 81-2, 271-2).

Hepatitis C

Hepatitis C virus (HCV) was identified in 1989 as the principal cause of post-transfusion non-A, non-B (NANB) hepatitis. Its clinical characteristics are summarised in Table V. HCV is also an important cause of chronic liver injury not transmitted via blood products. Those cases without an obvious parenteral exposure are called sporadic. The role of sexual transmission of HCV is controversial. As alcoholic liver disease has become the most prevalent diagnosis among patients undergoing liver transplantation in some centres, it should be stressed that HCV is a frequent infection in patients with alcoholic cirrhosis.

HCV RNA and its antigens are present in very small amounts in an HCV infected subject. Thus, measurement of HCV RNA or HCV proteins in serum or liver has proved difficult. The currently available clinical tests for HCV use measurement in serum of antibodies (IgG) to various epitopes encoded by HCV RNA. Both second generation RIBA (recombinant immunoblot assays) and ELISA (enzyme-linked immunosorbent assays) are more sensitive and specific than the original ELISA. However, until measurements of HCV RNA become readily available, either after amplification by polymerase chain reaction (PCR) or by other methodologies, the interpretation of anti-HCV antibody results remains a problem. At the time of writing, the following statements are true:

- Positive anti-HCV plus an abnormal liver biopsy usually indicates that HCV is present.
- Positive anti-HCV with normal liver tests may or may not be associated with the presence of the virus. A liver biopsy that shows even mild hepatitis or measurement of HCV RNA after PCR may clarify.
- A negative anti-HCV does not exclude HCV in an appropriate clinical setting. Anti-HCV may not be measurable for up to 6 months in a person who has acquired HCV that is progressing to chronic hepatitis. Similarly, intermittent disappearance of HCV RNA and anti-HCV has been recorded in a long term follow up after post-transfusion HCV infection.
- Although not all HCV infections become chronic, the frequency of acute HCV becoming chronic is unknown, and may be influenced by route of acquisition and inoculum size.
- Chronic HCV is usually a very slowly progressive disease. A 20–

30 year history from exposure to development of cirrhosis is not uncommon. A follow up study in 1992 of persons who developed acute post-transfusion NANB hepatitis between 1964 and 1980 found no increase in mortality compared to matched controls.

- HCV is emerging as an important aetiological factor in the development of hepatoma.

When a hepatitis C viraemic patient undergoes liver transplantation, infection of the graft by HCV is almost invariable.[36] No strategy to prevent HCV transmission by prior treatment with interferon has proved successful, although there are no large well-conducted studies. It is uncertain how frequently HCV acquisition at the time of transplantation, either from the donor organ or blood products, occurs.

Hepatitis D

Hepatitis D virus (HDV), which occurs in conjunction with HBV infection, may have important moderating effects on the outcome after liver transplantation. When patients infected by HBV and HDV undergo liver transplantation, HDV frequently infects the allograft. Initially, it may appear to be doing so independently of HBV and, indeed, unless HBsAg is expressed by the graft within a few months of transplantation, the subject will clear both viruses. The usual pattern is for the subject to develop HBV and HDV in the allograft. Curiously, allograft recipients infected with both viruses appear to have a more benign course than that observed in patients infected with HBV alone. It is presumed that the salutary effects of HDV arise from its inhibitory action on HBV replication. The only readily available serological tests for HDV are serum anti-HD antibody. Measurement of HDV RNA in serum or HDV antigen in liver tissue remains a research tool at present. Treatment before transplantation for HDV has not been attempted and, given the improved outcome of combined HBV and HDV, therapy aimed at the HDV may seem foolhardy.

Hepatitis E

Hepatitis E virus (HEV) is uncommon outside the less developed world, but may occasionally be encountered in the developed world in someone who has recently travelled from an endemic area. It has a predilection for causing fulminant hepatic failure in pregnant women. It does not seem to be a cause of non-A, non-B, non-C fulminant hepatic failure in the USA or the UK. Serological tests for anti-HE have been developed but are not in general clinical use at this time.

Alcoholic liver disease

Defining alcoholic liver disease

Alcohol is the most common aetiological factor implicated in end stage liver failure occurring in North America and western Europe. Alcoholic cirrhosis accounts for more than 10 000 deaths annually in the USA alone. However, alcoholic liver disease is not a homogeneous entity. Ingestion of alcohol may lead to variety of distinct abnormalities in the liver; these include alcoholic fatty liver, acute alcoholic hepatitis, and cirrhosis. Frequently, these entities overlap in the same individual and, furthermore, the interaction of alcohol with genetic and environmental factors in the pathogenesis is becoming increasingly recognised. A good example is the frequent association of alcoholism and hepatitis C virus in persons with putative alcoholic liver disease. Finally, it should be noted that histological features consistent with a diagnosis of alcoholic liver disease, such as Mallory's hyaline inclusions, peristellate fibrosis, and macrovesicular fat deposits, do not inevitably mean an alcoholic aetiology. Occasionally, these features may be due to other causes: post-jejunoileal bypass, medications such as amiodarone or perhexaline, or even for unclear reasons in persons who do not drink. The last syndrome has been called non-alcoholic steatohepatitis (NASH), and it affects particularly middle-aged women with diabetes mellitus. Occasionally, it may lead to end stage liver failure.

Assessment for liver transplantation

Psychiatric assessment

In the past, there has been considerable controversy regarding the probity of offering liver transplants to alcoholic patients.[37,38] A reasonable consensus is that few programmes now exclude liver transplantation in alcoholics, but almost all consider assessment of

---

BOX A   CAGE questions

1 Have you ever felt you should **C**ut down on your drinking?
2 Have other people **A**nnoyed you by criticising your drinking?
2 Have you ever felt bad or **G**uilty about your drinking?
4 Have you ever taken a drink first thing in the morning (**E**ye opener) to steady your nerves or get rid of a hangover?

---

the prognosis for sobriety after transplantation as a key component of the psychiatric assessment of alcoholic candidates. At the University of Michigan, the team have developed a system of close cooperation between the psychiatrist(s) and other members of the evaluation team. All persons referred for evaluation are screened for covert alcholism by use of the CAGE questions as shown in Box A. Two or more positive answers are considered to be a useful marker for alcoholism. All patients with a positive CAGE screen, plus all who carry a diagnosis of alcoholic liver disease, are referred for a formal psychiatric review. When psychiatric assessment confirms a diagnosis of alcohol abuse or dependence, attempts are made to determine likelihood of future sobriety. In common with many programmes, a fixed period of abstinence has been abandoned as a marker for future sobriety. Rather the Michigan Alcoholism Prognosis Scale has been devised as shown in Table VIII. This takes into account the patient's insight into alcoholism, and the presence of factors drawn from other studies which appear to predict that the patient is likely to remain off all alcohol after receipt of the transplant. Contrariwise, Beresford[39] has described five characteristics which portend poor prognosis for sobriety – shown in Box B. The data used to make this prognostic assessment must be corroborated by family members and others close to the patient such as alcoholism counsellors. Implicit in this approach is the view that continued alcohol use by the alcoholic patient with a liver transplant would be detrimental to the graft, and that patients and their families must acknowledge that abstinence for life is the best policy. The prognosis scale and the poor prognostic factors are used as guidelines for the final judgement regarding the probability of abstinence. Indeed, the final decision as to whether the patient should be placed on the transplant list remains a clinical one which is best made when there is close communication among members of

TABLE VIII—*The University of Michigan Alcoholism Prognosis Scale for candidates for major organ transplantation*

Factor		Points on scale		
Acceptance of alcoholism				
Patient and family	4			
Patient only	3			
Family only	2			
Neither	1			
Prognostic indices				
Substitute activities	Yes	3	No	1
Behavioural consequences	Yes	3	No	1
Hope/Self-esteem	Yes	3	No	1
Social relationship	Yes	3	No	1
Social stability				
Steady job	1			
Stable residence	1			
Does not live alone	1			
Stable marriage	1			

Reproduced from Lucey *et al.*,[9] with permission.

the evaluation team. In the programme at Michigan, selected patients undergo alcoholism rehabilitation before or after transplantation depending on their medical well being. This psychiatric review process is described in Chapter 3.

Medical assessment

The decision to place a patient on the transplant waiting list requires estimation of the patient's prognosis using medical/surgical management in the absence of transplantation. This poses special problems in alcoholic liver disease. In both acute alcoholic hepatitis and alcoholic cirrhosis, liver failure may have been precipitated by recent drinking. It is often difficult to predict the recuperative

BOX B Negative prognostic factors
- Pre-existing psychotic disorder
- Unstable character disorder
- Unremitted polydrug abuse
- Multiple alcohol rehabilitation attempts
- Social isolation

powers of the patient once alcohol has been withdrawn, especially in the case of acute alcoholic hepatitis. The risks of expectant medical management are compounded by the difficulty in estimating the length of waiting time until a suitable liver becomes available. Thus, it is sometimes necessary to place an alcoholic patient who is in extremis on the liver transplant list and subsequently to remove him or her when a recovery ensues. Because of this, a period of observation is sometimes advocated, especially in acute alcoholic hepatitis, in order to allow the patient to recover.

Extrahepatic manifestations of alcoholism

Table IX lists some common extrahepatic manifestations of alcoholism. Although up to 30% of alcoholics have significant cardiomyopathy in some studies, at Michigan we have been surprised how infrequently this problem is encountered. The policy at Michigan is to subject all alcoholics to careful cardiac evaluation including a stress test and an echocardiogram. Occasional patients require cardiac catheterisation. The major neurological dilemma in alcoholics (and indeed also in non-alcoholics with end stage liver disease) is distinguishing chronic encephalopathy from an organic brain syndrome. The waxing and waning quality of the signs usually provides a clear picture of chronic encephalopathy. In rare cases, where the signs appear constant, it may be impossible to tell whether the syndrome is chronic encephalopathy and potentially reversible with transplantation or a Wernicke–Korsakoff syndrome. In our experience, CT scanning of the brain, EEG, evoked potentials, or formal psychometric testing is of little help in solving this dilemma.

Infection must be carefully excluded in patients with alcoholic liver disease. As mentioned above, in some series 50% or more of patients with alcoholic cirrhosis are infected with HCV. Similarly, alcoholics, especially those with a history of intravenous drug abuse, may be carriers of HBV or HIV. Coincidence of HCV in an alcoholic is not sufficient to exclude transplantation. HBV infection, especially when accompanied by serum HBeAg or HBV DNA, is problematic. Alcoholics are also at risk of non-viral infections especially tuberculosis. All persons being evaluated for transplantation, but especially all alcoholics, should be skin tested for TB exposure. A positive result in a person who has not received prior BCG may be an indication for anti-tuberculous chemotherapy.

59

TABLE IX—*Some extrahepatic complications of alcohol damage*

Organ	Disease	Comment
Heart	Alcoholic cardiomyopathy	Appears to be uncommon in patients undergoing evaluation. Nevertheless, it is advisable that all alcoholics should have cardiac evaluation including stress test and echocardiography. Significant cardiomyopathy would constitute a reason to deny transplantation
	Ischaemic heart disease	History of smoking a risk factor
Muscle	Alcoholic myopathy	Muscle wasting commonly a feature in the cachectic alcoholic Rarely a factor in the decision to withhold transplantation
Pancreatitis	Alcoholic pancreatitis	Rarely requires specific investigation in the assessment before transplantation
CNS		Chronic encephalopathy is sometimes very difficult to distinguish for alcoholic organic brain syndrome. CT scans, or other investigations, do not predict whether the clinical syndrome will improve with improved liver function
Bone	Alcoholic osteopenia	Very few data on bone disease in alcoholics undergoing liver transplantation, on either incidence or response to the transplant organ. Osteopenia in alcoholics rarely requires specific organ investigation

TABLE X—*Primary tumours of the liver*

Benign	Malignant
Hepatocellular	
Adenoma	Hepatocellular carcinoma
	Fibrolamellar carcinoma
	Hepatoblastoma
Bilary	
Adenoma	Cholangiocarcinoma
Cystadenoma	Cystadenocarcinoma
Papillomatosis	
Mesodermal	
Haemangioma	
	Angiosarcoma
	Epithelioid haemangio-endothelioma
	Sarcoma

Transplantation for malignant disease

In the early days of transplantation, primary liver cancer was a major indication for liver transplantation (up to 34%). The reasoning for this was that such patients were ideal because operative mortality was low – patients were usually young to middle aged and otherwise fit and well, with disease confined to the liver and not complicated by the multi-organ involvement often seen with chronic liver diseases. Results were, however, poor with two year survival rates of only 31%[40] and the major cause of death was recurrent disease. This has brought the whole concept of transplantation as a treatment for cancer into question, and malignant liver disease still remains a controversial indication for transplantation.

Primary liver cancers (Table X)

Hepatocellular carcinoma

Hepatocellular carcinoma (HCC) is the most common primary malignancy in the liver on a world-wide basis (Table XI) and occurs most frequently in men with cirrhosis. Liver resection offers an opportunity for cure but, in the presence of decompensated underlying cirrhosis or because of the location of the tumour, resection may be technically impossible. Liver transplantation provides a logical alternative as total removal of the primary disease is obtained.

TABLE XI—*Incidence per 100 000 of liver tumours and cirrhosis*

Country	Liver tumour	Cirrhosis	Tumour/cirrhosis (%)
USA	1·4	22·5	6
UK	1·2	3·05	39
Australia	1·4	8·82	16
France	7·1	48·04	14
Italy	11·3	44·73	25
Japan	12·2	22·36	54

From Aoki.[41]

Survival figures for patient recovery on orthotopic liver transplantation (OLT) for HCC remain poor with only about a 18% five-year survival; death is usually from recurrent disease either in the graft or in the lungs.

This has led many centres to reconsider liver transplantation in the management of advanced HCC. Nevertheless, medical therapy for HCC remains largely ineffective, so surgery offers the best chance of a long term cure. Indeed, the longest survival in both the major series from Starzl and Calne was with patients with HCC.

The high rates of cancer recurrence following OLT is due to a number of factors including the following:

● Poor patient selection
● Circulating HCC cells and micrometastasis at the time of OLT.

The tumour growth-promoting effects of immunosuppressive agents, allowing rapid, unrestrained growth of any remaining tumour cells, have been questioned.

Thus improved survival following transplantation for HCC depends most importantly on better patient selection, on better modalities for eradication of circulating tumour cells and micrometastasis, and finally on better control and understanding of the relationship between immunosuppression and tumour recurrence – perhaps helped by newer immunosuppressive drugs.

Patient selection

In recent years attempts have been made to identify those patients with HCC who are likely to survive long term with OLT. Several features associated with a favourable prognosis have been identified:

TABLE XII—*TNM classification and stage grouping of HCC (UICC, 1987)*

Number	Size (cm)	Localisation	Vascular invasion		N0	N1	Established hepatic spread
Solitary	≤2		0	T1	I	III	IVB
Solitary	≤2		+	T2	II	III	IVB
Multiple	≤2	Unilobular	0	T2	II	III	IVB
Solitary	>2		0	T2	II	III	IVB
Solitary	>2		+	T3	III	III	IVB
Multiple	≤2	Unilobular	+	T3	III	III	
Multiple	>2		0,+	T3	III	III	
Multiple		Bilobular	+PV;HV	T4	IVA	IVA	IVB
					M0	M1	
						Metastases	

PV = portal vein. HV = hepatic vein.

- Unicentric tumours < 5 cm in size
- Absence of vascular invasion
- Presence of a pseudocapsule surrounding the lesion.

These prognostic parameters have recently been included in staging criteria for HCC by the International Union against Cancer (UICC) (Table XII). Using these criteria, patients with stage II disease have five-year survival rates of 60–75% (comparable with figures for transplantation for diseases such as PBC) compared to five-year survival rates of only 15–20% with stage III or IV disease.[42]

In addition to patients presenting with symptoms due to hepatoma, HCC may be diagnosed as a result of routine surveillance of cirrhotic patients, standard liver transplant evaluation, or on examination of the resected liver. Patients in the last two groups, who have what are termed 'incidental tumours', tend to have a longer survival after transplantation.

As a result of the risks of tumour seeding, biopsy of any tumour should be avoided in the situation where there is little doubt that the tumour is a hepatocellular carcinoma, such as in a cirrhotic liver, where there is a space occupying lesion and a rising serum α-fetoprotein. In the absence of elevated and rising serum α-fetoprotein levels, then histological or cytological examination should be sought to determine the nature of the tumour. Some forms of hepatocellular carcinoma may resemble pancreatic, renal, or colonic tumours.

Many centres have attempted to reduce the risk of tumour recurrence by a variety of therapeutic regimens before, during, or after surgery.[43, 44] Such approaches include use of chemotherapy, chemoembolisation, and radiotherapy with or without chemosensitisation. All these therapies have been restricted by the presence of preoperative liver dysfunction and hypersplenism, and by the systemic nature of HCC. At present, no clinical approach has achieved widespread acceptance and there remains a need for multicentre prospective studies. The role immunosuppression plays in the recurrence of HCC after OLT remains to be clarified.

HCC without cirrhosis

Up to 25% of patients with HCC do not have cirrhosis. Some of these patients have a fibrolamellar variant. In tumours that are non-resectable, OLT should be considered using the same staging and prognostic criteria as the above.

Fibrolamellar carcinoma

This is a malignant primary liver tumour affecting young people of either sex. There is a characteristic histological appearance with clumps of eosinophilic tumour cells containing hyaline and pale bodies interspersed with bands of mature fibrous tissue. The remaining liver is non-cirrhotic. It has been suggested that fibrolamellar carcinoma is an independent indicator of improved prognosis because of a relatively benign natural history. This has led to an aggressive surgical approach for resection. The evidence that survival following resection or transplantation for this tumour is better than for HCC arising in a non-cirrhotic liver is lacking.[45]

Data on transplantation for fibrolamellar carcinoma are few, but available figures for survival rates suggest a 55% five year survival following transplantation. The cause of death is recurrent disease in most cases.[45]

Hepatoblastoma

This is a rare tumour usually presenting in childhood, affecting females more than males. Characteristically, vascular encasement is seen early with this tumour which makes resection impossible in many cases. If resection is possible, the prognosis is better than with HCC – there is about a 36% five year survival.[7] Transplantation may be considered for non-resected tumours and where there is no evidence of extrahepatic spread. Unlike HCC, no clear guidelines or established prognostic factors exist. Published series show five year, tumour free survival approaching 50% following transplantation.[45, 46]

Cholangiocarcinoma

Results of transplantation for patients with cholangiocarcinoma are disappointing, and few centres will consider such patients to be suitable candidates. There is often extensive disease at diagnosis. In those who have been transplanted tumour recurrence is seen in up to 75%.[47] In one series of 109 patients undergoing transplantation for cholangiocarcinoma, only 17% of patients were alive at 5 years. As with hepatocellular carcinomas, cholangiocarcinoma may be symptomatic or incidental. As discussed elsewhere, in patients with primary sclerosing cholangitis (PSC), differentiation of benign and malignant structures may be very difficult. It is important, however, to identify early tumours. Starzl[48] reported a one year survival rate of patients with PSC of 85% compared to 72% in those with cholangiocarcinoma. A two year actuarial survival rate in those with pre-diagnosed cholangiocarcinomas was 29% compared to 55% in those in whom the tumour was found incidentally.[48]

Cystadenocarcinoma

This rare tumour occurs in adults, more often in females. The gross appearance of the liver shows multilocular cysts containing muddy, bile stained, mucinous material. Lesions tend to be large and multiple often making resection impossible. Isolated case reports on successful OLT for this tumour exist, but data on recurrence rates and survival are currently lacking.

Angiosarcoma

These tumours are rare and highly malignant. Tumours are usually multifocal and metastasise very early. Resection for tumours detected early may be possible. In the few patients who have been transplanted for this disease, recurrence is almost universal, with death occurring within two years of transplantation.

Epithelioid haemangio-endothelioma

This very rare tumour of adults is a slow-growing vascular tumour of low grade malignancy, usually presenting with multiple focal hypovascular lesions in both lobes of the liver. The intervening liver is normal. In patients in whom intrahepatic dissemination contraindicates resection and extrahepatic spread is absent, transplantation may be appropriate. Small series have produced encouraging results in transplantation for this tumour, showing 82% two year and 43% five year survival rates. Death is usually from recurrent disease.

Undifferentiated sarcoma of the liver

This tumour is highly malignant, running a rapidly progressive course, and with death usually occurring within two months of diagnosis. Transplantation is not an option to consider for this tumour; early lesions may be resectable but survival data are very poor.

Benign tumours of the liver

Most tumours do not require intervention and lesions are best left alone, but when producing severe symptoms they are best treated by resection. Transplantation is as an option in two circumstances:

- Where the benign tumour is so large (or multiple) that resection would leave insufficient functioning hepatic tissue.
- Multiple hepatic adenomatosis, where the liver contains simple adenomas. In advanced cases little functioning liver is left so that patients may be encephalopathic. Further, each adenoma has a

small risk of malignant transformation so the presence of dysplasia may be considered an indication for grafting.

Assessing suitability for transplantation for primary liver cancers

Once a diagnosis has been made and the histological type of tumour determined, the following questions need to be considered:

- Is the liver cirrhotic?
- Is the tumour single or multiple?
- What is the tumour size?
- Is the tumour surgically resectable?
- Is there any evidence of vascular invasion?
- Is there evidence of extrahepatic spread?

To answer these questions the following investigations may need to be performed:

- Ultrasound guided or laparoscopic biopsy of non-involved liver.
- Ultrasonography with Doppler studies of hepatic veins, portal vein, inferior vena cava, and hepatic arteries.
- CT scan with contrast enhancement.
- Dynamic CT scanning (CT portography) or Lipiodol scanning of suspicious lesions.
- Digital subtraction angiography for evidence of vascular invasion.
- Magnetic resonance imaging.
- Cytological examination of any ascitic or pleural fluid.

Extrahepatic spread almost inevitably precludes transplantation. Although current imaging techniques may miss even significant extrahepatic spread, metastatic deposits should be sought by CT examination of the chest, abdomen, and pelvis. Some centres also use bone scintigraphy. Laparoscopy is often helpful in diagnosing tumours that have spread though the liver capsule but minilaparotomy before transplantation is now rarely indicated because of the likelihood of causing metastasis. However, laparotomy at surgery before hepatectomy may reveal previously undetected tumour so that transplantation should be abandoned. Some centres arrange for a back-up in this situation. If the patient remains on the transplant list for more than a few weeks, re-evaluation of the tumour spread may be required.

If these investigations show the tumour to be stage II HCC or less, and unresectable, then transplantation should be considered.

Transplantation for hepatic metastasis

The liver is the most frequent site of blood-borne metastasis. Such metastases may only become apparent several years after apparently successful treatment of the primary tumour. For solitary metastases not suitable for resection, OLT has been considered and carried out. With the exception of carcinoid tumours (see later) data are very disappointing because of a rapid recurrence of the original disease or the discovery of distal metastases post-transplantation. Few centres will undertake transplantation for metastatic disease.

Carcinoid tumours

An aggressive surgical approach has been advocated for both primary and secondary hepatic carcinoid tumours after removal of the primary. This has included transplantation which has been successful in a number of series.

Less common indications

Budd–Chiari syndrome

Budd–Chiari syndrome (thrombosis of the hepatic veins) may present either acutely or with chronic liver disease. The acute presentation is with the triad of abdominal pain, ascites, and diarrhoea. In severe cases, there may be hepatic encephalopathy or variceal haemorrhage. The diagnosis is confirmed by demonstration using contrast enhanced CT or angiography, which shows a blocked hepatic vein. In about half the cases, it is possible to identify a cause, such as drugs (especially sex steroids), hypercoagulable states, or thrombocytosis.

When conditions permit, the treatment of choice is a surgical shunt or TIPS. Local infusion of thrombolytic agents has been tried with varying success in the acute phase of the illness. Transplantation should only be considered when such a shunt has failed or is not technically feasible.

Indications for surgery in *acute* Budd–Chiari syndrome are encephalopathy, jaundice, ascites, and abdominal pain. In *chronic* Budd–Chiari syndrome the usual indication is intractable ascites.

Conditions that justify consideration of liver transplantation include the following:

- Advanced cirrhosis on biopsy
- Occlusion of the retrohepatic vena cava
- Failed mesocaval shunt
- A primary thrombotic disorder (protein C, protein S, or antithrombin III deficiency).

In many cases of Budd–Chiari syndrome, there is no obvious underlying cause, although there are suggestions of an underlying myelodysplastic disorder, which may be detected by finding an abnormal erythrocyte colonisation factor. There are two implications:

- In such cases the patient will remain at risk of developing further thrombotic episodes and so should be maintained on warfarin (coumadin) anticoagulation
- Prolonged survival may be associated with the development of frank myelodysplasia.

Wilson's disease

Wilson's disease is due to a genetic defect localised to chromosome 13 which results in deposition of copper in various tissues, especially the liver and brain. The hepatic presentation may be either as an acute hepatic failure (although these patients almost always have an established cirrhosis at presentation), as chronic active hepatitis, or as end stage liver disease. The treatment of choice is copper chelation therapy. Instigation of treatment may be associated with neurological deterioration which, in rare instances, is permanent. However, even in many apparent end stage patients, there may be a dramatic response to treatment. In a newly diagnosed Wilson's disease patient, the indication for transplantation may be complications of end stage liver disease; the presence of neurological complications should not necessarily be a bar to transplantation

69

TABLE XIII—*Prognostic model of Nazer* et al.[49]

Score	Serum bilirubin (µmol/l)	Serum AST (IU/l)	PT prolongation (seconds)
0	<100	<100	<4
1	100–150	100–150	4–8
2	151–200	151–200	9–12
3	201–300	201–300	13–20
4	>300	>300	>20

AST = aspartate transaminase.
PT = prothrombin time.

because the neurological defect will usually improve as the graft adequately 'decoppers' the brain.

Liver transplantation, which is curative for Wilson's disease, is indicated: in patients presenting for the first time with fulminant hepatitis; for decompensated cirrhosis; and in some patients in whom neurological dysfunction is progressing despite optimal medical treatment, although this may also occur after transplantation.

Wilson's disease should be suspected as the cause of acute hepatitis under the following indications:

- Age 5–45 years
- Hepatitis accompanied by haemolysis (but consider also hepatitis A viral infection and drugs)
- Ascites, splenomegaly, and signs suggestive of cirrhosis accompanying acute hepatitis
- Low serum alkaline phosphatase
- Unusually deep jaundice
- Low serum ceruloplasmin
- History of hepatitis or behaviour/neurological disorder in a sibling.

Nazer *et al*[49] have developed a prognostic model for identification of patients with Wilson's disease who are potential transplant candidates (Table XIII). A total score of 7 or more was associated with a fatal outcome (in the absence of transplantation).

Kayser–Fleischer rings, discernible with slit-lamp examination of the eye, are frequently absent in teenagers who represent the peak age group in which Wilson's disease presents as hepatitis.

All patients with Wilson's disease must be referred urgently for transplantation, before the onset of encephalopathy if possible.

Graft versus host disease

Liver transplantation is indicated for graft versus host disease (GVHD) under the following conditions:

- The prognosis for cure from the disease which has been treated by bone marrow transplantation is excellent.
- GVHD has produced advanced and irreversible liver disease, usually involving the vanishing bile duct syndrome with progressive ductopenia involving more than 80% of portal tracts.
- GVHD involvement of tissues other than the liver is well controlled.

Haemochromatosis

Haemochromatosis is a disorder of iron metabolism, where iron is deposited in many tissues and in the liver leading to a cirrhosis; most other organs are affected, including heart, pancreas, skin, and brain. There is also an increased tendency to neoplasia. Medical treatment is iron removal, ideally by venesection.

Liver transplantation for haemochromatosis is indicated when the patient has decompensated cirrhosis or early primary liver cancer discovered during serial screening of serum α-fetoprotein and liver ultrasonography.

Contraindications include cardiomyopathy, and diabetic microvascular disease or advanced atheroma.

Protoporphyria

Patients with protoporphyria do rarely develop progressively deepening jaundice leading to liver failure. Once encephalopathy has developed, survival is most improbable without urgent liver replacement. Such patients should therefore be referred when it is recognised that they have progressively deepening jaundice. Referral is urgent when liver failure becomes manifest with prolongation of the prothrombin time or pre-coma. Muscular weakness also occurs in the later phases of deterioration due to a porphyric neuromyopathy which can seriously compromise recovery post-transplantation.

71

FULMINANT AND SUBACUTE HEPATIC FAILURE

DAVID MUTIMER

Liver transplantation has become an established treatment for patients with fulminant hepatic failure (FHF) and subacute hepatic failure (SAHF) (see Box C for definitions).[50] Improving results in this setting probably reflect the growing experience of specialist liver units in the management of patients with FHF/SAHF, and the application of transplantation in this setting.

Early recognition of poor prognostic features, followed by prompt referral and safe transfer to a specialist unit, improves patient outcome. Delayed consultation and late transfer reduce the chance of locating a suitable donor organ before the development of complications in the recipient such as renal failure and cerebral oedema. Furthermore, patients who are transferred in grade III/IV encephalopathy have a significant risk of developing irreversible complications, which preclude a successful outcome. Patients with FHF must be accompanied on transfer by experienced medical staff, who should be alert to the dangers of cerebral oedema, aspiration, and hypoglycaemia (Box D). Liver transplantation may no longer be an option for patients who develop these complications during transfer.

Subacute hepatic failure

Subacute or late onset hepatic failure carries a uniformly poor prognosis. There is a prolonged interval (>8 weeks) between the onset of jaundice and encephalopathy. Characteristically, the patient

---

BOX C   Definitions

Fulminant hepatic failure: the development of hepatic encephalopathy within 8 weeks of the onset of symptoms in a patient without previous liver disease

Subacute hepatic failure: the development of hepatic encephalopathy within 6 months, but after 8 weeks from the onset of symptoms. This is sometimes referred to as late onset hepatic failure (LOHF) or subacute hepatic necrosis

---

BOX D   Safe transfer of patients with acute liver failure

- Transfer high risk patients prior to the development of hepatic encephalopathy
- Endotracheal intubation of all patients with advanced or rapidly advancing encephalopathy prior to transfer
- Central venous lines should be inserted prior to transfer – permits administration of 50% glucose (avoiding large volumes of crystalloid solutions), and ensures adequate (but not excessive) intravascular volume replacement
- The patient should be accompanied by an experienced anaesthetist

---

is female, middle aged, with no definable risk factors. The disease has a typical fluctuating course, with the liver progressively shrinking and ascites developing. Although jaundice tends to increase, the prothrombin time is often not greatly prolonged. Encephalopathy occurs late and is a poor prognostic factor. Organ non-specific antibodies, including anti-liver or anti-kidney microsomal and antinuclear antibodies, may be present but the response to corticosteroids is poor.

Because of the fluctuating nature of the disease, the decision to refer for transplantation is often considered but deferred until the patient becomes ungraftable as a result of sepsis. Thus in those patients with SAHF, once encephalopathy has developed, suitable patients should be referred urgently.

Management before transfer

Hypoglycaemia may complicate FHF/SAHF and may occur suddenly. Blood sugar should be assessed 2-hourly and hypoglycaemia corrected with an infusion of 50% dextrose. Cimetidine or other H_2-receptor blockers should be given to reduce the risk of gastrointestinal bleeding. As patients rarely develop complications from the impaired clotting, and as laboratory variables of clotting are the most useful prognostic indicators, correction of coagulation should be undertaken only for specific clinical indications.

The major causes of death of patients with FHF are sepsis, cardiovascular instability, and cerebral oedema. Thus patients require intensive monitoring, together with early recognition and aggressive treatment of complications.

Lactulose, which is of established value in chronic encephalopathy, is of less importance in patients with FHF. Lactulose and magnesium sulphate enemas may be of benefit in the early stages of encephalopathy in FHF but should be avoided in patients with grade III/IV encephalopathy.

Placing on transplant list

It is important to consider not only when patients should be placed on the waiting list, but also when a patient should be withdrawn from the list. It is preferable to list the patient as soon as the early prognostic signs suggest a poor outcome. The decision whether to proceed to transplantation can be made when a suitable liver becomes available. Patients can be removed from the transplant list if they either show improvement or develop complications that preclude a successful outcome; such complications include a persistent, severe reduction in cerebral perfusion pressure, unresponsive to therapy or evidence of irreversible cerebral damage, and cardiovascular instability or sepsis that is unresponsive to therapy (particularly fungal sepsis).

Management while on transplant list

While waiting for a transplant, the major considerations are:

- Rapid detection and treatment of hypoglycaemia
- Maintenance of fluid balance
- Early recognition and treatment of renal failure (using diuretics, intravenous dopamine, or renal support as appropriate)
- Early recognition and treatment of raised intracranial pressure (using clinical signs and pressure monitoring)
- Early detection and treatment of sepsis (bacterial and fungal)
- Correction of coagulopathy, only when clinically indicated
- Respiratory support, with early use of assisted mechanical ventilation
- Minimal patient disturbance.

Early total hepatectomy has been used in some cases. It may result in haemodynamic and metabolic stabilisation before a graft becomes available.

Specific causes of hepatic failure

The cause of FHF is an important prognostic factor (Figure 5); patients with paracetamol (acetaminophen) hepatotoxicity and hepatitis A viral infection have the greatest probability of spontaneous recovery. Individual causes of FHF are described below. It is important to exclude sepsis or malignant infiltration as a cause of FHF because clearly transplantation is not appropriate in these situations.

There are also many rarer causes of FHF (Box E), including the microvesicular fat disorders and *Amanita phalloides* poisoning. Some conditions, such as septicaemia and malignant infiltration, can present in FHF and transplantation is not indicated. An enlarged

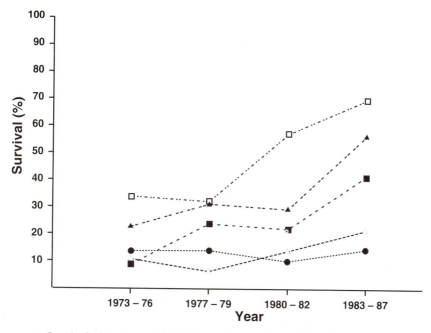

FIG 5—*Survival of patients with fulminant hepatic failure (FHF) at King's College Hospital showing improvement in survival with time, according to diagnosis.* □ *Hepatitis A;* ▲ *paracetamol (acetaminophen) poisoning;* ■ *hepatitis B;* △ *NANB hepatitis;* ● *halothane/drugs. (Reproduced with permission from O'Grady et al.[51])*

BOX E   Causes of fulminant hepatic failure

Drugs
  Paracetamol (acetaminophen)
  Halothane
  Anti-tuberculous therapy
  Many others

Toxins
  Amanita phalloides
  Other toxins as solvents

Viral
  Hepatitis A virus
  Hepatitis B virus
  Hepatitis D virus
  Hepatitis E virus
  Presumed non-A, non-B virus
  Herpes simplex virus
  Epstein–Barr Virus
  Cytomegalovirus

Other
  Fatty liver of pregnancy
  Budd–Chiari syndrome
  Sepsis
  Tumour
    malignant infiltration
    lymphoma: Hodgkin's/
      non-Hodgkin's
  Wilson's disease
  Veno-occlusive disease
  Hepatic vein thrombosis
  Hypotension/ischaemia
  Reye's syndrome
  Heat stroke

---

liver in FHF suggests malignant infiltration (cancer or lymphoma) and a tissue diagnosis should be considered before surgery is undertaken.

Paracetamol (acetaminophen) poisoning

Paracetamol poisoning is the most common cause of FHF in the United Kingdom. Most patients present within 12 hours of poisoning and are treated effectively with N-acetylcysteine. Late treatment (that is, after 12 hours have elapsed) with N-acetylcysteine may also improve survival,[52] but the likelihood of liver damage increases significantly as treatment becomes more remote from the time of poisoning. Specialist liver units ultimately see only a minority of all poisoned patients. Only 7 of 92 consecutive patients transferred to the Birmingham Liver Unit had presented within 12 hours of poisoning; four of these seven patients were not treated with N-acetylcysteine at presentation and two subsequently died (compared with all three treated patients who were successfully discharged from hospital). Physicians should be alert to the increasing likelihood of significant hepatotoxicity associated with late presentation. Analysis of prognostic factors in patients referred to Birmingham

---

BOX F   Paracetamol poisoning: indications for and timing of referral to specialist units

- The development of hepatic encephalopathy is an indication for urgent referral
- The following laboratory results should prompt referral before encephalopathy develops:
    Admission arterial pH $< 7 \cdot 35$ ($H^+ > 45$ mmol/l)
    Prothrombin time > 50 seconds (at any time after admission)
- Significant renal dysfunction rarely occurs in the absence of severe liver damage, and is rarely the sole indication for transfer

---

confirmed that those patients who subsequently died presented significantly later than those who survived to be discharged from hospital. Indications for transfer of patients with FHF due to paracetamol poisoning are shown in Box E. The two main indications are either the development of hepatic encephalopathy or the presence of adverse prognostic factors. In the Birmingham analysis, prognosis could also be related to degree of prolongation of pro-thrombin time (PT) at presentation, to arterial pH and serum creatinine at the time of admission to the liver unit, and to peak PT and peak creatinine. The findings are in keeping with analyses performed at King's College Hospital. Prognostic factors identified include: severity of coagulopathy, renal dysfunction, and metabolic acidosis.

Severity of coagulopathy

This is reflected by:

- Peak PT (PT > 100 seconds associated with 81% mortality rate)[51]
- PT still rising on day 4 (associated with 93% mortality rate)[53]
- Admission factor V levels (factor V < 10% associated with 91% mortality rate)
- Admission factor V/VIII ratio (ratio > 30 associated with 91% mortality rate).[54]

In practice, most hospitals will measure PT but not specific clotting factor levels. At Birmingham no deaths were observed in patients with a peak PT < 50 seconds (as measured in the UK) and we would suggest that patients are transferred to a specialist unit when the PT exceeds this value (Box F).

PT results may not be comparable between centres – most UK laboratories determine PT using human brain derived thromboplastin, which gives significantly longer times than does the rabbit brain derived thromboplastin used in US laboratories.

PT that improves and then deteriorates is suggestive of sepsis, either bacterial or fungal.

Renal dysfunction

A peak serum creatinine concentration of more than 300 μmol/l (3·8 mg/dl) is associated with an 80% mortality. The experience at Birmingham suggests that renal performance is frequently neglected in the time between presentation and transfer. A prerenal contribution to renal failure can be prevented by careful attention to fluid balance during this critical period. Renal damage may be prevented by early treatment with *N*-acetylcysteine, and physicians should be alert to the increasing probability of nephrotoxicity associated with late presentation. Significant renal dysfunction seldom occurs in the absence of severe liver damage, and is rarely the sole indication for patient transfer.

Metabolic acidosis

Admission arterial blood pH values of less than 7·30 is associated with an 85% mortality rate. Arterial pH is a time-dependent variable. Acidosis appears to be an early and transient phenomenon, and may have corrected spontaneously by the time of presentation in those patients presenting late. Acidosis at presentation (especially when severe and remote from the time of poisoning) has an excellent predictive value for poor outcome but has a poor sensitivity (that is, many patients with normal pH at admission will not survive). We recommend measurement of arterial pH at presentation in all patients. Patients with an arterial pH of less than 7·35 should be referred immediately to a specialist unit. Acidosis is often present before the development of encephalopathy and before the development of significant renal dysfunction or PT prolongation.

The potential influence of late and prolonged treatment with *N*-acetylcysteine upon the sensitivity and predictive value of these prognostic factors is not known.

Cerebral oedema may develop very early in the course of paracetamol induced FHF and is the principal cause of death in the first week after poisoning. The tendency to cerebral oedema may be aggravated by fluid overload, especially if renal failure is already established. These are important considerations for the patient who requires transfer to a specialist unit. Rapid deterioration in conscious state is frequently observed en route and in our experience at least 4 out of 92 patients have aspirated gastric contents during transfer. Aspiration pneumonitis precludes liver transplantation. Endotracheal intubation of all patients with advanced or rapidly advancing encephalopathy is recommended before transfer.

A central venous line should be inserted before transfer to assist adequate resuscitation, to prevent fluid overload, and to permit the administration of hypertonic glucose solutions. Vascular access can be safely achieved by experienced practitioners even in the presence of severe coagulopathy. The risks arising from inadequate monitoring are greater than those from complications of line insertion. These simple precautions (see Box D) result in optimal patient condition on arrival, and allow consideration of all treatment options including liver transplantation.

Intracerebral pressure

Cerebral oedema is a frequent cause of death in these patients. Raised intracerebral pressure (ICP) can be detected clinically, but in ventilated and paralysed patients, intracranial monitoring is helpful, although not free of complications. The cerebral perfusion pressure (mean arterial pressure – ICP) should be maintained above 6·65 kPa (50 mmHg). Raised ICP (> 3·36 kPa or 25 mmHg) can be treated by boluses of 10% or 20% mannitol, barbiturate infusion (phenobaritone or thiopentone), and hyperventilation. Mannitol administration can be repeated if there is adequate renal function or support, and hyperosmolality is avoided. Brain stem death can occur in the absence of raised ICP.

Psychiatric considerations

Most cases of paracetamol poisoning are due to deliberate overdose, and some patients clearly have serious premorbid psychiatric disturbance (but only 16 out of 92 consecutive admissions to the

Queen Elizabeth Liver Unit, Birmingham had significant past psychiatric problems, perhaps reflecting patient selection). Paracetamol overdose is usually an impulsive act precipitated by relationship or financial problems, and in these patients liver transplantation should be considered when prognostic factors predict a high likelihood of death with conservative management alone.

Successful rehabilitation is unlikely if the circumstances that led up to the suicide attempt are likely to persist after transplantation. Those factors that suggest repeat suicide attempts[54a,54b,54c] include:

- Substance abuse (alcohol and/or other)
- Previous suicide attempts
- Low social class
- Unemployment
- Previous inpatient psychiatric care
- Personality disorder
- Living alone
- Poor family support.

Results of transplantation for paracetamol poisoning in Birmingham

Seventeen of 92 patients with FHF following paracetamol overdose were 'listed' for, and 10 subsequently underwent, liver transplantation. Seven of 10 long term survivors have been followed for 8–30 months, and none has presented further significant psychiatric problems. Only one of seven patients who were listed but not transplanted survived to be discharged from hospital. The perioperative management of patients with paracetamol poisoning is focused upon the prevention and treatment of cerebral oedema. Patients remain at risk of this complication in the first 48 hours after transplantation and sedation and ventilation, and intracranial monitoring, should be maintained for at least 48 hours following transplantation. Although persisting neurological sequelae have been reported to occur in patients following transplantation for FHF, most patients will make complete neurological recovery. The syndrome of FHF is promptly and effectively reversed by liver transplantation, but renal failure may be slow to resolve. Seven of 10 patients transplanted for paracetamol induced liver failure had established renal failure (creatinine > 150 μmol/l or $1·9$ mg/dl) at the time of arrival on the Liver Unit and required haemodialysis before transplantation. Five of seven surviving patients required postoperative dialysis for a median period of 26 days (range 5–74 days) until recovery of renal function was observed.

Fulminant viral hepatitis

Viral hepatitis is the most common cause of FHF treated by liver transplantation. For the purpose of this discussion, sporadic, fulminant, non-A, non-B hepatitis (NANB) is assumed to be a viral disease.

Liver failure seldom complicates hepatitis A viral (HAV) infection, though the incidence of this complication may increase as primary exposure tends towards an older age group. The mortality rate of patients having fulminant HAV infection with grade III/IV encephalopathy and who have not undergone transplantation in two large reported series,[51, 55] was approximately 50%. Only 5% of all patients with FHF who undergo transplantation have a diagnosis of HAV infection.

Sporadic NANB hepatitis (or hepatitis of indeterminate aetiology) accounts for many patients transplanted for FHF. By definition, serological markers of acute hepatitis A virus (IgM anti-HAV) and hepatitis B virus (IgM anti-HBc) infection are absent. We, and others, have shown convincingly that fulminant NANB hepatitis is not due to hepatitis C viral (HCV) infection.[56] Hepatitis E viral (HEV) infection is a rare cause of liver failure in the Western World and should be considered in patients recently returned from countries such as Turkey, India, and the former Soviet Union, where this virus is endemic. Pregnant women, especially those in the third trimester, are at particular risk of FHF. NANB hepatitis, associated with either FHF or SAHF, has little chance of spontaneous resolution, and is associated with a mortality rate for those not undergoing transplantation of approximately 90%. NANB hepatitis may also be associated with aplastic anaemia which, if present before surgery, makes liver transplantation inappropriate. In some cases, aplastic anaemia develops after transplantation.

Fulminant HBV infection is rare in the UK but is the principal cause of acute liver failure in France, and is the most common indication for liver transplantation in patients with FHF in that country. Approximately 80% of patients with fulminant HBV will die without liver transplantation.[57] Co-infection of hepatitis D and B may result in FHF.

The indications for liver transplantation in patients with severe hepatitis complicated by liver failure have been defined by retrospective analysis of patients treated at King's College Hospital over a 14 year period (before the application of transplantation in this setting).[51] Poor prospects for spontaneous recovery are related to the following:

- Aetiology (NANB worse than HAV or HBV)
- Long duration (>7 days) of jaundice before onset of encephalopathy
- PT >50 seconds
- Bilirubin >300 μmol/l (16 mg/dl)
- Extremes of age (<10 or >40 years).

Bernuau et al prospectively validated a selection policy in the setting of severe viral hepatitis that required the presence of encephalopathy and clotting factor V levels of less than 20% in patients under 30 years of age (or less than 30% in older patients).[58] This study confirmed that factor V levels of less than 20% are predictive of death in patients with severe hepatitis.

The indications in this setting for patient transfer to a specialist liver unit are less well defined. The onset of hepatic encephalopathy is clearly an indication for prompt transfer. In addition, the development of poor prognostic factors (especially PT prolongation, in a patient with subacute NANB hepatitis) before the development of encephalopathy should prompt early consultation and transfer. Ascites and hepatorenal failure may develop prior to the onset of encephalopathy, especially in patients with SAHF,[59] and are an indication for patient transfer. Preoperative hepatorenal failure is strongly associated with a difficult course (and increased risk of death) following liver transplantation in this setting.

Recurrent infection of the graft

It has been claimed that anti-HBs immunoprophylaxis following liver transplantation reduces the incidence of graft HBV reinfection. Risk of HBV recurrence in patients receiving prophylaxis is related to the presence of viral replication (as reflected by either serum HBeAg or serum HBV DNA) at the time of grafting.[60] An accepted prophylactic regimen is the administration of anti-HBs (5000–10 000 units) during the anhepatic phase, repeated three times in the first postoperative week, and weekly for the first three months. The anti-HBs titre should be checked regularly and further anti-HBs should be given when serum levels fall below 100 units/l. There is no effective treatment for established recurrent HBV infection. Immunoprophylaxis should be abandoned if HBsAg reappears in the serum, as HBsAg recurrence is invariably followed by replicative infection with often severe graft hepatitis, and the results of retransplantation are discouraging.

NANB hepatitis may recur in the allograft. There is an increased incidence of chronic hepatitis in the graft of patients undergoing transplantation for fulminant NANB hepatitis.[61] Severe acute hepatitis is rare, and SAHF may occur due to apparent recurrent NANB infection. Although the short term results are excellent, the long term prognosis with respect to viral recurrence is still unknown.

Wilson's disease

The diagnosis of Wilson's disease should be considered in any patient under the age of 45 years presenting with FHF. The mean age at presentation is less than 18 years, and FHF rarely complicates Wilson's disease after the age of 30 years. Acute liver failure in Wilson's disease usually occurs on a background of undiagnosed but established cirrhosis. Clues to the diagnosis of Wilson's disease include the presence of intravascular haemolysis and renal failure. Cutaneous signs of chronic liver disease are rarely present. Kayser–Fleischer rings may be absent on eye examination of young patients with Wilson's disease.

Of the available diagnostic laboratory tests (including serum copper and serum ceruloplasmin), the measurement of urinary copper excretion provides the most sensitive test for confirming the diagnosis of fulminant Wilson's disease;[62] also serum alkaline phosphatase may be very low in such patients. Serum bilirubin is often high (sometimes $> 1000\,\mu mol/l$ or $55\,mg/dl$) as a result of the associated haemolysis and renal failure. A low ratio of alkaline phosphatase : bilirubin[63] is suggestive, but not diagnostic, of fulminant Wilson's disease.

Patients with suspected fulminant Wilson's should be referred urgently to a specialist liver unit. Attempts to treat this syndrome by cupriuresis are generally unsuccessful. Liver transplantation cures

TABLE XIV—*Results of liver transplantation for fulminant liver failure: the larger reported series*

Reference source	Period	Survivors/ total	Actuarial survival rate
Paris[65]	1986–90	62/92	70% 2 year
Birmingham[50]	1984–91	34/67	55% 1 year
			48% 2 year
Pittsburgh[66]	1980–87	21/42	60% 1 year
			46% 2 year
King's[67]	1982–88	21/33	Not reported
Omaha[68]	1986–88	14/24	58% 1 year

the metabolic abnormality or abnormalities responsible for the accumulation of copper in Wilson's disease. Family members should be screened for evidence of Wilson's disease.

Results of liver transplantation

Liver transplantation has clearly improved the prognosis of selected patients with FHF or SAHF. Before the use of liver transplantation in this setting, patients with fulminant NANB hepatitis and fulminant Wilson's disease rarely achieved hospital discharge. It seems unlikely that transplantation will ever be evaluated in a controlled study.[64] There is a lack of large series describing the outcome of patients transplanted for acute liver failure[65-68] (Table XIV). Reported actuarial survival figures will be influenced by a centre's initial (and often less successful) experience in liver transplantation in this setting. One year actuarial survival rate of 50–60% is reported by most centres. These results are clearly inferior to results reported in the transplantation of patients with chronic liver diseases, and most probably reflect the desperate preoperative condition of many patients with fulminant liver failure; however, the results of transplantation appear to be improving. Similar improvements have been observed in the results of transplantation for chronic liver disease. Improving results are probably due to better recognition of poor prognostic factors, earlier patient referral, and better perioperative management of special complications such as cerebral oedema and bleeding. Further improvement will depend in part on refinement of prognostic and better patient selection criteria. Further work is required to identify those patients with little hope of surviving liver transplantation. The establishment of such criteria will improve results and guarantee optimal usage of valuable donor organs.

PAEDIATRIC LIVER TRANSPLANTATION

DEIDRE A KELLY

The successful development of paediatric liver transplantation has dramatically changed the outlook for many babies and children dying of end-stage liver failure and is now accepted therapy for this condition (Figure 6).

Liver transplantation was pioneered in America and Europe in 1963. Although there were rapid advances in adult transplantation, successful paediatric liver transplantation was slower to develop, due to technical difficulties and donor shortages. By 1986, when adult units were achieving 80% one year survival rates, the average survival in children was only 60%.[69] Since then, there have been considerable advances in both medical and surgical management, and one year survival rates for paediatric liver transplantation are now between 85% and 90%.[70, 71] Of particular relevance to successful paediatric transplantation is the development of reduction hepatectomy.[72, 73] This innovation has not only increased the number of

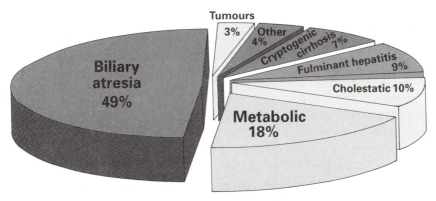

FIG 6—*Indications for liver transplantation in 1162 children under 15 years (European Liver Transplant Registry, 1991[76])*

donor grafts suitable for children, expecially young babies, but has greatly reduced the deaths on the waiting list.[74] The consequent improvement in survival rates has extended the range of indications for liver transplantation in children from terminally ill, high risk patients, to include semi-elective liver replacement and transplantation for metabolic liver disease.

The number of children receiving liver transplantation has increased rapidly; by 1990 over 1000 children had received liver grafts in the USA,[75] whereas a similar number had undergone transplantations in Europe by the end of 1991[76] (Figure 6). In Europe, 40% of transplantations were performed in children under 2 years of age, 50% in children aged 2–12 years, and 10% in children aged 12–15 years.[76]

Despite the recent success of liver transplantation, it remains an expensive procedure with enormous resource implications and an appreciable mortality; thus, careful consideration should be given to the selection of potential recipients.

Indications for liver transplantation

Liver transplantation is now accepted therapy for acute or chronic liver failure. Transplantation for metabolic liver disease without liver failure and for hepatic malignancy is more controversial.

In making the decision to recommend transplantation, the mortality and morbidity of the underlying disease must be balanced against the risk of the operation and its complications, including life long immunosuppression.

Chronic liver disease

Chronic liver failure is the most common indication for transplantation in children (Figure 6) and may arise from the following: neonatal liver disease, including biliary atresia; inherited metabolic liver disease, of which α_1-antitrypsin deficiency is the most common indication; familial cholestatic syndromes, such as Alagille's syndrome and Byler's disease; chronic hepatitis with cirrhosis; and less commonly from fibropolycystic liver disease or cystic fibrosis (Table XV).

TABLE XV—*Indications for liver transplantation in children*

Chronic liver failure
  Neonatal liver disease
    Biliary atresia
    Idiopathic neonatal hepatitis
  Inherited metabolic liver disease
    α_1-Antitrypsin deficiency – Niemann–Pick disease type B
    Tyrosinaemia type I
    Wilson's disease
    Cystic fibrosis
    Glycogen storage disease type I and type IV
  Cholestatic liver disease
    Alagille's syndrome
    Byler's disease
    Non-syndromic biliary hypoplasia
  Chronic hepatitis
    Postviral (hepatitis B, C, other)
    Autoimmune
    Idiopathic
  Other
    Cryptogenic cirrhosis
    Fibropolycystic liver disease ± Caroli's syndrome
Acute liver failure
  Fulminant hepatitis
    Viral hepatitis (A, B, other)
    Paracetamol poisoning
    Halothane exposure
    Autoimmune
    Drugs
  Metabolic liver disease
    Wilson's disease
    Tyrosinaemia type I
    Neonatal haemochromatosis
    Galactosaemia
    Fatty acid oxidation defects (eg, Reye's syndrome)
Inborn errors of metabolism
  Primary oxalosis
  Crigler–Najjar type I
  Familial hypercholesterolaemia
  Urea cycle defects
  Propionic acidaemia
Liver tumours
  Benign tumours replacing liver
  Unresectable malignant tumours
  Hepatic tumours secondary to:
    Tyrosinaemia
    α_1-Antitrypsin deficiency
    Glycogen storage disease type I

Neonatal liver disease

Biliary atresia remains the most common indication for liver transplantation in childhood, accounting for 70% of transplantation under the age of 2 years.[76] Although palliative surgery (Kasai portoenterostomy) may improve the initial outcome,[77] in practice few children are referred early enough for this form of surgery to be effective,[78] and urgent transplantation is indicated in children who do not achieve bile drainage following Kasai portoenterostomy.

Although 50–70% of children who develop neonatal cholestasis secondary to α_1-antitrypsin deficiency (phenotype protease inhibitor ZZ) will develop persistent liver disease progressing to cirrhosis, less than 25% will require transplantation in childhood.[79]

The outcome of Alagille's syndrome and other cholestatic liver diseases originating in infancy is variable. Liver transplantation may be indicated, not only for progressive liver disease but also to alleviate intractable pruritus, unresponsive to maximum medical therapy or biliary diversion, or the development of severe hyper-cholesterolaemia and xanthomas.[80]

Liver disease in children over the age of 2 years

The main indications for transplantation in older children include metabolic liver disease (22%) and cirrhosis secondary to biliary atresia (35%).[76]

Tyrosinaemia type I In this autosomal recessive disorder, tyrosine and methionine accumulate secondary to a deficiency of the hepatic enzyme fumaryl acetoacetase. The disease may present acutely in the neonate or with chronic liver failure in the older child. Hepatocellular carcinoma is an inevitable development; thus transplantation may be required either for hepatic failure or for prevention of hepatic malignancy. It is difficult to predict when hepatic malignancy may develop, but a rise in serum α-fetoprotein level, the appearance of hepatic nodularity on ultrasonography or on computed tomography (CT), or the detection of hepatic dysplasia on liver histological examination may be appropriate indications.[81]

Wilson's disease This is rarely diagnosed in children under the age of 3 years but may present with either acute or chronic liver failure. Liver replacement is appropriate if cirrhosis and portal hypertension are present at diagnosis, or if liver disease progresses despite penicillamine therapy.

Cystic fibrosis The improved outcome in children with cystic fibrosis has led to the identification of significant liver disease in approximately 20% of patients. Portal hypertension is usually severe and hepatic function remains adequate for many years. It is important to consider liver replacement only for those children with hepatic decompensation and to treat portal hypertension by other therapeutic means, such as sclerotherapy. If pulmonary disease is severe, these children should be considered for combined heart, lung, and liver transplants.

Liver function is usually normal in children with fibropolycystic liver disease even if they develop severe portal hypertension. Thus, liver replacement is only indicated when hepatic decompensation occurs with portal hypertension.

Timing of transplantation

As many children with cirrhosis and portal hypertension remain well compensated for many years, it may be difficult to estimate their need for liver replacement.

Attempts to predict decompensation with aminopyrine breath tests or caffeine clearance have been disappointing[82] but recent studies with lignocaine (lidocaine) metabolites in both adults and children have shown good correlation with liver function; some units consider that poor formation and excretion of the lignocaine metabolites are indications for liver transplantation.[83]

Malatack *et al.*[84] evaluated a combination of clinical and laboratory indices of hepatic decompensation to predict either death or the need for liver transplantation in children. Four factors were accurate predictors of death (Table XVI) and many centres have found these guidelines useful in selecting recipients.

As protein–energy malnutrition is an inevitable association of chronic liver disease in the growing child (Figure 7), a decrease in nutritional parameters may be a guide to early hepatic decompensation. Evidence of chronic malnutrition (reduced height for chronological age) is of no value in predicting potential need for liver transplantation, but evidence of acute malnutrition, ie, reduction in

TABLE XVI—*Indications for transplantation in chronic liver failure*

Clinical
    Severe portal hypertension
    Recurrent variceal bleeding
    Refractory ascites
    Intractable pruritus
    Growth retardation
    Unacceptable quality of life

Laboratory indices[83, 84]
    Serum cholesterol < 2·6 mmol/l (100 mg/dl)
    Indirect bilirubin > 100 μmol/l (6 mg/dl)
    Serum albumin < 35 g/l (3·5 mg/dl)
    Prothombin ratio (INR) > 1·4
    Poor formation of lignocaine (lidocaine) metabolites
    Portal vein < 4 mm on ultrasonography[73]

INR = international normalised ratio.

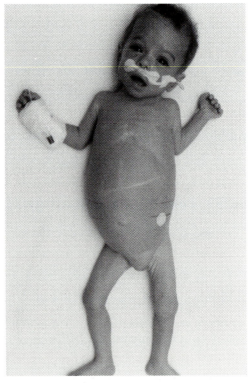

FIG 7—*Chronic liver failure secondary to biliary atresia, following an unsuccessful Kasai hepato-portoenterostomy in a 9-month-old girl. Note the malnutrition with loss of fat and muscle stores, distended abdomen with ascites and inguinal hernia, the nasogastric enteral feeding tube for nocturnal modular feed.*

fat stores (triceps skinfold) or protein stores (mid-arm muscle area) is a sensitive indicator of hepatic decompensation.[69]

Early referral should be considered for children with complex hepatic complications, such as ascites which is refractory to medical management, uncontrolled variceal haemorrhage, particularly if there are gastric varices, or persistent chronic hepatic encephalopathy.

Although psychosocial development in children with chronic liver disease has not been adequately studied, preliminary data suggest that there is a significant reduction in developmental motor skills which is reversed following liver transplantation.[85] Thus, any significant delay in developmental parameters is an indication for early transplantation.

In general, children with chronic liver disease should be referred for transplantation before the complications of their liver disease seriously impair the quality of their lives, and before growth and development are irreversibly retarded.

Acute liver failure

Acute liver failure is relatively rare in children but without transplantation it has a mortality rate of more than 70%.[86] The clinical presentation includes the combination of hepatic encephalopathy, coagulopathy, hypoglycaemia, and jaundice, but difficulties in appreciating this diagnosis mean that many children are referred too late for liver transplantation. Children with fulminant hepatitis secondary to drugs or infection (see Table XV) tend to present with a more acute illness than those with acute liver failure from underlying metabolic disease.

Fulminant hepatitis

Selection of recipients for liver transplantation in children with fulminant hepatitis is based on previous experience of mortality in the era before transplantation was common.[87] Prognosis is worst in children with non-A, non-B hepatitis – there is a rapid onset of coma with progression to grade III or IV hepatic coma, a diminishing liver size, falling serum transaminases in association with an increasing bilirubin, and persistent coagulopathy. These children should be referred early to a specialist centre for intensive care management and liver transplantation.

In practical terms, it is appropriate to place on the transplant list all children who have grade III hepatic coma, a persistent coagulopathy (international normalised ratio, INR > 4), and no evidence of irreversible brain damage from cerebral oedema or hypoglycaemia. As current management strategies for cerebral oedema are unsatisfactory and methods for determining irreversible brain damage imprecise, this may be a difficult decision. Careful management of cerebral oedema is critical and best monitored by measurement of intracranial pressure which improves the selection of recipients but not overall survival.[88] This monitoring should be done after transfer; assessment of cerebral blood flow is technically difficult, but assessment of cerebral perfusion pressure is more sensitive and useful. Cerebral CT scans will detect gross cerebral oedema, infarction, or intracranial haemorrhage. Serial electroencephalography (EEG) may indicate reduction in electrical activity and brain death, although care must be taken in interpreting these results, in ventilated patients, as the EEG tracing is affected by sedation and anaesthetic agents.

Paracetamol poisoning

Paracetamol (acetaminophen) poisoning in children has a bimodal presentation. In children aged 1–4 years accidental ingestion is likely, whereas in the adolescent self-poisoning is usual. The development of liver failure is dose dependent; hepatic failure is likely if the ingested dose is greater than 15 g. Children have a lower incidence of liver failure with paracetamol overdose than adults, perhaps because of the effect of age on glutathione production.[89] Hepatic enlargement and tenderness develop by the second day after ingestion, whereas jaundice, encephalopathy, and renal failure develop between the third and fifth days. Liver transplantation should be considered if there is a persistent coagulopathy (INR > 4), metabolic acidosis (pH < 7·3) and rapid progression to hepatic coma grade III.

Metabolic liver disease

Acute liver failure may be the presenting feature of inherited metabolic liver disease such as Wilson's disease or tyrosinaemia type I. The clinical presentation may be subacute and liver failure occurs in the presence of an underlying but undetected cirrhosis. It is unusual to detect a rapid decrease in liver size in these conditions.

Babies presenting with neonatal haemochromatosis do so within the first 6–8 weeks of life with severe coagulopathy and encephalopathy. In these neonates, liver transplantation may not be a viable option, because of their size, severity of illness, and the difficulty in obtaining suitable donor organs in time.

Inborn errors of metabolism

Liver transplantation may be indicated for inherited disorders in which the liver is functionally normal but deficiency of a hepatic enzyme may cause severe extrahepatic disease (see Table XV). In considering liver replacement for these disorders, it is particularly important to balance the potential mortality and morbidity of the primary disease with that of the complications of liver transplantation and life long immunosuppression.

The timing of transplantation in these disorders depends on the rate of progression of the disease, and the quality of life of the affected child. In general, it is important to perform liver transplantation before there is irreversible disease of other organs (for example, structural brain damage in Crigler–Najjar syndrome type I, or coronary artery disease in children with familial hypercholesterolaemia). If possible, transplantation should be delayed until the child is over 10 kg in weight to increase the probability of donor availability and to reduce surgical risks. In some cases, liver replacement should be combined with other organ transplantation – for example, renal transplantation for primary oxalosis.[81]

Liver tumours

There is little information about the outcome of transplantation for hepatic tumours in childhood, but indications include: unresectable benign tumours causing hepatic dysfunction; unresectable malignant tumours (hepatoblastoma or hepatocellular carcinoma), which are refractory to chemotherapy and radiotherapy without evidence of metastases; and hepatocellular carcinoma secondary to underlying liver disease, such as tyrosinaemia type I, α_1-antitrypsin deficiency, glycogen storage type I and hepatitis B, although the last named is associated with a high rate of recurrence of hepatitis B infection.

A recent series, which evaluated liver transplantation for hepatoblastoma in 12 children, found that there was a worse prognosis in children with extrahepatic metastases, multifocal tumours, or embyronal/anaplastic tumours. In contrast the prognosis was better in children who had unifocal tumours with predominantly fetal epithelium.[90] Thus the evaluation for transplantation should consider the histological grade of the tumour and a bone scan and chest radiograph should be obtained to exclude extrahepatic metastases.

Evaluation pre-transplantation

The evaluation process concentrates on:

- Assessing the need and urgency for transplantation
- Establishing technical feasibility
- Whether there are contraindications
- Whether it is appropriate for the child and the family
- Preparing both the child and the family for the child's transplantation.

Assessment pre-transplantation

On referral, the indication for transplantation should be critically evaluated as discussed above. It is particularly important to review the diagnosis, establish the prognosis of the disease, and consider whether alternative medical or surgical therapy is appropriate. It is essential to evaluate whether liver transplantation will improve the quality of life for both child and family.

Information on nutritional status and presence of hepatic complications is obtained from a clinical history and physical examination. Particular attention should be paid to the evaluation of cardiac and respiratory systems, neurological assessment, and dental examination.

Cardiac assessment

Many children with liver disease also have congenital cardiac disease, for example, atrial and ventricular septal defects are a feature of biliary atresia, whereas peripheral pulmonary stenosis is common in Alagille's syndrome. Careful assessment is required to establish whether cardiac function is adequate for transplantation or corrective surgery should take place before listing.

94

Respiratory assessment

A small percentage of children with end stage liver disease develop intrapulmonary shunts with or without pulmonary hypertension. Clinical signs of cyanosis and digital clubbing will indicate the need for pulmonary function studies or cardiac catherization.

Neurodevelopment assessment

In order to evaluate outcome or potential quality of life post-transplantation, it is necessary to determine the nature of any neurological defects and whether they are reversible. This is particularly important when considering transplantation for children with acute liver failure, or for those who have developed structural brain damage secondary to severe hypoglycaemia or anoxia. Chronic hepatic encephalopathy is usually reversible, and can be diagnosed clinically and confirmed by EEG.

Psychological or developmental assessments using standard tests (Griffiths Mental Development Scales or Stanford–Binet Intelligence Scale) provide baseline information with which to evaluate progress post-transplantation.

Dental assessment

Chronic liver disease has a devastating effect on the growth and development of young children which includes dentition. Dental problems pre-transplantation include hypoplasia, staining of teeth and gingival hyperplasia. It is important to establish good dental hygiene, even in very young children, particularly as gingival hyperplasia will be exacerbated by postoperative medications such as cyclosporin A, and the anti-hypertensive drug nifedipine.

Hepatic function

As discussed above, there are no reliable biochemical tests to evaluate hepatic function, and the decision to list transplantation is based on deterioration in standard liver function tests, with particular reference to prolonged coagulation indices unresponsive to vitamin K (see Table XVI). The severity of portal hypertension can be estimated by identifying oesophageal and gastric varices by gastrointestinal endoscopy; this will also detect gastritis or acid

TABLE XVII—*Evaluation for liver transplantation*

Clinical
  Nutritional parameters:
    Height, weight, triceps skinfold, mid-arm muscle area
  Identification of hepatic complications
  Dental assessment
  Cardiac assessment
    ECG, echocardiography, chest radiography
  Neurological and developmental assessment
    EEG
    Griffiths Mental Development Scales
    Stanford–Binet Intelligence Scales

Investigations
  Radiology
    Ultrasonography of liver and spleen for vascular anatomy
    Wrist radiograph for bone age and rickets
  Serology
    Cytomegalovirus
    Epstein–Barr virus
    Varicella-zoster
    Herpes simplex
    Hepatitis A, B, C
    HIV
    Measles
  Renal function
    Urea, creatinine, electrolytes
    Urinary protein/creatinine ratio
  Haematology
    Full blood count, platelets, blood group

peptic disease which are common complications in these children. If the histological diagnosis is not already apparent a liver biopsy may be required.

Renal function

Abnormalities of renal function are common in children with end stage liver disease, and include renal tubular acidosis, glomerulonephritis, acute tubular necrosis, and hepatorenal syndrome. Careful assessment of renal function is required not only to instigate specific therapy but to provide a baseline, from which to evaluate the potential nephrotoxic effects of post-transplant immunosuppression (Table XVII).

Haematology

Full blood count, platelets, coagulation indices, and blood group are obtained.

Serology

Immunity to previous infection is established (Table XVII) with particular reference to cytomegalovirus (CMV), as donor grafts are matched for CMV status where possible.

Radiology

Doppler ultrasonography of the liver and spleen will outline the vascular anatomy and identify whether the vessels are patent. It is important to examine the portal vein carefully to assess patency, direction of blood flow, and size. Although thrombosis of the portal vein is no longer a contraindication to transplantation, evidence of retrograde flow indicates severe portal hypertension as does decreasing size of the portal vein which is associated with an increase in perioperative technical problems.[73] Children with congenital liver disease, such as biliary atresia, have an increased incidence of abnormal vasculature. The hypovascular syndrome consists of an absent inferior vena cava, a preduodenal or absent portal vein, azygous drainage from the liver, and polysplenia syndrome; it is also often associated with situs inversus, dextrocardia, or left atrial isomerism. Recognition of these syndromes pre-transplantation should reduce technical complications during surgery.

Radiographs of the wrist or knee will determine bone age – an indication of nutritional status – and detect rickets secondary to vitamin D deficiency.

Contraindications to transplantation

As surgical skills have improved, the number of contraindications to transplantation have decreased. The main contraindications to transplantation include the following:

- Severe disease of another organ system which is not reversible after transplantation, such as severe cardiopulmonary disease not amenable to surgery or severe structural brain damage.
- The presence of severe systemic sepsis, particularly fungal sepsis,

at the time of operation. These children will not survive the operation and subsequent immunosuppression. Such infection should be vigorously treated and the transplantation deferred until sepsis is eradicated.

- Chronic hepatitis B (HBV) is likely to recur post-transplantation, especially in those who are HBV DNA positive. Although this is not an absolute contraindication, a guarded prognosis must be given. Hepatitis B does not usually recur following transplantation for fulminant HBV.
- Transplantation for HIV positive children remains controversial.
- The potential recurrence of malignant tumours post-transplantation may be a relative contraindication, and care should be taken to establish that there are no peripheral metastases prior to surgery.

At one time, babies under 1 year old, who weighed less than 10 kg, were not considered for transplantation because of the technical risks and shortage of available donors. With the development of innovative surgical techniques such as reduction hepatectomy and specialised medical and nursing management, there are now no specific contraindications related to age and size, although there may be difficulty in obtaining suitable donor livers for very small babies.

Preparation for transplantation

Immunisation

As live vaccines are contraindicated in the immunosuppressed child, every effort must be made to protect the child from infection post-transplantation. It is customary to ensure that routine immunisations are complete, such as diphtheria, pertussis, tetanus and polio, Pneumovax for protection against streptococcal pneumonia and Hib for protection against *Haemophilus influenzae* b. In children older than 9 months, measles, mumps, and rubella immunisation (MMR) should be offered. Some centres immunise against varicella-zoster, although currently in the UK this vaccine is available on a "named patient basis" only.

Management of hepatic complications

Preoperative management includes treatment of specific hepatic complications such as diuretic therapy for ascites, sclerotherapy for

TABLE XVIII—*Nutritional support pre-transplantation*

Energy intake
110–160% RDA

Modular feed
Carbohydrate
Glucose polymer (7–25%)
Protein   Oral or nasogastric
Whey protein (2–4%)   nocturnal feeding
Fat
Total fat 3–6%
MCT 1–3%
LCT 1–3%
Vitamins
Trace elements   8–6 g daily
Minerals

Vitamin supplements
Vitamin A   5000–15 000 units daily
Vitamin D   50 ng/kg (α-calcidol)
Vitamin E   50–200 mg daily
Vitamin K   2·5–10 mg daily

RDA = recommended dietary allowance.
MCT = medium chain triglyceride.
LCT = long chain triglyceride.

variceal bleeding, and vigorous treatment of any sepsis, particularly ascending cholangitis and spontaneous bacterial peritonitis. Retention of salt and water is a major problem which is managed with diuretics, fluid, and salt restriction. Restriction of fluids may create particular difficulties in providing adequate calories for babies whose enteral intake is dependent on milk feeds.

Haemodialysis or haemofiltration should be instituted if acute renal failure or hepatorenal failure develops, usually secondary to acute liver failure. Haemodialysis is rarely needed in chronic liver failure, unless there is acute decompensation.

Nutritional support

Nutritional support plays a major part in the preparation for transplantation, because at least 60% of children referred for transplantation are malnourished (see Figure 7),[69, 85] and effective therapy has been shown to reduce morbidity and mortality.[91]

The pathophysiology of protein–energy malnutrition in liver

disease is complex and not fully understood, but the aim of therapy is to provide sufficient calories to reverse malnutrition, and to overcome fat malabsorption and ongoing catabolism. A high calorie protein feed (110–160% recommended dietary allowance (RDA)), with sufficient medium chain triglycerides (MCTs) to reduce fat malabsorption, and long chain triglyceries (LCTs) to provide essential fatty acids, is used. It is difficult to provide this high energy intake with standard feeds, particularly in fluid restricted children; thus, a modular feed, in which individual components can be concentrated to maximise energy intake, is most appropriate for young babies (Table XVIII). It is optimistic to think that sick babies and children will take the large volume of concentrated feeds orally, and nocturnal nasogastric enteral feeding is usually necessary. A small percentage of children will not tolerate enteral feeds, because of either food intolerance or recurrent complications, and parenteral feeding is mandatory for these children. Generous oral, fat soluble, vitamin supplementation is essential but occasionally parenteral vitamins may be required (Table XVIII).

Psychological preparation

The importance of counselling and preparation of the child and family cannot be over-emphasised. A specialised multi-disciplinary team including medical, surgical, and nursing staff, a social worker, transplant coordinator, and play therapist is intrinsic to the success of this preparation. Parents and appropriate relatives should be fully informed of the necessity of liver transplantation in their child, the risks and complications, and the long term implications. Psychological preparation of children over 18 months of age is essential and can be successfully achieved through innovative play therapy and books suitable for children.

Particularly careful counselling is required for parents of children being considered for transplantation to correct inborn errors of metabolism, because they may find it difficult to accept the complications of the operation and the potential mortality. Likewise, the parents of children undergoing transplantation for acute liver failure are usually too shocked to understand the implications of transplantation fully. Children surviving liver grafting for acute liver failure should have postoperative counselling and play therapy.

The role of living related organ donation is discussed elsewhere.

References

1 European Liver Transplant Registry. Update 30/6/1992. Hôpital Paul Brousse, Villejuif, France.

2 Ghent CN. Selection of patients. *Transplant Proc* 1986; **18**: 160–2.

3 Van der Putten ABMM, Bijleveld CMA, Slooff MJH, Wesenhagen H, Gips CH. Selection criteria and decisions in 375 patients with liver disease, considered for live transplantation during 1977–1985. *Liver* 1987; 7: 84–90.

4 Samuel D, Benhamou J-P, Bismuth H, Gugenheim J, Ciardullo M, Saliba F. Criteria of selection for liver transplantation. *Transplant Proc* 1987; **19**: 2383–6.

5 Llach J, Rimola A, Arroyo V, *et al*. Transplante hepático: selección de candidatos y resultados obtenidos en un programa para pacientes adultos. *Med Clin (Barc)* 1991; **96**: 41–6.

6 Dindzans VJ, Schde RR, Gavaler JS, Tarter RE, Van Thiel DH. Liver transplantation. A primer for practicing gastroenterologists, part I. *Dig Dis Sci* 1989; **34**: 2–8.

7 Wood RP, Pikkers LF, Shaw BW, Williams L. A review of liver transplantation for gastroenterologists. *Am J Gastroenterol* 1987; **82**: 593–606.

8 Donovan JP, Zetterman RK, Burnett DA, Sorrell MF. Preoperative evaluation, preparation, and timing of orthotopic liver transplantation in the adult. *Semin Liver Dis* 1989; **9**: 168–75.

9 Lucey MR, Merion RM, Henley KS, *et al*. Selection for and outcome of liver transplantation in alcoholic liver disease. *Gastroenterology* 1992; **102**: 1736–41.

10 Lake JR, Wright TL. Liver transplantation for patients with hepatitis B: what have we learned from our results? *Hepatology* 1991; **13**: 796–9.

11 Llach J, Ginés P, Arroyo V, *et al*. Prognostic value of arterial pressure, endogenous vasoactive systems, and renal function in cirrhotic patients admitted to the hospital for the treatment of ascites. *Gastroenterology* 1988; **94**: 482–7.

12 Titó L, Rimola A, Ginés P, Llach J, Arroyo V, Rodés J. Recurrence of spontaneous bacterial peritonitis in cirrhosis: frequency and predictive factors. *Hepatology* 1988; **8**: 27–31.

13 Ginés P, Ginés A, Arroyo V. Prognisis of patients with cirrhosis and ascites. In: Rodés J, Arroyo A, eds. *Therapy in Liver Diseases*. Barcelona: Ediciones Doyma, SA, 1992: 166–72.

14 Pugh RNH, Murray Lyon IM, Dawson J, *et al*. Trans-section of the oesophagus for bleeding varices. *Br J Surg* 1973; **60**: 646–9.

15 Alwmark A, Bengmark S, Börjesson B, Gullstrand P, Joelsson B. Emergency and long-term transesophageal sclerotherapy of bleeding esophageal varices. *Scand J Gastroentrol* 1982; **17**: 409–12.

16 Barsoum MS, Bolous FI, El-Rooby AA, Rizk-Allah MA, Ibrahim AS. Tamponade and injection sclerotherapy in the management of bleeding oeseophageal varices. *Br J Surg* 1982; **69**: 76–8.

17 Westaby D, Macdougall BRD, Williams R. Improved survival following injection sclerotherapy for esophageal varices: final analysis of a controlled trial. *Hepatology* 1985; **5**: 827–30.

18 Söderlund C, Ihre T. Endoscopic esclerotherapy v. conservative management of bleeding oesophageal varices. A 5-year prospective controlled trial of emergency and long-term treatment. *Acta Chir Scand* 1985; **151**: 449–56.

19 Sauerbruch T, Weinzierl M, Köpcke W, Paumgartner G. Long-term sclerotherapy of bleeding esophageal varices in patients with liver cirrhosis. An evaluation of mortality and rebleeding risk factors. *Scand J Gastroenterol* 1985; **20**: 51–8.

20 DiMagno EP, Zinsmeister AR, Larson DE, *et al*. Influence of hepatic reserve and cause of esophageal varices on survival and rebleeding before and after the introduction of sclerotherapy: a retrospective analysis. *Mayo Clin Proc* 1985; **60**: 149–57.

21 Rigau J, Terés J, Visa J, *et al*. Long-term follow-up of 100 patients with portal hypertension treated by a modified splenorenal shunt. *Br J Surg* 1986; **73**: 708–11.

22 Garden OJ, Mills PR, Birnie GG, Murray GD, Carter DC. Propranolol in the prevention of recurrent variceal hemorrhage in cirrhotic patients. *Gastroenterology* 1990; **98**: 185–90.

23 Navasa M, García-Pagán JC, Bosch J, Rodés J. Valor pronóstico del aclaramiento del

101

verde de indocianina en pacientes con cirrosis hepática y hemorragia por varices esofágicas. *Med Clin (Barc)* 1992; **98**: 290–4.

24 Iwatzuki S, Starzl TE, Todo S, *et al.* Experience in 1000 liver transplants under cyclosporine–steroid therapy: a survival report. *Transplant Proc* 1988; **20**(suppl 1): 498–504.

25 Baliga P, Merion RM, Turcotte JG, *et al.* Preoperative risk factor assessment in liver transplantation. *Surgery* 1992; **112**: 704–11.

26 Christensen E, Neuberger J, Crowe J, *et al.* Beneficial effect of azathioprine and prediction of prognosis in primary biliary cirrhosis. *Gastroenterology* 1985; **89**: 1084–91.

27 Christensen E. Prognostication in PBC. *Hepatology* 1989; **10**: 111–13.

28 Markus B, Dickson ER, Grambsch P, *et al.* Efficiency of liver transplantation in patients with primary biliary cirrhosis. *N Engl J Med* 1989; **320**: 1709–13.

29 Klion F, Fabry TZ, Palmer M, Schaffner F. Prediction of survival of patients with primary biliary cirrhosis. *Gastroenterology* 1992; **102**: 310–13.

30 Hughes MD, Rasthino C, Pocock S, *et al.* Predictor of short term survivors with an application in PBC. *Statist Med* 1992; **11**: 1731–45.

31 Dickson ER, Murtaugh P, Wiesner R *et al.* Primary sclerosing cholangitis: refinement and validation of survival models. *Gastroenterology* 1992; **102**: 1893–901.

32 Lucey MR. Hepatic infection. In: Greenfield LA ed. *Surgery: Scientific Principals and Practice.* Philadelphia: JB Lippincott, 1992: 865–75.

33 Lucey MR, Martin P, Di Bisceglie A, *et al.* Recurrence of hepatitis B and delta hepatitis following orthotopic liver transplantation. *Gut* 1992; **33**: 1390–6.

34 Ottobrelli A, Marzano A, Smedile A, *et al.* Patterns of hepatitis delta virus reinfection and disease in liver transplantation. *Gastroenterology* 1991; **101**: 1649–55.

35 Hoofnagle JH, Di Bisceglie AM, Waggoner JG, Park Y. Interferon alpha for patients with clinically apparent cirrhosis due to chronic hepatitis B. *Gastroenterology* 1993; **104**: 1116–21.

36 Wright TL, Donegan E, Hsu HH, *et al.* Recurrent and acquired hepatitis C viral infection in liver transplant recipients. *Gastroenterology* 1992; **103**: 317–22.

37 Lucey MR, Beresford TP. Alcoholic liver disease: To transplant or not to transplant? *Alcohol Alcohol* **27**: 103–8.

38 Benjamin M, Turcotte JG. Ethics, alcoholism and liver transplantation. In Lucey MR, Merion RM, Beresford TP, eds, *Liver Transplantation and the Alcoholic Patient.* Cambridge: Cambridge University Press, 1994: in press.

39 Beresford TP. Psychiatric assessment of alcoholic candidates for liver transplantations. In Lucey MR, Merion RM, Beresford TP, eds, *Liver Transplantation and the Alcoholic Patient.* Cambridge: Cambridge University Press, 1994: in press.

40 Bismuth H, Castaing D, Ericzon BG, *et al.* Hepatic transplantation in Europe. First report of the European Liver Transplant registry. *Lancet* 1987; **ii**: 674–9.

41 Aoki K. *World Health Statistical Report* no. 31 1978; 28–50.

42 Iwatsuki S, Starzl TE, Sheahan DG, *et al.* Hepatic resection versus transplantation for heptocellular carcinoma. *Ann Surg* 1991; **214**: 221–9.

43 Stone MJ, Klintmalm GBG, Potter D, *et al.* Neoadjuvant chemotherapy and liver transplantation for liver hepatocellular carcinoma: results in 20 patients. *Gastroenterology* 1992; **103**: 196–202.

44 Ringe B, Pichlmayr R, Wittekind C, Tusch G. Surgical treatment of hepatocellular carcinoma: experience with liver resection and transplantation in 198 patients. *World J Surg* 1991; **15**: 270–85.

45 Penn I. Hepatic transplantation of primary and metastatic cancers of the liver. *Surgery* 1991; **110**: 726–35.

46 Sherlock S. Hepatic tumours. In: *Diseases of the Liver and Biliary System,* Blackwell Scientific, Oxford, 1989: 584–617.

47 Iwatsuki S, Gordon RD, Shaw BW, *et al.* Role of liver transplantation in cancer therapy. *Ann Surg* 1985; **202**: 401–9.

48 Abu-Elmhed KM, Selby R, Iwatsuki, S, *et al.* Cholangiocarcinoma and sclerosing cholangitis: clinical characteristics and effect on survival after liver transplantation. *Transplant Proc* 1993; **25**: 1124–5.

49 Nazer H, Ede RJ, Mowat A, Williams R. Wilson's disease: clinical presentation and use of prognostic index. *Gut* 1986; **27**: 1377–81.

50 Mutimer DJ, Elias E. Liver transplantation for fulminant hepatic failure. *Progress in Liver Diseases*, 1992; **10**: 349–67.

51 O'Grady JG, Alexander GJM, Hayllar KM, Williams R. Early indicators of prognosis in fulminant hepatic failure. *Gastroenterology* 1989; **97**: 439–45.

52 Harrison PM, Keays R, Bray GP, Alexander GJM, Williams R. Improved outcome of paracetamol-induced fulminant hepatic failure by late administration of acetyl cysteine. *Lancet* 1990; **335**: 1572–3.

53 Harrison PM, O'Grady JG, Keays RT, Alexander GJM, Williams R. Serial prothrombin time as prognostic indicator in paracetamol induced fulminant hepatic failure. *BMJ* 1990; **301**: 964–6.

54 Pereira LMMB, Langley PG, Hayllar KM, Tredger JM, Williams R. Coagulation factor V and V/VIII ratio as predictors of outcome in paracetamol induced fulminant hepatic failure: relation to other prognostic indicators. *Gut* 1992; **33**: 98–102.

54a Hawton K, Fagg J, Platt S, Hawkins M. Factors associated with suicide after parasuicide in young people. *BMJ* 1993; **306**: 1641–4.

54b Nordentoft M, Breum L, Munck LK, *et al.* High mortality by natural and unnatural cancer. *BMJ* 1993; **306**: 1637–40.

54c Morgan G. Long term risks after attempted suicide. *BMJ* 1993; **306**: 1626–7.

55 Bernuau J, Rueff B, Benhamou JP. Fulminant and subfulminant liver failure: Definitions and causes. *Semin Liver Dis* 1986; **6**: 97–106.

56 Mutimer DJ, Shaw JC, Young L, Neuberger JM, Elias E. Hepatitis C in fulminant and subfulminant non-A, non-B hepatitis. Presented at the meeting of the IASL, Brighton 1992.

57 Bernuau J, Goudeau A, Poynard T, *et al.* Multivariate analysis of prognostic factors in fulminant hepatitis B. *Hepatology* 1986; **6**; 648–51.

58 Bernuau J, Samuel D, Durand F, *et al.* Criteria for emergency liver transplantation in patients with acute viral hepatitis and factor V below 50% of normal: A prospective study. *Hepatology* 1991; **14**: 49A.

59 Gimson AES, O'Grady J, Ede RJ, Portman B, Williams R. Late onset hepatic failure: Clinical, serological and histological features. *Hepatology* 1986; **6**: 288–94.

60 Samuel D, Bismuth A, Matthieu D, *et al.* Passive immunoprophylaxis after liver transplantation in HBsAg-positive patients. *Lancet* 1991; **337**: 813–15.

61 Hubscher SG. Chronic hepatitis in liver allografts. *Hepatology* 1990; **12**: 1257–8.

62 Sallie R, Katsiyiannakis L, Baldwin D, *et al.* Failure of simple biochemical indexes to reliably differentiate fulminant Wilson's disease from other causes of fulminant liver failure. *Hepatology* 1992; **16**: 1206–11.

63 Berman DH, Leventhal RI, Gavaler JS, Cadoff EM, Van Thiel DH. Clinical differentiation of fulminant Wilsonian hepatitis from other causes of hepatic failure. *Gastroenterology* 1991; **100**: 1129–34.

64 Chapman RW, Forman D, Peto R, Smallwood R. Liver transplantation for acute hepatic failure? *Lancet* 1990; **335**: 32–5.

65 Samuel D, Bismuth H. Selection criteria and results of orthotopic liver transplantation in fulminant and subfulminant hepatitis. In: Williams R, Hughes RD, eds. *Acute Liver Failure*. Proceedings of the Eleventh BSG Smith, Kline and French International Workshop, 1990: 73–7.

66 Iwatsuki S, Steiber AC, Marsh JW, *et al.* Liver transplantation for fulminant hepatic failure. *Transplant Proc* 1989; **21**: 2431–4.

67 O'Grady JG, Alexander GJM, Thick M, Potter D, Calne RY, Williams R. Outcome of orthotopic liver transplantation in the aetiological and clinical variants of acute liver failure. *Q J Med* 1988; **69**: 817–24.

68 Schafer DF, Shaw Jr BW. Fulminant hepatic failure and orthotopic liver transplantation. *Semin Liver Dis* 1989; **9**: 189–94.

69 Shaw BW, Wood PR, Kelly DA, *et al.* Liver transplantation in children. In: Lebenthal E, ed. *Textbook of Gastroenterology and Nutrition in Infancy*, New York: Raven Press, 1989: 1045–70.

70 Salt A, Noble-Jamieson G, Barnes ND, *et al*. Liver transplantation in 100 children: Cambridge and King's College Hospital Series. *BMJ* 1992; **304**: 416–21.

71 Broelsch CE, Whitington PF, Emond JC. Evolution and future perspectives for reduced-size hepatic transplantation. *Surg Gynecol Obstet* 1990; **171**: 353–60.

72 Bismuth H, Houssin D. Reduced size orthotopic liver grafts in hepatic transplantation in children. *Surgery* 1984; **95**: 367–70.

73 Badger IL, Czerniak A, Beath S, *et al*. Hepatic transplantation in children using reduced size allografts. *Br J Surg* 1992; **79**: 47–9.

74 Langnas A, Wagner C, Marujo W, *et al*. The results of reduced-size liver transplantation including split livers in patients with end-stage liver disease. *Transplantation* 1992; **53**: 387–91.

75 Alexandria BA. *Nachri Reports*, National Association of Children's Hospitals and Related Institutions. June 25 1990.

76 European Liver Transplant Registry. Hôpital Paul Brousse, Villejuif, France: December 1991.

77 Ohi R, Nio M, Chiba T, Endo N, Goto M, Ibrahim M. Long-term follow-up after surgery for patients with biliary atresia. *J Pediatr Surg* 1990; **25**: 442–5.

78 Hussain M, Howard ER, Mieli-Vergani G, Mowat AP. Jaundice at 14 days of age – exclude biliary atresia. *Arch Dis Child* 1991; **66**: 1177–9.

79 Hussain M, Mieli-Vergani G, Mowat AP. Alpha-1-antitrypsin deficiency in liver disease: clinical presentation, diagnosis and treatment. *J Inherited Metab Dis* 1991; **14**: 497–511.

80 Whitington PE, Balistreri WF. Liver transplantation in pediatrics: Indications, contra-indications and pre-transplant management. *J Pediatr* 1991; **118**: 169–77.

81 Burdelski M, Rodeck B, Latta A, *et al*. Treatment of inherited metabolic disorders by liver transplantation. *J Inherited Metab Dis* 1991; **14**: 604–18.

82 Baker A, Kotak EA, Schoeller D. Clinical utility of breath tests for the assessment of hepatic function. *Semin Liver Dis* 1983; **3**: 318–29.

83 Oellerich M, Burdelski M, Lautz HU, Schultz M, Schmidt SW, Herrmann H. Lidocaine metabolite formation as a measure of liver function in patients with cirrhosis. *Ther Drug Monit* 1990; **12**: 219–26.

84 Malatack JJ, Schald DJ, Urbach AH, *et al*. Choosing a pediatric recipient of orthotopic liver transplantation. *J Pediatr* 1987, **112**: 479–89.

85 Beath S, Pearmain G, Kelly DA, *et al*. Liver transplantation in babies and children with extra hepatic biliary atresia: Pre-operative condition, complications, survival and outcome. *J Pediatr Surg* 1993; in press.

86 Kelly DA. Fulminant hepatitis and acute liver failure. In: Buts JP, Sokal EM, eds. *Management of Digestive and Liver Disorders in Infants and Children*. Amsterdam: Elsevier Science, 1933: 551–68.

87 Psacharopoulos HT, Mowat AP, Davies M, Portmann B, Silk DB, Williams R. Fulminant hepatic failure in childhood. *Arch Dis Child* 1980; **55**: 252–8.

88 Lidofsky SD, Bass NM, Prager MC, *et al*. Intracranial pressure monitoring and liver transplantation for fulminant hepatic failure. *Hepatology* 1992; **16**: 1–7.

89 Lauterberg BH, Vaishnar Y, Stillwell WB, Mitchell JR. The effects of age in glutathione depletion on hepatic glutathione turnover in vivo determined by acetaminophen probe analysis. *J Pharmacol Exp Ther* 1980; **213**: 54–8.

90 Koneru B, Wayneflye M, Busuttil RW, *et al*. Liver transplantation for hepatoblastoma. *Ann Surg* 1991; **213**: 118–21.

91 Moukarzel AA, Najm I, Vargas J, McDairmid J, Busuttil RW, Ament ME. Effective nutritional status on outcome of orthotopic liver transplantation in paediatric patients. *Transplant Proc* 1990; **22**: 1560–2.

III: Management on the waiting list

5: Management of the end stage liver disease patient

SUZANNA I PARK

Introduction

Patients on the liver transplant waiting list require special management to maintain clinical stability and ensure survival to the time of transplantation. Such individuals are typically frail, precariously existing on minimal hepatic reserve and at high risk of dying from complications of liver disease. When complications arise, they may delay or prevent the procedure. Management of these patients is challenging. Advanced liver disease often confers a cloak of false stability so that affected individuals may not manifest on-going sepsis, electrolyte disturbance, gastrointestinal bleeding, or other serious pathology until severe morbidity is present and the threat to life is real. Astute clinical vigilance is therefore important to detect and treat decompensation. Intense and often heroically aggressive measures must be taken to restore stability and fitness for transplantation. This chapter will focus on general aspects of medical care as well as the specific liver disease complications commonly encountered in this unique patient population.

General approach to patient management

Outpatient care (Table I)

The stable patient on the transplant waiting list is able to live outside the hospital with the assistance of medication, close

TABLE I—*Management of the end stage liver disease patient while on the liver transplant waiting list: outpatient care*

Astute vigilance to detect and treat complications early:
    Spontaneous bacterial peritonitis
    Variceal haemorrhage
    Renal failure
    Hepatic encephalopathy
    Malnutrition
    Sepsis

Avoid iatrogenic complications from medications:

Drug	*Complications*
Non-steroidal anti-inflammatory agents, aspirin	Gastrointestinal bleeding
	Renal failure
	Fluid retention
Sedative medications, opiates	Hepatic encephalopathy

Prophylactic medical therapy to prevent:
    Spontaneous bacterial peritonitis (norfloxacin)
    Variceal haemorrhage (β-blockers)

Optimise nutritional status

Maintain close ongoing communication with transplant centre regarding patient's status

---

physician supervision, and family support. The primary objective in caring for these individuals is to maintain clinical stability so that liver transplantation can be accomplished successfully. This is achieved through:

- Early detection and treatment of complications of liver disease
- Avoidance of iatrogenic misadventures to which these patients are highly susceptible
- Prophylactic measures to prevent complications and decompensation.

To ensure optimal physical condition, nutritional deficiencies should be corrected as far as possible before transplantation, to increase the probability of a successful outcome.

Patients and their families should be educated about the clinical signs of deterioration and the need to notify physicians early and/or to transport the patient to the closest emergency room when deterioration occurs. Patients should be instructed to avoid any medication other than that prescribed by the physician. In many centres patients with a history of spontaneous bacterial peritonitis are maintained on antibiotic prophylaxis using medications such as norfloxacin to prevent recurrence of this process, which is often fatal.[1]

It is the practice at Cincinnati to give prophylaxis to those individuals with ascites but without a history of spontaneous bacterial peritonitis who are deemed to be at high risk as a result of low ascitic fluid albumin and peripheral hypoalbuminaemia. Individuals with large oesophageal varices, with or without a history of bleeding, should be considered for prophylactic β-blocker therapy to lower portal hypertension and diminish the risk for fatal variceal bleeding.

Antibiotic prophylaxis should be administered when cirrhotic patients develop gastrointestinal haemorrhage.[2] It is essential to have close on-going communication with physicians and co-ordinators at the transplant centre regarding the clinical condition of these patients. Deterioration in clinical status may affect timing of transplantation for the individual patient and therefore the allocation of organs on a national level.

The hospitalised patient (Table II)

Patients on the liver transplant waiting list frequently require hospitalisation for complications of liver disease or other related medical problems. When this occurs, the physicians at the transplant centre should be notified. If the patient is not hospitalised in the transplant unit, early transfer to the transplant centre should be considered. These patients are often critically ill and can be optimally managed by the transplant team, who are experienced in the care of patients with severe end stage liver disease. Furthermore, timing of transplantation can be better assessed. Inpatient management of these extremely ill patients is a multidiscplinary team effort involving transplant hepatologists, transplant surgeons, relevant medical and surgical specialists, and transplant coordinators, social workers, dieticians, and psychiatrists. A heightened vigilance should be maintained both to prevent iatrogenic complications and to monitor for decompensation. Iatrogenic complications can occur during routine daily care of these patients. Central intravenous line

TABLE II—*Management of the end stage liver disease patient while on the liver transplant waiting list: inpatient care*

Avoid iatrogenic complications from the following:
   Excessive hypertonic intravenous fluids
   Central line placement
   Medications

Drug	*Complication*
Opiates, sedatives	Hepatic encephalopathy
Aminoglycoside antibiotics	Renal failure
Heparin, warfarin (coumadin)	Bleeding
Non-steroidal anti-inflammatory	Renal failure
agents	Fluid retention
	Gastrointestinal bleeding

   Intramuscular injections (haematoma)
   Hospital induced malnutrition

Preserve anatomical integrity of left axilla and left groin for impending venovenous bypass

Optimise nutritional status

Early subspecialty consultation to assist in management of relevant medical problems

Vigilant attention to detect decompensation

---

placement, intravenous fluid administration, and medication prescription can all result in complications. If these patients require central intravenous lines or other invasive vascular procedures, the procedure should be performed by experienced physicians because of the high risk for life threatening bleeding complications (these patients often have coagulopathy and thrombocytopenia) or organ perforation. Intravenous lines and phlebotomy, in the region of the left axilla or left groin, should be avoided if possible. Vessels in these two anatomical areas are used in venovenous bypass. Intravenous fluids, especially those with a high sodium concentration, should be minimised to prevent worsening ascites and oedema. A thoughtful approach should be taken when medication orders are prescribed. Opiate or sedative medications, aminoglycoside antibiotics, heparin or warfarin (coumadin), and non-steroidal anti-inflammatory medications should be avoided because of the increased risk of adverse effects from these drugs in this patient population. Intramuscular injections should be avoided because of the risk of inducing haematoma.

BOX A   Management of ascites in the patient pre-transplantation

- Conservative palliation with moderate diuretics and/or therapeutic paracentesis
- Monitor electrolyte and renal function carefully while on diuretic therapy
- Sodium restriction
- Avoid peritoneovenous shunts

Common complications of liver disease

This section discusses management of common end stage liver disease complications including ascites, spontaneous bacterial peritonitis, hepatic encephalopathy, fluid and electrolyte disturbances, and malnutrition in the patient awaiting liver transplantation.

Ascites (Box A)

Most patients with end stage liver disease have ascites resulting from a combination of hyperaldosteronism, hypovolaemia, abnormal renal retention of sodium, and altered hepatic lymph flow.[3] It is often unrealistic and potentially dangerous to attempt to rid the patient entirely of ascites. Aggressive diuretic therapy or excessive paracenteses will place the patient at high risk for complications of renal failure, volume depletion, hepatic encephalopathy, paracentesis complications, hyponatraemia, and other electrolyte disturbances. The goal of ascites management in this patient population is conservative palliation. These individuals should be kept comfortable on judicious doses of diuretic agents. Large volume paracenteses (with simultaneous albumin infusion to prevent volume depletion)[4] should be used with patients who become symptomatic due to, for example, significant dyspnoea or abdominal discomfort. Sodium restriction to 1–2 g/day is advised. While on diuretics, periodic renal profiles should be obtained to monitor serum sodium, potassium, urea, and creatinine. For those patients who are unable to tolerate diuretic medications because of renal insufficiency, large volume paracentesis can be performed on a more scheduled basis to control ascites.

Peritoneovenous shunts should be avoided in patients pre-trans-

TABLE III—*Management of spontaneous bacterial peritonitis: University of Cincinnati protocol*

Early detection: suspect diagnosis of spontaneous bacterial peritonitis when the
  following signs/symptoms appear:
  Abdominal discomfort
  Worsening ascites
  Fever
  Malaise, non-specific deterioration
  Hepatic encephalopathy
  Leucocytosis

Diagnosis: diagnostic paracentesis
  Ascitic fluid neutrophil count $> 250 \times 10^6/l$
  or culture/microscopy positive

Treatment: duration of 5–7 days
  Cefotaxime or
  Vancomycin/aztreonam for penicillin allergic patients

Institute follow up indefinite
  Antibiotic prophylaxis for spontaneous bacterial peritonitis with oral norfloxacin
  400 mg once daily

Can re-list for transplantation after 2–3 days of intravenous antibiotics

plantation because abdominal surgery may interfere with the impending abdominal surgical procedure for transplantation. In addition, peritoneovenous shunts offer no significant advantage over diuretic therapy and large volume paracentesis, both of which can effectively control this problem during the waiting period pre-transplantation. Peritoneovenous shunts also expose the patient to such complications as infection and disseminated intravascular coagulation.[5–7]

Spontaneous bacterial peritonitis (Table III)

Spontaneous bacterial peritonitis (SBP) is a common cause of morbidity and mortality in the period pre-transplantation. It is a poor prognostic sign for survival in the patient with end stage liver disease, indicating a severely compromised individual with impaired immunity.[8] Diagnosis of this condition necessitates a delay in transplantation until the infection is controlled, so that immunosuppression can be safely administered. It is important to remember that spontaneous bacterial peritonitis usually has a subtle rather than an overt presentation. Such non-specific manifestations as worsening ascites, slight deterioration in clinical status or hepatic function, hepatic encephalopathy, mild fever, mild leucocytosis, and abdominal discomfort can be the presenting features of this disorder. Frank peritonism is rarely present. When any of these non-specific clinical signs is present, the diagnosis should be considered and immediately confirmed or excluded objectively with a diagnostic paracentesis. Spontaneous bacterial peritonitis is present if the neutrophil count on an ascitic fluid sample is greater than $250 \times 10^6/l$.[9] Ascitic fluid should be cultured in blood culture bottles at the bedside (rather than delaying inoculation by sending the specimen to the laboratory to be plated) in order to improve the chance of defining the infection.[10] Usual aetiological organisms in SBP include *Streptococcus* spp. and Gram-negative organisms. These are ideally treated with cefotaxime which provides excellent coverage with minimal adverse effects in cirrhotic individuals.[11] Penicillin allergic patients may be treated with vancomycin and aztreonam.[12] Aminoglycosides should be avoided because of the increased risk of nephrotoxicity associated with their use in liver disease patients. Most patients are adequately treated with a 5–7 day course of antibiotics.

Failure to improve after a few days of antibiotics suggests secondary rather than spontaneous bacterial peritonitis and requires diagnostic testing to search for intestinal perforation. Additional clinical clues to secondary peritonitis include marked neutrophilic leucocytosis on ascitic fluid cell counts (ie, $> 5 \times 10^9/l$) and positive ascitic fluid cultures with polymicrobial or anaerobic organisms. Patients who are awaiting transplantation can be relisted for transplantation after the infection is under control with 3–4 days of intravenous antibiotics. Postoperative antibiotics may, however, be continued for a full seven day course to assure clearance of the infection.

Once the patient has recovered from spontaneous bacterial peritonitis, he or she should be placed on prophylactic antibiotics such as norfloxacin until the time of transplantation to prevent recurrence of spontaneous bacterial peritonitis, and the attendant morbidity associated with it.[1]

> ## BOX B   Fluid and electrolyte disorders in end stage liver disease
>
> - Dilutional hyponatraemia
> - Primary respiratory alkalosis with metabolic compensation
> - Renal insufficiency
>   Hepatorenal syndrome
>   Prerenal azotaemia from volume depletion
>   Acute tubular necrosis

Fluid and electrolyte disturbances (Box B)

Fluid and electrolyte abnormalities can be seen in end stage liver disease. It is important to be aware of these so that erroneous diagnoses are avoided and inappropriate therapeutic manipulations are not prescribed. These abnormalities include hyponatraemia, primary respiratory alkalosis with metabolic compensation, and renal insufficiency.

Hyponatraemia

Hyponatraemia in liver disease is a dilutional phenomenon and occurs as a consequence of impaired free water excretion by the kidney. A state of relative intravascular volume depletion is present in end stage liver disease and is related to extravascular sequestration of fluids. This stimulates compensatory mechanisms which result in high renin levels, hyperaldosteronism, increased antidiuretic hormone (ADH) levels, enhanced thirst, and increased proximal tubular absorption with impaired delivery of glomerular infiltrate to the distal tubule.[13] Free water excretion is secondarily and chronically impaired, and a dilutional hyponatraemia ensues. The serum sodium usually does not fall below 125 mmol/l in this setting.[13] In general, the hyponatraemia of liver disease is asymptomatic and requires no specific intervention. Free water restriction should be avoided if possible because it may be punitive to the patient and can lead to significant dehydration. Serum sodium levels of less than 125 mmol/l often indicate a superimposed insult such as excessive diuretic therapy or administration of excessive hypotonic intravenous fluids. If the serum sodium is less than 120 mmol/l, diuretics should be withheld and free water restriction should be instituted until the serum sodium level improves.

114

Hypokalaemia should be corrected as this may improve the serum sodium level via a shift of potassium intracellularly in exchange for sodium movement into the extracellular fluid.[13]

Primary respiratory alkalosis with metabolic compensation

When patients with end stage liver disease develop hepatic encephalopathy, hyperventilation and primary respiratory alkalosis with metabolic compensation may be observed simultaneously. This is thought to be related to direct stimulation of the medullary respiratory centre by retained amines and toxins which are normally cleared by the liver.[14] This acid–base disturbance requires no specific therapy other than that for the hepatic encephalopathy. It is important, however, to consider and exclude other more serious causes of primary respiratory alkalosis such as early bacterial sepsis or acute cerebrovascular injury.

Renal insufficiency

Renal insufficiency is a common problem in end stage liver disease and may stem from functional renal failure (also known as the hepatorenal syndrome) or acute tubular necrosis resulting from drugs or severe volume depletion. It may be difficult to define the specific cause even using standard clinical criteria of urine : plasma creatinine ratio, urinary sodium level, and volume of urine.[15] When renal insufficiency occurs in the patient before transplantation, it is important to discontinue all potentially nephrotoxic drugs and address any possible underlying volume depletion with an empirical trial of gentle volume repletion. Swan–Ganz catheterisation with pulmonary capillary wedge determination may be required to determine the status of intravascular volume accurately. If renal insufficiency is progressive, aggressive supportive measures such as continuous arteriovenous filtration (CAVHD) or haemodialysis should be instituted to support the patient through transplantation. Renal failure due to hepatorenal syndrome generally resolves after liver transplantation.

Hepatic encephalopathy (Table IV)

Hepatic encephalopathy may present in two ways in patients with end stage liver disease:

115

TABLE IV—*Management of hepatic encephalopathy:*

Acute hepatic encephalopathy:
 Exclude other causes of acute mental status deterioration
  Central nervous system injury
  Central nervous system infection
  Drug overdose

 Identify and correct any possible precipitants:
  Spontaneous bacterial peritonitis
  Gastrointestinal bleeding
  Sepsis
  Sedative medications
  Metabolic alkalosis
  Renal insufficiency
  Hypokalaemia
  Constipation
  Excessive oral protein intake
  Medical non-compliance
  Deterioration in hepatic function due to superimposed hepatic injury

 Empirical therapy:
  Cleansing tap water enema
  Lactulose
  Temporary dietary protein restricted to 20 g/day
  Aspiration precautions
Chronic hepatic encephalopathy:
 Assess compliance with lactulose therapy
 Optimise lactulose dosage
 Mild dietary protein restriction
 Consider adjuvant therapy with metronidazole

- Acute encephalopathy presenting as a sudden deterioration in mental status in a patient with otherwise normal mental status.
- Chronic encephalopathy in those with particularly severe disease manifesting as continuous mild dysfunction[16] (such as minor memory impairment, difficulty concentrating) or overt impairment with lethargy, impaired ability to interact with others and perform activities of daily living.[17]

The syndrome of acute hepatic encephalopathy arises when an inciting agent precipitates the development of or a quantitative increase in hepatically cleared toxins which impair brain function via poorly defined mechanisms. Specific aetiological factors include gastrointestinal bleeding, sedative drugs, infection, constipation, hypokalaemia, metabolic alkalosis, renal impairment, excessive dietary protein intake, hypoxaemia, dehydration, medical non-compliance, and a deterioration in hepatic function due to superimposed injury from such entities as viral hepatitis or hepatocellular carcinoma.

Management of the individual with acute hepatic encephalopathy is straightforward and has changed little over the years.

- It is necessary to exclude other serious disorders that cause acute mental status deterioration such as central nervous system injury, meningitis/encephalitis, or drug overdose.
- A thorough search must be made to identify and correct aggressively any possible precipitating factors. If ascites is present, a diagnostic paracentesis should be performed to exclude spontaneous bacterial peritonitis as a cause.
- Empirical therapy for hepatic encephalopathy should be initiated. This consists of gut lavage with a cleansing tap water enema (this removes excessive stool from the colon and alleviates any underlying constipation), and/or oral lactulose (initially at high doses, 30–60 ml every hour until producing a stool, followed by a reduction in dosage to 30 ml every 6–8 hours, titrating to produce two to three soft formed stools each day), and dietary protein restriction to 20 g/day. If the patient is unable to take oral lactulose, it may be administered as an enema.

In the early stages of treating hepatic encephalopathy in patients at risk, it is very important to institute precautions against aspiration with head-of-bed elevation and frequent clearing of secretions. Mental status typically improves and normalises within 24–36 hours after initiating this treatment regimen. Failure of the mental status to improve suggests one of the following:

- Incorrect diagnosis
- Inadequate therapy
- Failure to correct precipitating factors (usually latent sepsis)
- Marked deterioration in hepatic function due to a superimposed injury.

Once acute hepatic encephalopathy resolves, the patient and his or her family should be re-instructed regarding lactulose therapy and the importance of compliance. Measures should be taken to prevent the recurrence of precipitating factors. Dietary protein should be reintroduced and increased over 3–4 days to at least 60–80 g/day to avoid catabolism. Most patients are able to tolerate this level of protein intake if compliance with lactulose is adequate.

The patient with chronic hepatic encephalopathy represents a true challenge. A careful assessment of compliance with lactulose therapy should be made. Many patients have difficulty taking this sweet syrupy medication, are non-compliant, and may deceptively appear to be refractory to lactulose. In these patients, lactitol may be a better alternative. In those who are deemed compliant but still encephalopathic, adjuvant therapy with metronidazole (at a dose adjusted for hepatic insufficiency)[17] or neomycin may be attempted. Chronic metronidazole therapy should, however, be avoided because of the risk of peripheral neuropathy. Dietary protein restriction can be instituted but should not be so severe that the diet is unpalatable with the consequence that nutrition is compromised.

Several other potential therapeutic agents for hepatic encephalopathy have been proposed over the years and include benzodiazepine antagonists, zinc therapy, and vegetable protein diets.[18–21] Conclusive evidence regarding safety and efficacy of these is not yet available. They should be considered experimental therapy at the present time.

Varices (Table V)

Oesophageal and/or gastric varices are frequently present in patients with end stage liver disease and significant underlying portal hypertension. Rupture and bleeding of these varices are a feared complication associated with a high morbidity and mortality in patients on the transplant waiting list. Numerous treatment modalities (both prophylactic and therapeutic), with variable success rates, have arisen over the years in an attempt to prevent and control this difficult problem. It is helpful to approach the management of varices in the liver transplant candidate with regard to the status of bleeding:

- Patients who have never bled
- Patients who are experiencing their first variceal bleed
- Patients with recurrent variceal bleeding.

Patients who have never experienced variceal bleeding

In patients who have never bled but who have documented varices, prophylactic β-blocker therapy should be considered if

118

TABLE V—*Management of varices in the end stage liver disease patient awaiting transplantation**

Never bleed: Prophylactic β-blocker therapy
First bleed: Aggressive resuscitation with blood and volume replacement Correct coagulopathy Diagnostic upper endoscopy to confirm source of bleed Sclerotherapy or rubber band ligation

Recurrent variceal bleeding:
Institute *second line therapy* with intravenous vasopressin (plus nitroglycerin) or
    somatostatin, with balloon tamponade if necessary
If this fails, consider *third line therapy* with:
    Radiological modalities:
      1 Transjugular intrahepatic portosystemic shunts
      2 Coronary vein embolisation
    Surgery:
      Distal splenorenal shunt

*This is according to status of bleeding.

there are no contraindications, in an attempt to lower portal pressure and therefore reduce the risk of variceal rupture and bleeding. This therapy is particularly important in those individuals who are at high risk for variceal bleeding, namely those with large varices or those whose varices have such stigmata as red weals or haemocystic spots on endoscopic examination. Propranolol and nadolol (at a dose to reduce the heart rate by 25%) are effective in preventing first bleeding and reducing the mortality rate from gastrointestinal bleeding in patients with cirrhosis.[22]

Prophylactic oesophageal sclerotherapy has no role.

Patients who are experiencing their first variceal bleed

Patients who are experiencing their first bleed should be treated with aggressive resuscitative measures and should have adequate blood and volume replacement. An attempt should be made to correct any coexisting coagulopathy with vitamin K, fresh frozen plasma, and platelet transfusions if the platelet count is below $50 \times 10^9/l$. This should be followed by early diagnostic oesophago-gastroduodenoscopy to confirm oesophageal varices as the source of bleeding. Sclerotherapy or rubber band ligation should be administered at the time of endoscopy. If this controls bleeding, a protocol for an oesophageal variceal obliteration protocol with sclerotherapy or further rubber band ligation should be instructed. When the bleeding episode has subsided and the patient is stable, β-blocker therapy can be introduced. Sucralfate (4 g daily) may ameliorate sclerotherapy ulceration.

Patients with recurrent variceal bleeding

Recurrent variceal bleeding is associated with a high mortality. Patients with this complication pre-transplantation often die before operation. When sclerotherapy fails to control the first bleed, or if the patient rebleeds after sclerotherapy, second line therapy with intravenous vasopressin (combined with nitroglycerin to reduce mesenteric ischaemia)[23] or somatostatin[24] (both of which lower portal pressure and therefore pressure in the varices theoretically to allow an adequate clot to form at the site of the variceal rupture) is instituted. Local tamponade using a Sengstaken–Blakemore tube or Minnesota tube should also be instituted if necessary. When oesophageal tamponade is planned, the patient should usually be intubated prior to placement of the tamponade balloon to protect the airway and reduce the risk of aspiration. Tamponade should be used for a maximum of 24 hours after which the balloons should be deflated. While intubated many of these patients require intravenous sedation. Care should be taken to use short acting benzodiazepines in minimal amounts to avoid hepatic encephalopathy or coma related to sedative drug use. Continuous intravenous infusions of sedative drugs should be avoided because these individuals have impaired hepatic metabolism and may suffer prolonged drug-induced hepatic coma. After the balloons are deflated, repeat upper gastrointestinal endoscopy with sclerotherapy may be performed. On occasion, as a result of severe portal hypertension, a patient will fail to respond to these manoeuvres and further third line treatment options must be pursued in an attempt to save the individual's life. These include radiological treatment modalities such as (1) transjugular intrahepatic portosystemic shunt (TIPS) placement, a nonsurgical portosystemic shunt between the portal vein and the hepatic vein,[25,26] and (2) coronary vein embolisation which obliterates blood flow to the oesophageal and gastric varices, and surgical venous shunting.

BOX C   Nutritional management of the end stage liver disease patient: University of Cincinnati protocol

- Formal consultation with dietician should be obtained for all patients on liver transplant waiting list
- Optimise dietary protein intake
- Aim for 35–50 kcal/kg ideal body weight per day including 1·3–1·5 g protein/kg body wt
- For those unable to meet energy and caloric needs:
  Enteral supplementation with standard adult formulations, commercial "instant breakfast" formulae, or individualised, supplemented "milkshake" recipes designed by dietician

---

Formal surgical venous shunting should be avoided if at all possible because of the risks associated with anaesthesia and surgery in the end stage cirrhotic individual as well as the fact that abdominal surgery may impede future transplant surgery. If surgical shunting is absolutely necessary, however, the shunt of choice is a distal splenorenal shunt because this avoids the hepatoportal area where orthotopic liver transplantation is performed.[27]

Malnutrition (Box C)

Malnutrition is a highly prevalent but frequently overlooked problem in patients on the transplant waiting list. It is evident in the cachectic, muscle wasted physical appearance of these individuals and can be confirmed through such objective parameters as skinfold thickness determinations and short turnover protein assessments. End stage liver disease causes malnutrition through several mechanisms which include diminished oral intake of calories, malabsorption, and impaired incorporation of nutrients at a biochemical level.[28] In the face of poor nutrition, energy and protein requirements are increased in liver disease. These needs often cannot be met by the patient. Because of this, a catabolic state arises whereby the body breaks down muscle mass for a protein source. This leads to a downward spiral of further cachexia and uncontrolled catabolism. Iatrogenic or hospital associated malnutrition contributes to the problem when meals are missed for diagnostic tests or when unpalatable, restricted diets are ordered.

It is important to address the problem of malnutrition and to treat aggressively. Uncorrected malnutrition may have serious negative consequences for the patient. Nutritional deficiencies are associated with impaired immunity, a diminished ability to heal wounds, diminished resilience, and generalised muscular weakness. Although data from confirmatory trials are not available, it has been the experience at Cincinnati that severe malnutrition is a poor prognostic sign for survival in the period before transplantation. In addition, malnutrition may increase morbidity in and prolong hospitalisation of the patient after transplantaion. Aggressive and often prolonged nutritional intervention measures must be instituted in cachectic patients to improve physical strength, resilience, and sense of well-being to the point that these individuals can complete inpatient rehabilitation and be safely discharged home.

A careful assessment and optimisation of nutritional status should therefore be considered a standard part of all evaluations before liver transplantation. A dietician who is familiar with the problems of end stage liver disease and transplantation should be consulted to assist in this regard. Each patient requires individualised attention and dietary prescription. In the unit at Cincinnati for most patients the aim should be 145–210 kJ/kg (35–50 kcal/kg) ideal body weight (about 8370–12 550 kJ (2000–3000 kcal)) including 1·3–1·5 g/kg ideal body weight protein per 24 hours to prevent further catabolism and to achieve a positive nitrogen balance.[28]

Palatability of the diet should be optimal. Patients and their families should be carefully instructed on the requirements of the diet, and compliance should be assessed and brought to the best level on an ongoing basis.

Although significant protein restriction is frequently necessary in patients with acute bouts of hepatic encephalopathy, it should be discontinued as soon as the episode is resolved.

Dietary protein should be made available up to the patient's tolerance level because it will improve palatability of the food and, therefore, caloric intake. Despite availability of dietary protein, some patients simply cannot meet their own needs through oral intake and require some form of supplementation. This can be done through the enteral or the parenteral route. The enteral route is the preferred method because it is physiological and safer than intravenous supplementation which is associated with risks of central line placement and catheter sepsis.

With regard to formulations, no specific formula is ideal for the end stage liver disease patient. The prescription should be individualised for the patient. Some may require low salt, low protein, low volume regimens, whereas others may tolerate standard formulations for adult supplementation without difficulty. In addition, special milkshakes containing protein and milk powder supplements prescribed by the dietician can be easily made at home, or "instant breakfast" formulations can be incorporated at minimal expense to the patient. Formulations of branched chain amino acids are probably no better than standard formulations and are more expensive.

Conclusion

In summary, the patient on the liver transplant waiting list with severe end stage disease is at high risk of dying from complications and may not survive to reach transplantation. The goal of management of these patients is to maintain clinical stability and survival until transplantation can take place. Managing these individuals requires astute clinical vigilance to detect and treat complications in their earliest stages, care to avoid iatrogenic complications or activities that may interfere with transplant surgery, and reaching an optimal clinical status for surgery and recovery post-transplantation. Close communication should be maintained at all times with the transplant centre about the status of these candidates, because any deterioration may affect timing of transplantation for the individual patient as well as allocation of organs on a national level.

References

1 Gines P, Rimola A, Planas R, *et al*. Norfloxacin prevents spontaneous bacterial peritonitis recurrence in cirrhosis. *Hepatology* 1990; **12**: 716–24.
2 Soriano G, Cuarner C, Tomas A, *et al*. Norfloxacin prevents bacterial infection in cirrhotics with gastrointestinal hemorrhage. *Gastroenterology* 1992; **103**: 1267–72.
3 Arroyo V, Gines P, Jimenez W, *et al*. Ascites, renal failure, and electrolyte disorders in cirrhosis. Pathogenesis, diagnosis, and treatment. In: McIntyre N, Benhamou J-P, Bircher J, Rizzetto M, Rodes J, eds. *Oxford Textbook of Clinical Hepatology*. Oxford: Oxford University Press, 1991: 427–71.
4 Tito L, Gines P, Arroyo V, *et al*. Total paracentesis associated with intravenous albumin in the management of patients with cirrhosis and ascites. *Gastroenterology* 1990; **98**: 146–51.
5 Berhnhoft RA, Pellegrini CA, Way LW. Peritoneovenous shunt for refractory ascites. Operative complications and long-term results. *Arch Surg* 1982; **117**: 631–5.

6 Laveen HH, Vujic I, D'Ovidio NG, et al. Peritoneovenous shunt occlusion. Etiology, diagnosis, therapy. Ann Surg 1984; 200: 212–23.

7 Harmon DC, Demirjian Z, Ellman L, et al. Disseminated intravascular coagulation with the peritoneovenous shunt. Ann Intern Med 1979; 90: 774–6.

8 Runyon BA. Spontaneous bacterial peritonitis: an explosion of information. Hepatology 1988; 8: 171–5.

9 Jones SR. The absolute granulocyte count in ascites fluid. An aid to the diagnosis of spontaneous bacterial peritonitis. West J Med 1977; 126: 344–6.

10 Hoefs JC, Runyon BA. Spontaneous bacterial peritonitis. Disease of the Month 1984; 31–9.

11 Felisart H, Rimola A, Arroyo V, et al. Cefotaxime is more effective than ampicillin-tobramycin in cirrhotics with severe infections. Hepatology 1985; 5: 457–62.

12 Ariza J, Xiol X, Esteve M, et al. Aztreonam versus cefotaxime in Gram negative spontaneous peritonitis in cirrhotic patients. Hepatology 1991; 14: 91–8.

13 Rose BD. Clinical Physiology of Acid–Base and Electrolyte Disorders, 2nd Ed. New York: McGraw-Hill, 1984: 515–48.

14 Kartezky MS, Mithoefer JC. The cause of hyperventilation and arterial hypoxia in patients with cirrhosis of the liver. Am J Med Sci 1967; 254: 797–804.

15 Diamong JR, Yoburn DC. Nonoliguric acute renal failure associated with low fractional sodium excretion. Ann Intern Med 1982; 96: 597–600.

16 Gitlin N. Subclinical portal–systemic encephalopathy. Am J Gastroenterol 1988; 83: 8–11.

17 Morgan MY. The treatment of chronic hepatic encephalopathy. Hepato-gastroenterology 1991; 38: 377–87.

18 Morgan MH, Read AE, Speller DC. Treatment of hepatic encephalopathy with metronidazole. Gut 1982; 12: 1–7.

19 Jones EA, Basile AS, Mullen KD, et al. Flumazenil: potential implications for hepatic encephalopathy. Pharmacol Ther 1990; 43: 331–43.

20 Reding P, Duchateau J, Bataille C. Oral zinc supplementation improves hepatic encephalopathy: results of a randomized controlled trial. Lancet 1984; ii: 493–5.

21 Uribe M, Marquez MA, Ramos GG, et al. Treatment of chronic portal–systemic encephalopathy with vegetable and animal protein diets. Dig Dis Sci 1982; 27: 1109–16.

22 Poynard T, Cales P, Pasta L, et al. Beta-adrenergic-antagonist drugs in the prevention of gastrointestinal bleeding in patients with cirrhosis and esophageal varices. N Engl J Med 1991; 324: 1532–8.

23 Gimson AES, Westaby D, Hegarty J, et al. A randomized trial of vasopressin and vasopressin plus nitroglycerin in the control of acute variceal hemorrhage. Hepatology 1986; 6: 410–13.

24 Kravetz D, Bosch J, Teres J, et al. Comparison of intravenous somatostatin and vasopressin infusions in the treatment of acute variceal hemorrhage. Hepatology 1984; 4: 442–6.

25 Ring EJ, Lake JR, Roberts JP, et al. Using transjugular intrahepatic portosystemic shunts to control variceal bleeding before liver transplantation. Ann Intern Med 1992; 116: 304–9.

26 Crass RA, Keeffe EB, Pinson W. Management of variceal haemorrhage in the potential liver transplant candidate. Am J Surg 1989; 157: 476–8.

27 Munoz SJ. Nutritional therapies in liver disease. Semin Liver Dis 1991; 11: 278–81.

28 Morgan MY. Nutritional aspects of liver and biliary disease. In: McIntyre N, Benhamou P, Bircher J, Rizzetto M, Rodes J, eds. Oxford Textbook of Clinical Hepatology. Oxford: Oxford University Press, 1991: 1339–88.

IV: Management in the transplant unit

6: Donor organ retrieval, allocation, and logistics

JEREMIAH G TURCOTTE, JAMES NEUBERGER

Introduction

With the increasing success of liver transplantation, systems have been developed for fair and appropriate allocation of what is becoming an increasingly scant resource. Different countries have developed their own system of allocation of donor livers. As the UNOS system in North America covers the largest single group, this chapter will concentrate on the organ system allocation used and developed in the USA. Clearly, different systems apply in other countries but, for the point of view of this chapter, in the interests of brevity, these will not be discussed in depth.

Liver transplantation in the USA

In the USA a national system has been instituted for retrieving and distributing donor organs for transplantation. The "system" or network is a blending of local and private initiative with state and federal regulation. Government involvement began in earnest with the implementation of the End Stage Renal Disease (ESRD) Program, and was later extended to extrarenal transplantation when heart and liver transplantation became more successful and widespread. The development of policies for establishing the network required enabling legislation and has renewed interest in the bioethical principles underlying the logistics of the sharing process.[1,2] Allocation policies specific for each type of donor organ have been mandated. Leadership has been provided in large part by transplant surgeons and other health care professionals. The introduction of

---

BOX A   Landmark events in the history of the organ procurement and distribution system in the USA

End Stage Renal Disease (ESRD) Program – 1972
   Provides federal funding through Medicare for kidney
      transplantation and dialysis
Uniform Anatomical Gift Act
   A model for state laws establishing legality of donating body
      parts and defining neurological death
Organ Procurement Organizations (OPOs)
   Evolved from hospital and regional kidney procurement
      agencies
   Eligible for ESRD funding in 1972
National Organ Transplant Act – 1984
   Legal basis for the Organ Procurement and Transplant Network
      (OPTN) and the Scientific Registry
   Requires certification of OPOs by the Federal Government
United Network for Organ Sharing (UNOS) – 1984
   Awarded contracts for OPTN and Scientific Registry in 1986
Omnibus Budget Reconciliation Act of 1986
   Transplant programme, OPOs, and histocompatibility
      laboratories must be members of OPTN

---

changes necessary to achieve relative uniformity throughout the system has at times been controversial, especially when considering life conserving procedures such as liver transplantation.

History and philosophy

In 1972 the federal government implemented the ESRD Program (Box A). This programme partially funds almost all dialysis and kidney transplantation, and also pays the costs associated with organ retrieval. The ESRD Program made it imperative that personnel and facilities associated with cadaveric kidney retrieval should be organised into Organ Procurement Agencies, although the initial concern was to ensure that the expenditure of funds and audit procedures conformed to ESRD regulations.

As extrarenal transplantation expanded in the early 1980s, the Organ Procurement Agencies (later named Organ Procurement Organizations or OPOs) also assumed the task of coordinating multi-organ retrieval, including procurement of donor livers. The government did not adopt a special funding programme comparable to ESRD for extrarenal transplantations because of the huge costs that had been incurred by the so-called categorical funding for dialysis and renal transplantation. The government and others did express great concern about convenient and fair access to donor organs, the efficient use of these scarce organs, and related issues such as preferential use of cadaveric organs for foreign nationals. Congress responded to these concerns by passing the National Transplant Act in 1984. This legislation called for a national task force to study the issues and the establishment of a National Organ Procurement Network (OPTN).[3] After 18 months of study by the task force, the United Network for Organ Sharing (UNOS), a private non-profit-making corporation, was awarded a contract to implement the OPTN and a related Scientific Registry.[4] In a subsequent law, the Omnibus Budget Reconciliation Act of 1986, Congress required that all transplant programmes, OPOs, and transplant tissue typing laboratories must be members of the OPTN. Hospitals were required to work with certified OPOs when cadaveric organs became available.

This federal legislation specified a national computerised list of patients awaiting cadaveric organ transplantation should be maintained by OPTN, and that there should be an organ placement centre to match donor organs and recipients. The purpose of the system is to ensure equitable patient access to organs and to guarantee that organs are recovered and used safely and efficiently. The Division of Organ Transplantation within the Health Resources Services Administration was established to administer the OPTN contract. UNOS was awarded the contract initially for one year and then for three years with competitive renewal for the contract required every three years.

Thus a national system based on principles of equitable patient access to organs, and safe and efficient use of organs, was put in place. Government regulations required major changes for many transplant programmes and their affiliated OPOs. Many OPOs had been associated with a single transplant centre or region and had considered their responsibilities to extend only to the patients served by that centre or region. The task of translating these principles of equity, efficiency, and safety into a national system was in effect delegated to a private group through a contract – an unusual arrangement for the implementation for a federal regulatory law.

Organ Procurement Organizations

In the late 1960s organisations began to appear whose purpose was to assist kidney retrieval, sharing, and distribution (Box A). Frequently these were simply hospital based administrative units. When several transplant programmes were served, an independent legal entity, such as an incorporated tax free foundation, proved to be a useful vehicle for coordinating and governing a multicentre enterprise. Early examples are the New England Organ Bank (founded in 1968) which now serves 15 transplant centres throughout New England and the Transplantation Society of Michigan (founded in 1971) which now serves all nine transplant centres in Michigan.[5]

Currently there are 65 OPOs distributed throughout the USA, and number 66 is in Puerto Rico.[6] According to UNOS, 18 of the OPOs are hospital based and serve a single transplant centre; the others are sometimes referred to as Independent OPOs (IOPOs), and serve more than one transplant centre. Although OPO service areas have been designated, donor hospitals are free to work with any certified OPO. The government has frequently indicated a preference for fewer OPOs with larger service areas. Reimbursement for the costs of providing extrarenal organs is obtained from the transplant hospitals who, in turn, recharge the usual array of third party insurance carriers or the recipients themselves. Costs for donor kidneys continue to be reimbursed by ESRD. The Association of Organ Procurement Organizations reported that in 1991 the standard acquisition charge for livers ranged from \$6000 to \$23 000.

Most OPOs are responsible for many related activities.[7] These activities may include a 24-hour communication service, organ preservation services, coordination of donor teams, provision of transportation for donor retrieval teams, public and professional education, tissue typing and cross-matching, maintenance of a central serum repository for cross-matching, viral serology and other laboratory studies, and the retrieval of bone and other tissues. Table I summarises these activities for 1992.

The United Network for Organ Sharing (UNOS)

The origin of UNOS can be traced to the Southeastern Regional Organ Program (SEROPP), a programme initially designed to tissue

TABLE I—*Results for 1992 reported to the Association of Organ Procurement Agencies by 65 OPOs**

	Number
Donors recovered	4 549
Organs recovered	15 216
Livers recovered	3 290
Livers used in transplantation	3 029

	Livers/million population
Retrieved	14·3
OPO median	20·0
OPO range	33·3–5·0
Used in transplantation	13·2

*Puerto Rico is not included.

type and share kidneys among eight transplant centres as part of a National Institutes of Health multicentre study.[4] To accommodate an increase in member programmes and activity the South-Eastern Organ Procurement Foundation (SEOFF) was incorporated in 1975. SEOFF became the largest organ-sharing organisation in the USA.

UNOS is a large organisation with an annual budget of several million dollars. By early 1993, over 30 500 patients had been registered and listed in the UNOS computer as potential candidates for a cadaveric organ transplantation (Table II) of which 2526 were registrations for liver transplantation. Two government contracts and patient registration fees are the major sources of financial support, with the current fee for registering a patient for receipt of a donor organ being $264.

Details of the members of UNOS are given in Boxes B and C, and the 11 UNOS regions are shown in Figure 1. These regions provide important geographical donor organ allocation criteria.

UNOS liver allocation criteria and the logistics of distribution

The OPTN contract requires that organs be allocated, retrieved, and distributed to accomplish equitable access and safety for patients and efficient use of organs. It should be noted that equitable

131

TABLE II—*Data on organ transplantations (1991) in the USA as reported by UNOS in March 1993*

Organ	Number of transplant programmes	Number of patients registered	Number of transplantations performed in 1991
Kidney	240	23 129	10 051
Liver	109	2 526	2 953
Pancreas	103	131	533
Kidney–pancreas		839	
Heart	159	2 809	2 126
Heart–lung	87	185	51
Lung	102	1 048	403
Totals	800*	30 667	16 117

*The 800 individual organ programmes are located in 268 separate institutions.

BOX B   UNOS institutional membership (March 1993)

Transplant centres	268
Consortium members	4
Independent Organ Procurement Organizations (IOPOs)	51
Voluntary health organisations	9
Independent tissue typing laboratories (TTLs)	49
General members of the public	11
Professional organisations	24
Total	416

---

access to organs for *transplant centres* is not a criterion.[1,8] The requirement for efficient use of organs often restricts policies intended to assure equitable access. For instance, taking histocompatibility match into account when allocating kidneys may achieve longer average graft survival, but may also favour patients who have inherited those histocompatibility antigens more commonly present in the donor organ pool. Likewise, medical requirements, such as relatively short safe preservation times, may restrict the organ allocation formula. The UNOS Ethics Committee considered these matters in depth, and published their conclusions.[2] A major conclusion was that matters of access (distributive justice) and matters of

BOX C   Composition of the 32 Member UNOS Board of Directors (March 1993)

UNOS officers	5
Regional councillors	11
Heart transplant representative	1
Histocompatibility representatives	2
IOPO representatives	2
Transplant coordinator representatives	2
General public representatives	2
Voluntary health organisation representatives	4
Medical/scientific organisation representatives	3

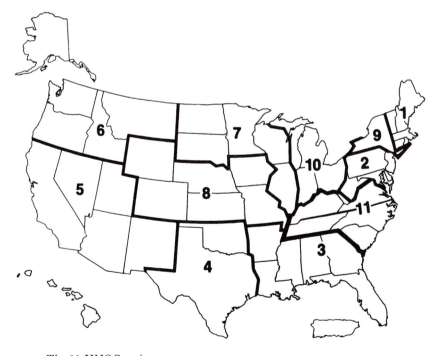

FIG 1—*The 11 UNOS regions*

133

efficiency (beneficence or medical utility) should be given equal weight.

The major criteria included in UNOS organ allocation policies are:[1,8]

- medical urgency
- waiting time
- histocompatibility match
- ABO red blood cell type
- distance between donor hospital and transplant centre.

Organs are first offered to patients listed by the OPO that retrieved the organ. If no candidate is available in the local area, then the organ is offered to patients in the UNOS region and finally the organ is offered nationally. Allocation of six antigen matched (O antigen mismatched) kidneys is the major exception to this three tiered geographical scheme; such kidneys are distributed nationally whenever such a good match is identified. The specific allocation criteria differ for each organ, eg histocompatibility match is not a criterion for liver allocation.

Policies that tend to direct organs to specific centres, such as assigning extra points to a particular transplant centre's patient if the donor hospital is near that transplant centre, are currently being re-examined. Such policies will probably be prohibited unless some documented patient benefit or increase in organ retrieval rate results from the policy. Individual transplant centres or recipients are not required to accept an organ. Individual transplant programmes may have varying indications for accepting patients for transplantation. Recently Medicare and many private insurance companies have designated preferred centres (sometimes called "centres of excellence"). The need to travel long distances to these preferred centres may restrict access for some patients, and such a system is not synchronous with the UNOS three tiered geographical distribution of donor organs.

The specific policies for allocation of donor livers according to current UNOS policies are summarised in Table III. The policies take into account the lack of numbers of donor livers available for all qualified candidates, and that, sadly, no matter what allocation scheme is designed some patients will die while waiting for a liver transplantation. The policies also recognise that it is not reasonable or fair that most patients wait until they are acutely ill before they

TABLE III—*UNOS liver allocation policies, March 1993*

Status	Condition	Points
Medical urgency		
0	Temporarily inactive	0
1	Home, good function	6
2	Continuous care, mostly at home	12
3	Continuously hospitalised	18
4	In intensive care unit, critically ill, maximum 14 days as status 4	24
Time waiting	Points depend upon duration of waiting time. Status 4 patients have separate waiting time ranking	0–10
ABO match	Identical	10
	Compatible	5
	Incompatible	0
Other factors		
Centre acceptance	Livers will not be offered if donor or liver is outside a centre's acceptance criteria	
Donor weight	Liver will not be offered if donor weight is outside the range indicated by listing centre	
Distance	Distance between donor hospital and transplant centre is no longer a criterion for liver allocation	
Histo-compatibility	Not a criterion for liver allocation	
Local	Either an individual transplant centre list or the donor OPO service area. May be modified	
Alternative point systems	UNOS may accept alternative point systems for transplant centres or OPOs if approved by the Organ Procurement and Donation Committee and the Board	

are likely to receive a donor organ – it is recognised that the risks of success are often less with acutely ill patients. Thus there is an attempt to balance a just distribution of livers to patients with an efficient use of the donor liver. The policy that organs are first distributed locally, then regionally, and then nationally is the major balancing factor, permitting a liver to be used for transplantation in elective circumstances in one local area or region even though acutely ill patients with more points for medical urgency are listed in other areas.

The UNOS Scientific Registry reported that, in 1992, 1165 (38·5%) of liver transplant recipients were out of the hospital (status 1 and 2) at the time the transplant organ became available, 453

(15·0%) were in the hospital but not in the intensive care unit (status 3), 517 (17·1%) were in the intensive care unit (status 4), and the status of 889 (29·4%) was not reported. Thus, of those whose status was known there is a relatively equal distribution of more elective (status 1 and 2) with more urgent (status 3 and 4) circumstances at the time of transplant availability. Of patients listed for a liver transplantation, 7·9% died while waiting. This may be an under-estimate of deaths because patients may be taken off the list when they are still alive but have become too ill to be at reasonable risk. Their deaths at a later time may not be recorded in the Scientific Registry of UNOS.

Some of the liver allocation policies are framed to facilitate administration and auditing of the system, for example, it is much easier to verify that a patient is in the intensive care unit than to verify specific physical findings indicating acute illness. When patients are listed as status 3 or 4, the highest priority medical urgency categories, a form indicating conformance to the criteria must be completed and signed by a responsible transplant surgeon or physician. This form is sent to UNOS within 24 hours. UNOS also conducts telephone and on site audits to verify adherence to the policies. This auditing system is very important in maintaining confidence in and cooperation with the allocation system. An Ad hoc Liver Committee meets twice yearly to review the system and make recommendations to the UNOS Organ Procurement and Distribution Committee. Policy changes must be approved by the Board of Directors. All major policies must be published in the Federal Register, circulated for public comment, reapproved or modified by the Board, and finally be approved by the Health Care Financing Administration. As experience is gained and data are collected, the allocation formula has been modified on an almost yearly basis.

When an organ donor is identified, the usual sequence of events is the following: the donor hospital notifies the local OPO. Most OPOs send a transplant coordinator to the donor hospital to assist with the donation and management of the donor. Frequently, the transplant coordinator has given in-service seminars at the hospital and is well known to the hospital staff. The OPO forwards the required donor information to UNOS. Most OPOs are linked by computer for two way communication with the central UNOS Organ Bank in Rich-mond. The UNOS computer prints out a list of potential recipients in priority order on the local OPO terminal. The OPO notifies local transplant programmes with high priority transplant recipients about the potential availability of a donor organ and serves as a communication centre to coordinate the multiple individuals involved in the procurement and transplant operations. Usually the details of the medical condition of the donor and the suitability of each donor organ for transplantation are discussed with the appropriate individual transplant surgeon. OPOs frequently provide an organ perfusion technician and supplies, arrange for transportation of the retrieval team and the organ, and may perform histocompatibility testing and viral serology. After the donation, the OPO will frequently make a goodwill visit to the donor hospital to encourage identification of future donors.

Conclusion

The OPTN, as administered by UNOS, has made the organ distribution system in the USA more visible and accountable. A governing mechanism, the Board of Directors of UNOS, has also been established which incorporates broad representation and facilitates cooperation, modification, and improvement of the system. The Scientific Registry, for the first time, provides outcome and other data for all transplant operations in the USA. The system has also added significant expense. The goal of equitable access to organ donors has been pursued and is more uniform than previously. Whether the system brings more efficiency or equity is difficult to determine because comprehensive records of the previous system were not kept, although most observers are of the opinion that it has. The ability to match organs on the basis of histocompatibility is an obvious accomplishment; another strength of the system is the contractual linking of the private and public sectors to achieve a common goal. The unique features of the system could have application in many other areas of health care in the USA and in other countries.

Liver graft allocation in the UK

In the UK, a special authority was established by the Secretary of State for Health to provide an efficient support system for the transplant centres in the UK and the Republic of Ireland. This support agency, the United Kingdom Transplant Support Services Authority (UKTSSA),[9] is responsible for coordinating not only liver but other organ allocation.

The liver allocation scheme was set up and agreed by the liver users and has been in operation since October 1992.

Liver allocation scheme

Once the Authority is notified of a possible organ donor, one of the liver transplant centres is contacted and invited to retrieve the donor organ. At present, this is done on a rotation scheme among the designated liver transplant centres. However, this scheme does not take into account the number of patients on the waiting list at each centre, so that a centre with a small number of patients on the waiting list may receive disproportionately more offers.

Patients are placed in one of two categories: super urgent or routine. The super urgent liver exchange scheme was agreed as some patients are likely to die within a very short period unless they receive a graft. The principle was that those patients who were thought to be unlikely to survive for more than 3 days without a graft could be placed in this category. The three diagnoses that were felt to be compatible with this indication were: those requiring emergency regrafting, those with fulminant hepatic failure, and those with total absence of liver function (for example, following total hepatectomy). The patients are registered and, to prevent any abuse of the system, anonymous clinical details are faxed to all other transplant centres. If any clinician in the transplant centres wishes to discuss any aspect of registration he or she may do so within 24 hours. Patients are ranked in order of length of time on the super urgent waiting list; the sequence of offers depends on the length of time on the waiting list and the blood group of the patient. Blood group identical patients take priority over blood group compatible ones. If there are no patients on the super urgent list for whom a graft is available, then the routine patients will be considered.

The determination of priority order is achieved through the rotation of the designated transplant centres. Offers are made in the following order of priority:

1 NHS eligible super urgent patients registered in a designated centre in the UK or Republic of Ireland.

2 Other NHS eligible patients registered in a designated centre in the UK or Republic of Ireland.

3 NHS eligible patients registered in a non-designated centre in the UK or Republic of Ireland.

4 NHS non-eligible patients registered in a designated centre in the UK or Republic of Ireland.

5 NHS non-eligible patients registered in a non-designated centre in the UK or Republic of Ireland.

The designated centres are those centres that are supported by the Department of Health to carry out a liver transplant programme. At present these include the Queen Elizabeth Hospital, Birmingham; Addenbrooke's Hospital, Cambridge; King's College Hospital, London; The Royal Free Hospital, London; St James' Hospital, Leeds; Freeman Hospital, Newcastle upon Tyne; and the Edinburgh Royal Infirmary, Edinburgh. St Vincent's Hospital in Dublin performs transplantations in the Republic of Ireland.

The factors that are taken into account in selecting the patients for donor eligibility include ABO blood group compatibility, paediatric recipients (for paediatric donors), and patient eligibility.

Zoning

Changes are being proposed to the liver allocation system and these are due to be in place at the end of 1993.

The UK will be divided into zones and each of the supraregionally funded and recognised transplant centres will be responsible for harvesting all donor livers offered in their zone. The size of the zone is proportional to the number of liver transplantations that the transplant centre is contracted to perform with the Department of Health. When a potential donor organ becomes available, the UKTSSA is informed and, wherever possible, the harvest team for the donor region will collect the liver. In principle, paediatric donors (ie, donors of less than 40 kg body weight or less than 16 years of age) will be used for paediatric recipients. If there is a suitable recipient outside the region who is in the super urgent category, then that liver may be 'exported' to the super urgent patient. Otherwise, the harvesting centre will have the first call on the liver. If there is no suitable recipient, the donor liver will be offered to the other transplant centres, using the sequence outlined

139

above. Those harvest teams that export more livers than they import will have priority in the use of livers from outside their zone.

The proposed system has many advantages, not least that the harvest centre can develop close contact with hospitals within its region and so, it is hoped, increase the donor rate.

ABO blood group

Livers are transplanted into ABO compatible patients and most centres will endeavour to use ABO identical grafts. Nevertheless, it is not the role of the UKTSSA to identify which patients may be selected for grafting by the transplant centre.

Paediatric recipients (aged 16 years or less)

Such patients are given priority within the rota for donors defined as paediatric by the donating unit or if the offer was specifically for a paediatric liver patient.

Patient eligibility

All livers donated in the UK and Republic of Ireland have first to be offered to NHS eligible patients. The eligibility criteria, as defined by the Department of Health, broadly include UK and Republic of Ireland nationals, patients registered at UK or Republic of Ireland centres, and European community E112 reciprocal health arrangements.

Other considerations

At present there is no clear evidence that the presence of panel reactivity (PRA), HLA identity between donor and recipient, and absence of a positive lymphocyte cross-match cytotoxicity significantly affects graft outcome. Because of the enormous logistic problems that would be required to match donors and recipients with respect to any of these parameters, no attempt is made to provide HLA identity or prospectively to cross-match.

At present, the unit which will use the liver is responsible for harvesting the organ. However, there are currently plans to alter this

TABLE IV—*Cadaveric organs donated for transplantation (reported to UKTSSA): results for 1991*

Organ	Number
Kidney	1840
Heart	283
Heart–lung	88
Lung	100
Liver	449*
Pancreas	36
Liver/million population	
Range (by region)	4·8–13·9
Median	6·8

*Of the livers 15 were not used (for a variety of reasons).

TABLE V—*Numbers on waiting lists reported to UKTSSA in 1991*

	New patients	Deaths awaiting transplantation
Heart	374	69
Heart–lung	147	41
Lung	101	16
Liver	379	15

system so that certain zones within the UK would be covered by local transplant centres.

The use of organs within the UK for 1991 is shown in Tables IV and V.

Acknowledgement

The data and analyses reported in the Annual Report of the US Scientific Registry for Organ Transplantation and the Organ Procurement and Transplantation Network, 1990, have been supplied by United Network for Organ Sharing (UNOS), Richmond, Virginia, and the Division of Organ Transplantation, Health Resources and Services Administration, Bethesda, Maryland. The authors alone are responsible for the reporting and interpretation of these data and thank the UNOS, the Association of Organ Procurement Organizations, the Transplant and Health Policy Center, the Organ Procurement Agency of Michigan, and the New England Organ Bank, for providing much of the data included in this chapter.

References

1 Benjamin M, Turcotte JG. Organ procurement: Supply, demand and ethics. *Transplant Proc* 1992; **24**: 2139–237.
2 Burdick JF, Turcotte JG, Veatch RM. Principles of organ and tissue allocation and donation by living donors. *Transplant Proc* 1992; **24**: 2226–37.
3 Organ Transplantation: Issues and Recommendations. Report of the Task Force on Organ Transplantation. US Department of Health and Human Services, April 1986.
4 Pierce GA. UNOS history. In: Phillips MG, ed. *UNOS: Organ Procurement, Preservation and Distribution in Transplantation*. Richmond, VA: The William Byrd Press, 1991: 1–3.
5 Broznick BA, Johnson HK. History of Organ Procurement Organizations. In: Phillips MG, ed. *UNOS: Organ Procurement, Preservation and Distribution in Transplantation*. Richmond, VA: The William Byrd Press, 1991: 21–22.
6 1992 AOPO Year End Voluntary Fax Survey on Local Organ Donor Activity. Association of Organ Procurement Organizations. Falls Church, Virginia.
7 1991 Annual Survey. *Solutions for Healthcare*. Association of Organ Procurement Organizations. Coopers & Lybrand.
8 Turcotte JG, Benjamin M. Selection criteria in transplantation: The critical questions. *Transplant Proc* 1989; **21**: 3377–445.
9 United Kingdom Transplant Services Support Authority. *First Annual Report*. HMSO: London, 1991.

7: Surgical aspects

XAVIER ROGIERS, CHRISTOPH E BROELSCH

Liver transplantation is the ultimate therapeutic intervention in the treatment of hepatic disease. The surgical feasability of liver replacement was demonstrated in the 1950s and refined in the 1960s. In 1963 the first human liver transplantation was attempted by Starzl. Progressively the results have improved and the number of liver transplantations performed has increased. In 1991 more than 4000 liver transplantations were performed with 1 year survival rates in excess of 70%. In this chapter the standard procedure for liver procurement, preservation, and transplantation is described as well as the most important technical variants.

The standard procedure

Liver procurement and preservation

Liver procurement from heart-beating cadaveric donors can safely be performed without jeopardising the procurement of other organs. The abdominal and thoracic cavities are entered through a mid-line thoraco-abdominal incision. The abdomen is inspected to exclude the presence of any unexpected infectious or neoplastic disease. The texture and colour of the liver are evaluated to determine its suitability as a transplant. The hepatoduodenal and gastroduodenal ligaments are explored for the presence of replaced hepatic arteries. The aorta is encircled just above its bifurcation and below the diaphragm. Usually the portal vein is cannulated, for instance through the inferior mesenteric vein. Dissection of the hepatoduodenal ligament is optional. After heparinisation, a cannula is inserted in the infrarenal aorta. The infradiaphragmatic aorta is cross-clamped and the inferior vena cava is opened at its entrance in the heart; then in situ core cooling is performed by infusion of cold preservation solution through the aorta and the portal vein after which the liver, pancreas (or liver and pancreas *en bloc*), and kidneys are removed in this sequence. Detailed descriptions of the technique of organ procurement can be found elsewhere. The iliac arteries and veins should be procured because they may be required for performing vascular reconstructions.

Different solutions have been used for cooling and preservation of the liver. The Euro-Collins solution and the University of Wisconsin solution are the best known. Their use has accomplished better organ preservation and longer preservation times. The University of Wisconsin solution (UW solution) permits safe liver preservation for up to 24 hours. Recent publications, however, have suggested that long preservation times may be associated with late bile duct complications, prompting surgeons to transplant the liver as soon as possible after procurement. During the time between procurement and transplantation the liver is stored in its preservation solution at 4°C in sterile plastic bags.

Orthotopic liver transplantation

The standard operation for replacement of the liver is the orthotopic liver transplantation. In this operation the whole diseased liver is removed and replaced by a cadaveric liver in the same position. The different stages or phases in the procedure are described below.

The pre-anhepatic phase

The abdomen is entered through a bilateral subcostal incision with median extension to the xyphoid process. The gastroduodenal ligament is dissected by trans-section and ligation of bile duct and arteries as close to the liver as possible, leaving only the portal vein intact. The left and right lobes of the liver are mobilised, and the posterior surface of the interior vena cava freed. Dissection around the diseased liver may be very difficult because of the presence of extensive venous collateral circulation resulting from chronic portal hypertension. This part of the operation can be particularly bloody and challenging in the presence of previous surgery in the upper abdomen.

The anhepatic phase

After clamping the supra- and infrahepatic vena cava and the portal vein, the liver is removed together with its retrohepatic vena caval segment.

Most transplant surgeons use venovenous bypass during the anhepatic phase in selected patients over 40 kg in weight. The inferior vena cava is cannulated through the saphenous or femoral vein in addition to the portal vein. Using a pump, the blood is re-fed into the axillary vein, providing portal and systemic venous decompression.

The vascular anastomoses are usually performed in the following sequence: the suprahepatic and the infrahepatic inferior vena cava, artery, and portal vein. Before reperfusing the liver the UW solution is flushed out of the liver using 500 ml 5% albumin solution infused through the portal vein and recovered through a catheter in the inferior vena cava.

Variations of the vasular anastomoses are possible in special situations. Sometimes interposition of donor iliac artery or vein is used in order to reach the infrarenal aorta with the artery or to bridge a thrombosed portal vein with the vein (Figure 1).

The post-anhepatic phase

The liver is reperfused by removal of the vascular clamps. This critical phase of the operation demands close circulatory monitoring by the anaesthetic team because of the potentially lethal consequences of releasing cold, hyperkalaemic fluid into the systemic circulation.

After a first check for causes of surgical bleeding, the venovenous bypass is taken down. Usually at this time there is a waiting period to allow the patient to warm up and for coagulation to improve.

Biliary reconstruction is performed by end-to-end choledochocholedochostomy, with or without T tube, or by a Roux-en-Y hepaticojejunostomy.

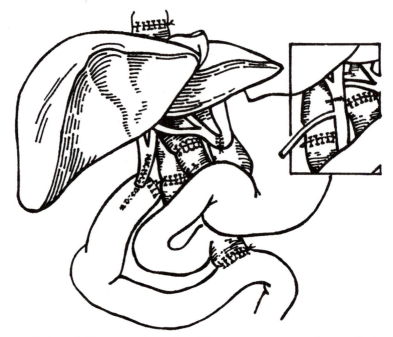

FIG 1—*Orthotopic liver transplantation: biliary tract reconstruction usually involves choledochojejunostomy (to a Roux limb) or (inset) choledocho-choledochostomy, which is stented with a T tube. (Redrawn with permission from Georg Thieme)*

Auxiliary orthotopic and heterotopic transplantation

Auxiliary transplantation means the transplantation of a liver without the complete removal of the diseased liver. In auxiliary heterotopic liver transplantation the liver is positioned as an extra liver in the right paravertebral gutter. In auxiliary orthotopic liver transplantation a left lateral hepatectomy is first performed, thus creating space for transplantation of a left lateral segment in its normal position (Figure 2).

Problems of auxiliary transplantation include the risk of development of a tumour in the remaining cirrhotic liver, the competition between the two livers for the portal blood with its hepatotrophic factors, and the lack of space (especially in the heterotopic auxiliary liver transplantation).

Promising results have recently been obtained with auxiliary liver transplantation for acute hepatic failure and for enzyme deficiency diseases.

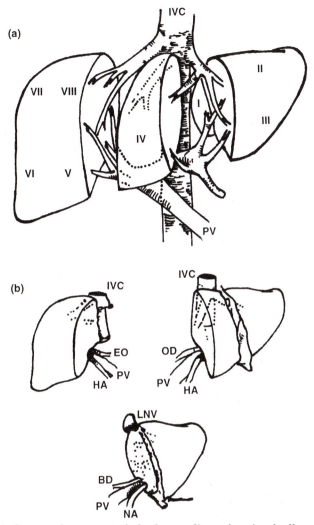

FIG 2—(a) Segmental anatomy of the human liver: functional allografts can be constructed from segments that have discrete vascular supply and bile drainage. (b) In practice, the right lobe graft consists of segments V–VIII, the left lobe graft of segments I–IV, and the left-lateral segment graft of segments I–III. IVC = inferior vena cava; PV = portal vein; HA = hepatic artery; LHV = left hepatic vein; BD = bile duct. (Redrawn with permission from Emond et al[1])

Reduced size, split and living related liver transplantation

In paediatric liver transplantation organ availability is critical. This is mainly due to the disparity in size between most paediatric

TABLE I—*Types of reduced size liver grafts*

Graft type	Segments*	Donor: Recipient ratio
Right lobe	V,VI,VII,VIII	2:1
Left lobe	(I),II,III,IV	4:1
Left lateral lobe	II,III	10:1

*Figure 3.

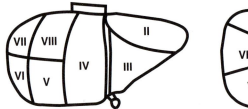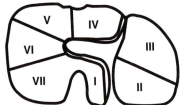

FIG 3—*Lobes of the liver.*

candidates for transplantation (>50% in those less than 2 years of age) and paediatric donors. Mortality rates for children on the transplant waiting list of 25% were not uncommon.

Reduced size liver transplantation

Knowledge of the segmental anatomy of the liver has allowed surgeons to modify liver grafts so as to allow transplantation in smaller recipients.

Several types of reduced size liver grafts can be performed, as shown in Table I. In the case of a left lateral lobe transplant, the donor's retrohepatic cava is left in place, allowing end-to-side implantation of the donor left hepatic vein on it.

The results of reduced liver transplantation have been at least as good as those of whole organ transplantation.

Split liver transplantation

With reduced size liver grafting proving successful it became conceivable that using the remaining portion of the liver for a second

148

transplantation could also be achieved successfully. Split liver transplantation allows one donor organ to be used for two smaller recipients; this would prove even more efficient by achieving the goal of reducing the paediatric donor shortage. The results of split liver transplantation, however, have been inferior to those of whole or reduced organ transplantation. This is related to technical problems (such as biliary leaks due to devascularisation of the bile duct during graft preparation) and to the more frequent use of split liver transplantation for emergency transplantations.

The increasing shortage of organs prompts transplant surgeons once again to take up the theme of split liver transplantation. It is hoped that with increased experience the results of this procedure will approximate the results of other types of transplantation.

Living related liver transplantation

The concept of living related liver transplantation has its basis in two observations. The experience with split liver transplantation proved that it was possible to procure a segment of the liver, suitable for transplantation, without jeopardising the function of the remaining liver. Also, the growing experience with liver resection has demonstrated that the procurement of such a segment can be performed with a maximum of safety and with minimal blood loss.

Usually segments II and III are procured from the donor. In order to do this the vessels for the left lateral liver segments are isolated (left artery, left portal vein, left hepatic vein). After transsection of the parenchyma, which can usually be performed with minimal blood loss and without vascular occlusion, the vessels can simply be clamped, and the liver segment taken out and perfused with UW solution. Vascular reconstructions are necessary to elongate the portal vein and the hepatic artery. The operation for the recipient is similar to that of the cadaveric left lateral segment transplantation.

More than 100 living related liver transplantations have been performed world wide, and donor mortality or major morbidity has not been reported.

The advantages of living related transplantation are linked to the quality of the graft and to the elective nature of the procedure. First, because the graft is procured from a perfectly healthy donor, and with an almost non-existent warm ischaemia time, an excellent

149

initial graft function can be guaranteed. In fact primary non-function of the graft has not been observed. Second, the permanent availability of a graft for transplantation makes it possible to perform the operation electively, at the optimal time for the recipient. Consequently a potentially long waiting time, during which the recipient's health deteriorates, can be avoided.

These advantages are well illustrated by the results obtained in Hamburg. Of 20 recipients 14 were transplanted as an elective procedure: of these 13 survived (93%). Of six urgent cases only one (17%) survived, revealing that the advantage of living related transplantation is lost in these cases. Further development of living related liver transplantation for use in adult recipients is likely in the near future.

Combined organ transplantation

The liver can be transplanted together with any other organ. Multivisceral transplantation (liver, pancreas, and bowel *en bloc*) is probably the most daring example of this. It can be used in the treatment of short bowel syndrome with associated liver failure. Starzl also performed this procedure after cluster resection of the upper abdominal organs for right upper quadrant malignancy.

Conclusion

Liver transplantation as a surgical procedure has evolved considerably over the last few years. A liver can be transplanted as a whole, as a reduced or split cadaveric organ, and, in addition, as a living related graft. Transplantation of the liver in combination with many other organs has been performed successfully. Further advances such as xenotransplantation of the liver or hepatocellular transplantation are to be expected.

References

1 Emond JC, Whitington PF, Thistlethwaite JR, Alonso EM, Broelsch CE. Reduced-size orthotopic liver transplantation: use in management of children with chronic liver disease. *Hepatology* 1989; **10**: 867–72.

8: Problems before discharge

JOHN A C BUCKELS

This chapter is concerned with the postoperative in-hospital course of liver transplant recipients and deals with the probable complications and ways in which these can be either prevented or effectively treated. There are differences in complications between patients grafted for chronic and those grafted for acute fulminant liver failure. Most patients transplanted for chronic disease now have a smooth postoperative course and can expect to go home within 2–3 weeks. For others, the road to recovery can be very rocky with prolonged periods in intensive care, multiple surgical procedures, and a total hospital stay of several months. Patients are more likely to recover quickly if grafted at optimum time before the ravages of advancing liver failure produce a pre-terminal state. Thus, timely referral as discussed earlier in Part II is important in both humane and economic terms. Although protocols vary between centres, in this chapter a broad consensus approach is presented.

Routine postoperative management

Following liver grafting patients are routinely ventilated on the intensive care unit. They can usually be extubated within 24 hours, provided that they are haemodynamically stable with satisfactory liver function, urine output, and blood gases. For patients with acute fulminant hepatic failure, encephalopathy may persist for several days and so these patients may also need ventilation for several days. Doppler ultrasonography of the graft is performed in all patients on the first postoperative day, to demonstrate patency of the vessels; this is repeated whenever clinically indicated.

Biliary drainage is established in most adults during surgery by a duct-to-duct anastomosis over a latex rubber T tube, but those with an abnormal biliary tree (such as patients with primary sclerosing cholangitis) require a Roux-en-Y jejunal loop. Bilary complications are common and several workers have advocated changes in practice such as the universal use of Roux-en-Y jejunal loops, the avoidance of T tubes in duct-to-duct anastomoses, or the retention of the gall bladder with an indwelling catheter, leaving the bile duct anastomosis unsplinted. There are no controlled trials as yet to indicate which method is best.

Advantages of a T tube include the ability to observe the quality of bile as an indication of early liver function, an opportunity to perform minimally invasive cholangiography, as well as a source of bile for bacteriological culture. The T tube is normally left on drainage for the first week when a cholangiogram is performed and, if satisfactory, the tube is clamped. Cholangiography carries a risk of cholangitis and should be covered by two doses of broad spectrum antibiotics – one before and one after the examination. Cholangiography can be repeated when indicated clinically (see biliary complications later) and always before T tube removal at 2–3 months.

Daily tests of liver function, including asparate transaminase, prothrombin time, bilirubin, and alkaline phosphatase, are needed during the early postoperative period. Initially the transaminases are significantly elevated (between 500 units/l and 2000 units/l) though these fall rapidly, usually halving each day until normal values are obtained. Patients with cholestatic diseases soon become less jaundiced as the excess bilirubin is excreted by the liver, and good quality bile from the T tube is a sign of satisfactory early graft function. Patients with non-cholestatic disease, and who are not icteric before transplantation, paradoxically often become jaundiced in the early postoperative period; this is probably a result of preservation injury, but soon settles with adequate graft function. The prothrombin time often remains elevated (international normalised ratio, INR, up to two to three times normal) for the first few days after grafting. Unless there is active bleeding, correction is unnecessary and may mask deteriorating graft function which warrants further assessment. Spontaneous improvement implies improving liver function. Other signs of satisfactory graft function include correction of the acidosis, which usually develops during

152

BOX A   Complications after liver transplantation

Immediate
- Haemorrhage
- Primary non-function
- Acute renal failure

Early
- Primary poor function
- Acute rejection
- Massive haemorrhagic necrosis
- Chronic rejection
- Hepatic artery thrombosis
- Portal vein thrombosis
- Cholangitis
- Bile leakage
- Biliary obstruction
- Biliary sludge
- Non-anastomotic biliary stricture
- Graft versus host disease
- Bacterial infection
- Opportunistic infection (viral, fungal)

---

surgery, and maintenance of normoglycaemia in the absence of glucose support.

Enteral feeding through a fine bore nasogastric tube is instituted if oral intake cannot be resumed within 2–3 days and gastrointestinal function is adequate. Abdominal drains and vascular access lines are usually removed within a few days. In some units, the T tube, if used, is irrigated daily with sterile saline until its removal at three months. Many patients are well enough to be mobilised within the first few days and are able to spend time out of hospital within 2–3 weeks. Recovery can, however, be prolonged in some patients, particularly if acute renal failure requiring dialysis has occurred, or in those grafted for fulminant liver failure.

The problems that occur in liver transplant recipients prior to discharge (or death) can be classified as immediate (intensive care phase) or early (Box A).

Problems before discharge

Immediate problems after surgery

Immediate problems after liver transplantation are haemorrhage, primary non-function, and acute renal failure. These are greatly

153

influenced by the transplant operation itself and the quality of the newly inserted liver.

Haemorrhage

Hepatectomy in the recipient can be a difficult procedure in patients with severe portal hypertension, especially if there has been previous surgery around the liver. Haemostasis is usually possible using a variety of approaches, including correction of clotting abnormalities, adequate warming of blood and blood products, venovenous bypass for decompression during the anhepatic phase, and the local control of bleeding points including suture ligation, use of fibrin glue, and diathermy. The use of the thromboelastograph, which measures the quality of blood clot rather than individual clotting factors, allows a dynamic evaluation of the coagulation status of the patient in the operating room. This is usually performed by the anaesthetist who is responsible for the transfusions of clotting factors, and enables a judgement to be made of which factors are required – platelets, fresh frozen plasma, or cryoprecipitate. The thromboelastograph can detect fibrinolysis which can be corrected or prevented by an infusion of aprotinin which is used routinely by many centres.[1]

In some patients, full haemostasis may not be possible and options include introduction of haemostatic packs or application of externally applied abdominal binders. Both can be effective, although control of bleeding is very dependent on early function of the new liver with production of clotting factors. Ongoing haemorrhage on the intensive care unit, despite replacement of blood and clotting factors, indicates a need for re-exploration. Usually no focal bleeding point is found, but removal of blood clot is effective by stopping the ongoing fibrinolysis which potentiates this bleeding. Provided the liver is working well, further haemorrhage is uncommon. Bleeding after uneventful surgery in patients who were dry at time of closure is always an indication for exploration, and a specific bleeding point will usually be found and controlled.

Primary non-function

Primary non-function is when the new liver fails to work, defined as unexplained failure of graft function in the first 24 hours of surgery. This may be the result of pre-existing factors in the donor,

154

poor graft preservation, or injury caused by reperfusion at implantation. The occurrence of non-function is often unpredictable and the exact cause difficult to identify, and it may result from a combination of factors. During and following surgery the patient develops a progressive and severe acidosis, renal failure, and all other features of fulminant hepatic failure. Haemodynamic instability and death ensue unless re-transplantation is undertaken urgently. Earlier reports of reversing non-function with prostaglandins have not been confirmed.[2] Haemodynamic instability may be improved by doing a total hepatectomy and portocaval shunt while waiting for a new liver. Although primary non-function is rare in most centres, poor function does occur in around 5–10% of cases. These patients may display some features of acute liver failure including renal dysfunction, encephalopathy, cholestasis, and an elevated prothrombin time. Liver biopsy taken at implantation in such cases may show excess fat or centrolobular necrosis (so-called preservation injury). Microvesicular fat in donor livers is common and probably reflects pre-terminal starvation in the donor. Macrovesicular fat is more serious and is associated with a high early failure rate. Thus, livers that appear fatty at time of removal should, if possible, be checked histologically before insertion or discarded. Grafts that are slow to function usually improve within a couple of weeks. Although the fitter transplant recipients may cope well with a liver that is slow to function, such dysfunction can be life threatening to the sickest recipients when regrafting might be the only chance for recovery.

Renal failure

Some evidence of renal dysfunction is seen in most liver transplant recipients and is characterised by a period of oliguria and rise in serum creatinine for 2–3 days after surgery. Oliguria will usually respond to correction of any fluid deficit and an infusion of dopamine. Acute renal failure requiring dialysis is uncommon in patients transplanted for chronic liver disease unless they have hepatorenal failure, or if surgery involved significant hypotension or haemorrhage. Patients transplanted for acute fulminant hepatic failure have often become dialysis dependent before grafting. Dialysis for all these patients is best performed as continuous arteriovenous haemodialysis (CAVHD) using a dedicated large-bore double-lumen central line or a peripheral arteriovenous shunt. Most patients establish a diuresis within two weeks although if longer treatment is necessary intermittent haemodialysis is more appropriate for a patient with increasing mobility.

Early complications after surgery

Potential complications after liver grafting are legion, and the learning curve for liver transplantation is long and arduous. The advantage for larger units is that having seen most of the common complications, problems can be pre-empted by the early recognition of clinical patterns, and it is hoped that potential disasters can be averted. The most common problems are rejection, infection, graft ischaemia, biliary tract obstruction or leakage, and psychological.

Rejection

Hypoacute rejection is a rare form of rejection occurring immediately after grafting, and may be associated with pre-formed antibodies.

Despite early reports (based on animal studies) that the liver is an immunologically privileged organ, cellular rejection is a major problem after liver grafting. The clinical and histological features of acute cellular rejection are discussed on pages 180–188 and 301–303. High dose immunosuppression will reduce rejection but may lead to unacceptable risks from infection.

The introduction of cyclosporin A (cyclosporine) coincided with a significant improvement in the results of liver grafting. Nevertheless, a continuing high incidence of rejection episodes led several centres to give "triple therapy" using a combination of low dose cyclosporin A, azathioprine, and steroids. Standard doses of immunosuppressive agents together with drugs employed for prophylaxis against infection and peptic ulceration are given in Box B. Episodes of acute rejection are treated with high dose oral or intravenous corticosteroids such as oral prednisolone or methylprednisolone (200–1000 mg daily for three days). One problem with cyclosporin A is that, as it is fat soluble, bile is required for its absorption. Thus, if rejection is the cause of the liver dysfunction (with increasing cholestasis), further reduction in cyclosporin A levels due to poor absorption may compound the situation. FK506 (troleandomycin) does not have this problem. Moreover liver dysfunction may in-

---

BOX B   Immunosuppression and prophylactic drug regimens: The Birmingham Protocols

Immunosuppressant drugs:
- Intravenous hydrocortisone 200 mg daily converted to prednisolone 20 mg daily after oral feeding commences. Steroids reduced by 5 mg every three weeks and stopped at three months
- Azathioprine 1·5–2·0 mg/kg daily: initially intravenously, converted to oral once oral feeding commences
- Cyclosporin A initially 2 mg/kg per day as a slow intravenous infusion in divided doses converted to 10 mg/kg per day once oral feeding commences but adjusted to give therapeutic blood levels

Prophylaxis for infections (stopped at three months):
- Broad spectrum intravenous antibiotics (stopped at 48 hours)
- Co-trimoxazole, 1 tablet alternate days
- Amphotericin lozenge, suck 1 daily
- Nystatin suspension 5 ml four times daily via nasogastric tube or orally
- Ranitidine 50 mg intravenously three times daily, then 150 mg twice daily orally
- Acyclovir 200 mg five times daily if receiving cytomegalovirus positive graft
- Isoniazid 200 mg daily plus pyridoxine in patients at risk of tuberculosis, ie, Asians, some alcoholics

---

crease blood levels of FK506 and this can be beneficial if the cause of the liver dysfunction is immunological. The results of controlled trials comparing FK506 with conventional immunosuppression are awaited.

The role of anti-thymocyte or anti-lymphocyte globulin or monoclonal antibodies such as OKT3 in liver transplantation remains uncertain. Attempts to induce immunosuppression with OKT3 immediately after grafting, followed several days later by conventional immunosuppression (so-called sequential therapy), have not shown any survival advantage.[3] There is evidence, however, that OKT3 may be helpful in patients with acute rejection that is proving resistant to high dose steroids, although at the cost of an increased incidence of infection, particularly with viruses such as cytomegalovirus (CMV).[4]

Early acute rejection occurs in up to 80% of liver grafts[5] and is usually associated with deteriorating graft function (rising bilirubin, liver enzymes, and prothrombin time). Other common causes of dysfunction may mimic the biochemical changes in rejection and these include bacterial infection (such as cholangitis), viral infection (such as CMV hepatitis), ischaemia, and biliary obstruction which should be excluded before additional immunosuppression is given. Thus, whenever possible, histological confirmation of rejection should be sought. Late acute rejection is uncommon and doses of immunosuppressant drugs can be progressively reduced in most patients with a reduction in the risks of infection. Corticosteroids are discontinued at three months in some centres. Long term maintenance is with a combination of steroids, azathioprine, and cyclosporin A.[6] If later acute rejection is seen, factors such as poor absorption due to gastroenteritis or poor compliance should be considered.

A rare complication after liver transplantation is acute graft necrosis and failure in the absence of vascular obstruction. This occurs in livers that initially function well but then fail acutely. Histological features include widespread haemorrhage and infarction, and the syndrome has been described as massive haemorrhagic necrosis.[7] This is considered by some to be an acute immunological event, and if suspected and treated early it may be reversed by high dose steroids. In most patients, however, massive haemorrhagic necrosis requires emergency re-transplantation.

Chronic or ductopenic rejection in the liver initially presents as a biliary phenomenon rather than the vascular process as seen in renal or heart transplantation. The small bile radicals are destroyed (leading to a vanishing bile duct syndrome, VBDS) and this process is usually irreversible.[8] This occurs in less than 10% of grafted livers and may be detected very early after transplantation. This is in contrast to the progressive (vascular) chronic rejection eventually producing graft failure in most renal and heart grafts. The fact that the liver has a dual blood supply may account for some of this difference. Vanishing bile duct syndrome, as seen on biopsies, is a focal phenomenon and demonstration on subsequent biopsies is needed to establish this diagnosis definitely. Regrafting is the only definitive option although there may be recurrence of the syndrome in some cases leading Starzl to call such patients "liver eaters".

One final immunological event of note is the occurrence of massive haemolysis if grafts that are ABO blood group compatible but non-identical are used. In this situation the recipient might be blood group A, B, or AB. In the first two, a blood group O liver or, in the case of an AB recipient, an A, B, or even O liver is implanted which then produces antibodies to the A and B antigens on the host red cells. This is followed by massive haemolysis with a rapidly falling haemoglobin and a rapidly rising serum bilirubin. If the liver is functioning well the bilirubin is mainly conjugated which might mislead the unwary. A blood film shows fragmented red blood cells and the direct Coombs' test is positive. This haemolysis usually occurs around the seventh to the tenth postoperative day and is usually self-limiting. Knowledge about the non-identity of the graft and recipient blood groups should enable early diagnosis. To prevent the dangers of ongoing haemolysis, any anaemia should be corrected by the administration of blood that is only of the donor group.

Early infection

The most common bacterial infections after liver transplantation are those of the respiratory and the biliary tract. The combination of postoperative ventilation, a painful upper abdominal wound, and a high incidence of pleural effusions contributes to respiratory impairment. Adequate analgesia and frequent physiotherapy are necessary to prevent underventilation and subsequent pulmonary infection. Larger pleural effusions should be aspirated, particularly if symptomatic.

Most patients rapidly develop colonisation of the bile with pathogenic bacteria, and thus cholangitis as a source of infection or liver dysfunction is often difficult to prove. A combination of fever, bactobilia, and altered liver function in the presence of a relatively normal biopsy supports the diagnosis of cholangitis and indicates the need for antibiotic therapy. Cholangitis is more probable with biliary obstruction, so allowing free drainage from the T tube can be helpful both in reaching a diagnosis and in resolving any fever. Attempts to sterilise the bile by repeated antibiotic therapy is likely to lead to suprainfection with either resistant bacteria or fungi. Early biliary obstruction or leakage as a cause of cholangitis can be detected by cholangiography through the T tube and this is considered below.

Opportunistic infections are an inherent risk to all immunosuppressed patients. Those commonly seen after liver replacement are CMV and fungal infections. *Pneumocystis carinii* was seen in early series but has been eradicated by the use of co-trimoxazole – one tablet taken orally on alternate days. Severe CMV infections are invariably primary infections rather than reactivation, and theoretically they might be avoided by the use of CMV matched donors. Many units are, however, not able to obtain CMV tested blood and blood products that are often required in sufficient quantities to make CMV liver matching superfluous. CMV usually presents with fever, malaise, and leucopenia.

The more severe infections cause gastrointestinal upset, pneumonia, encephalopathy, and hepatitis. Even without a rise in serum transaminases, the liver tests may be abnormal with a cholestatic pattern. Prompt diagnosis is imperative. Serological confirmation often takes time although newer tests such as polymerase chain reaction can give early results. Tissue diagnosis (liver biopsy, or rectal or gastric biopsies in patients with gastrointestinal symptoms) is often the quickest way to reach a diagnosis. Clinical infections are treated with ganciclovir supplemented with hyperimmune globulin if severe. In all clinical infections, baseline doses of immunosuppressant drugs should be reduced. The use of acyclovir as prophylaxis against CMV in patients given CMV positive grafts has only been partially effective through reduction of the incidence and severity of attacks.

Fungal colonisation is common in patients with end stage liver disease. Prophylaxis with oral nystatin and amphotericin can reduce oral and oesophageal candidiasis. Invasive fungal infections can be difficult to diagnose and may only come to light *post mortem*; thus, they should be treated on suspicion with specific therapy together with a reduction in immunosuppression. Patients at greatest risk for fungal infections include those requiring prolonged ventilation and patients receiving repeated high dose immunosuppression for rejection.

Finally, tuberculosis is a risk in patients from the Asian subcontinent who receive transplants. This is a reactivation of primary infections and carries a grave prognosis even with adequate therapy and cessation of immunosuppressant agents. Prophylaxis with isoniazid (plus pyridoxine) for 3–6 months is effective. Other patients at risk of this complication include some patients who undergo transplantation for alcoholic liver disease.

Graft ischaemia

Graft ischaemia due to hepatic artery thrombosis can be a devastating complication. This occurs most frequently in the first postoperative month and leads to graft necrosis, intrahepatic abscess, and infarction of the bile ducts with bile leakage. The incidence varies between series but is higher in children (up to 25%) than in adults (up to 10%). Infarction is often heralded by massive rises in the liver enzyme levels but should also be suspected in any case of acute graft failure, biliary problems, and Gram-negative septicaemia. In all these situations urgent Doppler ultrasonography is performed which should be confirmed by arteriography if thrombosis is suggested. Early thrombosis is an indication for urgent regrafting although patients with late thrombosis may survive with satisfactory graft function. Even though technical factors are important, there is an increased incidence of hepatic artery thrombosis in patients with an elevated haematocrit ($>44\%$) in the early postoperative period; thus, the postoperative maintenance of a low haemoglobin (<11 g/dl) and haematocrit ($<35\%$) is advocated.[9]

Thrombosis of the portal vein is rare and usually presents with variceal bleeding in the early postoperative period. Such bleeding is highly suggestive of portal vein thrombosis which should be urgently investigated by means of Doppler ultrasonography and angiography. Emergency thrombectomy is usually effective and graft loss is uncommon.

Biliary obstruction and leakage

The biliary anastomosis has aptly been called the "Achilles heel" of liver transplantation. In the absence of ischaemia due to arterial thrombosis, four patterns of biliary problems are seen:

- Leakage from the anastomosis or T tube insertion site
- Stenosis of the anastomosis
- Non-anastomotic strictures of the donor bile duct
- Biliary sludge.

If biliary problems are suspected, Doppler ultrasonography is always indicated to confirm patency of the vessels. This might also detect intra-abdominal bile collections or intrahepatic duct dilatation if present. For patients with a T tube, cholangiography is the most useful investigation. Minor leakage around the T tube or from the anastomosis will often settle by placing the T tube on drainage. Any significant intra-abdominal collection can be aspirated percutaneously. During this period, special care is needed to maintain cyclosporin A levels in the therapeutic range, and intravenous administration may be needed. Although late anastomotic obstruction of the biliary anastomosis can be dilated at endoscopic retrograde cholangiopancreatography or by the transhepatic route, early obstruction requires surgical correction. This is best carried out as a Roux-en-Y choledochojejunostomy.

Non-anastomotic strictures of the donor ducts are rare but usually affect the confluence. Prolonged preservation times have been suggested as a cause but this has not been confirmed. Surgical correction can be successful though some patients require re-transplantation. Biliary sludge is a common problem and probably represents a degree of ischaemic injury to the biliary tree at time of implantation. The sludge often settles after T tube removal and might be helped by the oral administration of ursodeoxycholic acid. Patients without a suitable recipient bile duct (such as those with primary sclerosing cholangitis) have bile drainage established at transplantation by means of a Roux jejunal loop without a T tube. Suspected biliary problems can be investigated by means of ultrasonography to detect obstruction or collections. Additional information on biliary drainage can be gained with iodine isotope scanning even in the presence of a high serum bilirubin or by percutaneous transhepatic cholangiography. Again, biliary obstruction requires surgical revision as does major bile leakage, although minor leaks can be effectively treated with percutaneous drainage.

Psychological problems

The careful counselling of patients before the operation should help reduce psychological problems in the early postoperative period. Nevertheless, liver transplantation is probably the most stressful event in the life of such patients and psychological problems do occur. Almost all patients exhibit a degree of euphoria in the early phase (that they have survived the operation!) which can rapidly turn to depression over the coming weeks. Family and pastoral support should be encouraged. Patients with recurrent rejection and those requiring multiple grafts need additional support and care, and even brief visits home can be beneficial when feasible. Patients who undergo transplantation for acute fulminant hepatic failure usually do not remember being admitted to hospital and certainly do not feel better for having received a transplant because they were fit before their illness. These patients require special counselling which needs to extend well beyond the period of hospitalisation.

Ascites

Although it might be anticipated that liver replacement would rapidly restore normal portal pressure and liver function, it is recognised that those patients who, at transplantation, have significant ascites will remain with ascites for several months after surgery. Studies have shown that although portal pressure does normalise, liver blood flow remains increased.[10] The ascites usually persists for several weeks. If drain tracts or drains remain the ascites will leak out. It is important to ensure that hydration remains adequate. Use of intravenous colloid is often necessary. If there is no external drainage, the ascites should be treated in the conventional way, with salt restriction, diuretics, and drainage if clinically indicated.

Neurological problems

Neurological problems after transplantation may occur especially in patients grafted for fulminant hepatic failure and with multiple organ failure. Seizures may be related to cyclosporin A therapy, electrolyte disturbance (particularly calcium and magnesium), infections (especially fungal), and other medications. Central pontine myelinolysis may be associated with a rapid change in serum sodium. Confusion and psychosis may also occur but usually resolve with time (see Chapter 14).

Early postoperative mortality

Mortality in the first postoperative month depends on the underlying indication, the stage of disease at transplantation, the quality of the grafted liver, and the precision of the surgical technique. Significantly higher mortality is seen in patients grafted for acute fulminant hepatic failure compared to those with chronic liver

TABLE I—*Causes of early (30 day) mortality**

Cause	No	(%)
Multiple organ failure/sepsis	16	(33)
Bleeding	9	(19)
Cerebral (mainly in acute fulminant failure)	6	(13)
Primary non-function	5	(10)
Vascular occlusion	5	(10)
Cardiac	4	(8)
Rejection	1	(2)
Other		
Massive haemorrhagic necrosis and pulmonary oedema	2	(4)

*Data derived from an analysis of 48 deaths (13·6%) within 30 days in a consecutive series of 353 patients undergoing transplantation in Birmingham between January 1990 and December 1992.

BOX C   Indication for re-transplantation

- Primary non-function
- Early arterial thrombosis
- Massive haemorrhagic necrosis
- Acute drug resistant rejection
- Established chronic rejection
- Major non-anastomotic biliary stricture

---

disease; cerebral events account for much of this difference. Furthermore, patients with acute liver failure have an increased incidence of sepsis, probably related to the loss of function of Kupffer's cells as part of the organ failure. As mentioned earlier, patients grafted in the agonal stages of chronic liver disease have a worse outcome with an increased incidence of renal failure and sepsis. A list of the causes of the 30 day mortality in the Birmingham series over the last three years is given in Table I.

Re-transplantation

Approximately 15% of patients will suffer graft loss and need re-transplantation, the incidence being higher in children than in adults. Indications for regrafting are given in Box C. Early retransplantation is usually technically straightforward and long term survival exceeds 50%. An aggressive approach to re-transplantation was a significant factor in the improvements in survival pioneered by the Pittsburgh group.[11] Chronic ductopenic rejection is the usual indication for late re-transplantation which can be difficult due to dense adhesions around the liver.

References

1 Mallett S, Rolles K, Cox D, Burroughs A, Hunt B. Intraoperative use of aprotinin (Trasylol) in orthotopic liver transplantation. *Transplant Proc* 1991; **23**: 1931–2.
2 Greig PD, Woolf GM, Abecassis M, *et al.* Treatment of primary liver graft non-function with prostaglandin E₁ results in increased graft and patient survival. *Transplant Proc* 1989; **21**: 2385–8.
3 McDiarmid SV, Busittil RW, Levy P, Millis MJ, Terasaki PI, Ament ME. The long-term outcome of OKT3 compared with cyclosporin prophylaxis aftger liver transplantation. *Transplantation* 1991; **52**: 91–7.
4 Cosimi AB, Cho SI, Delmonico FL, Kaplan MM, Rohrer RJ, Jenkins RL. A randomised clinical trial comparing OKT3 and steroids for treatment of hepatic allograft rejection. *Transplantation* 1987; **43**: 91–5.
5 Kirby RM, McMaster P, Clements D, *et al.* Orthotopic liver transplantation: postoperative complications and their outcome. *Br J Surg* 1987; **74**: 3–11.
6 Padbury RTA, Gunson BK, Dousset B, *et al.* Long-term immunosuppression after liver transplantation: are steroids necessary? *Transplant Int* 1992; **5**(suppl 1): 470–2.
7 Hubscher SG, Adams DH, Buckels JAC, McMaster P, Neuberger J, Elias E. Massive haemorrhagic necrosis of the liver after liver transplantation. *J Clin Pathol* 1989; **42**: 360–70.
8 Hubscher SG, Buckels JAC, Elias E, McMaster P, Neuberger J. Vanishing bile-duct syndrome following liver transplantation—is it reversible? *Transplantation* 1991; **51**: 1004–10.
9 Buckels JAC, Tisone G, Gunson BK, McMaster P. Low haematocrit reduces hepatic artery thrombosis after liver transplantation. *Transplant Proc* 1989; **21**: 2460–1.
10 Hadensue A, Lebrec D, Moreau R, *et al.* Presence of systemic and splanchnic hyperkinetic circulation in liver transplant patients. *Hepatology* 1993; **17**: 175–8.
11 Shaw BW, Gordon RD, Iwatsuki S, Starzl TE. Retransplantation of the liver. *Semin Liver Dis* 1985; **5**: 394–401.

V: After discharge

9: Survival after transplantation

JAMES NEUBERGER, MICHAEL R LUCEY

Since the initial human liver transplantation by Dr Starzl in 1963 there has been a slow but steady increase in the number of transplant operations performed. However, in the last decade, there has been a dramatic increase in liver transplant activity. In the USA, 15 liver allografts were carried out in 1980; as shown in Figure 1, this number had increased to 2656 by 1990.[1] In the same period, the number of centres carrying out liver transplantation has grown from 1 to 85, with each centre doing an average of 31 liver grafts annually.[1] Coincident with this growth of transplant services and activity, the numbers of patients on liver transplant waiting lists have shown a commensurate increase (Table I). By the end of 1991, the United Network for Organ Sharing (UNOS) reported that 2327 patients were on the US National Waiting list; the median waiting time had increased from 33 days in 1988 to 67 days in 1991.[2]

The pattern in Europe is similar: between 1968 and 1972, 30 grafts were performed and, yet, in 1991 alone over 2200 grafts have been performed (Figure 1). In addition, the number of transplant centres undertaking transplantation has also shown a major increase (Figure 2). The number of transplant centres per 10 million of the population within Europe varies from 0·7 in the UK to 4·6 in France. Clearly the number of centres within any country is dependent not only on the size of population, and the prevalence and incidence of liver disease, but also on geographical considerations so that patients do not have to travel great distances to the local transplant centre. There are also regional differences in the number of transplantations performed. Thus, according to European Transplant Registry Data, the number of liver transplantations per million of the population in 1992 ranged from 2·1 to 13·7. The average rate

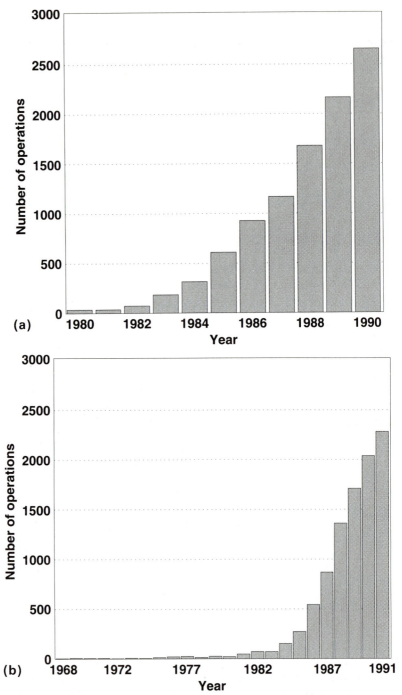

FIG 1—*Annual number of liver transplantations carried out in the USA, Series 1 (a) and Europe (b). (Data from UNOS and European Liver Transplant Registry)*

TABLE I—*Number of waiting list registrations and waiting time for liver recipients in the USA*

Year	Number	Waiting time (days)
1988	2110	33
1989	2829	39
1990	3587	44
1991	4097	67

Data from UNOS.

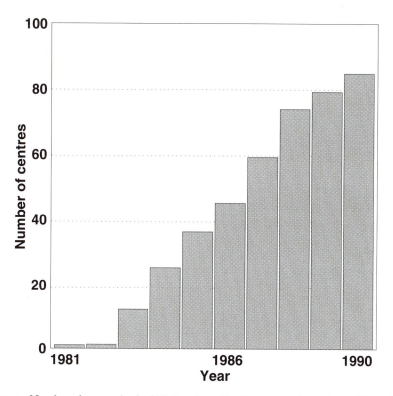

FIG 2—*Number of centres in the USA undertaking liver transplantations. (Data from Series 1, UNOS)*

in Europe as a whole is 5·9 per million of the population. These figures contrast with the rate in the USA of 11·0 per million in 1990. Current evaluation suggests that the actual need varies between 10 and 20 per million.

Results of transplantation

Knowlege of the survival rates achieved in different centres is essential not only for audit but also for justification of continued support. It is customary to consider results of transplantation in one year survival figures, although it is clear that in order to justify the enormous resources of a liver transplantation programme, there must be good five and ten year survival results. It is important that survival rates of different centres are not compared directly because there is great potential for error. First, survival rates depend on the indication for transplantation: patients with chronic liver disease tend to have a better one year survival than those with fulminant hepatic failure. Second, within individual disease categories, it is possible to identify those factors that are associated with poor outcome – for example, the presence of renal impairment appears to be a major prognostic factor. One centre may be grafting patients at a relatively early stage of their disease and therefore a greater probability of surviving one year would be anticipated than if the patient had a transplantation in a pre-terminal condition. Thus, for comparison of results between different centres, it is important that all these factors are taken into account; indeed, one centre with one year survival rates of 80% may actually be doing better than another with survival rates of 90%, if the former is operating on higher risk patients.

Overall survival

Survival after liver transplantation has increased in the last decade. In 1983, Scharschmidt[3] reported combined survival data from four centres in the USA and Europe which showed a 50% one year survival among 200 patients grafted for non-malignant disease between 1980 and 1983. In 1991, the cumulative 12 month survival from all centres in the USA was 74%. Of the factors that influence outcome, two have been readily identified in most series: the date of transplantation and the disease indication (Figures 3 and 4).

An example of this is shown by the Birmingham Liver Unit, where methods of immunosuppression and surgery have not altered greatly during the lifetime of the Unit; however, survival results have shown a significant but progressive improvement with time (Figure 3a), and similar results are seen both in Europe and in the

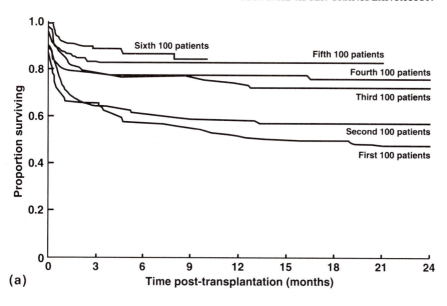

(a)

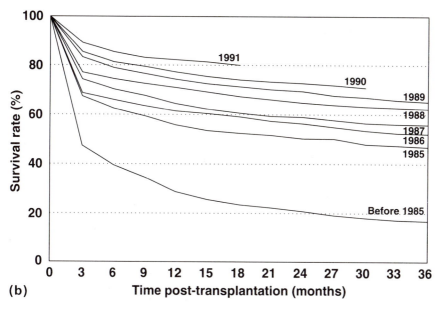

(b)

FIG 3—*Survival curves for patients receiving a liver transplant in (a) Birmingham, UK and (b) Europe. (Data from the European Liver Transplant Registry)*

173

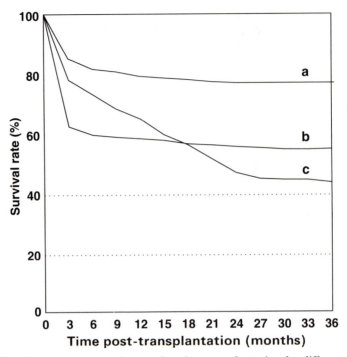

FIG 4—*Survival curves for patients undergoing transplantation for different indications. (a) Primary biliary, (b) hepatocellular, (c) fulminant liver disease. (Data from the European Liver Transplant Registry)*

USA (Figure 3b). Historical controls should not therefore be used to determine the efficacy or otherwise of new immunosuppressive treatments or other techniques.

The disease for which the patient is undergoing transplantation can also affect survival figures (Figure 4). Thus, those undergoing transplantation for fulminant hepatic failure tend to do less well than those having the operation for chronic liver disease. The results for primary liver cancers are of greater importance. Although such patients usually survive the operation, later there is attrition due to recurrence which may occur three or more years after grafting.

The goals of research into improving the results of liver transplantation must include the improvement of survival. The 20% mortality in the first year remains unacceptably high. Furthermore, clinicians must go beyond consideration of survival, and take into account the morbidity and quality of life after surgery. This broad area includes reducing the unwanted risks of medication, achieving

174

more targeted immunosuppression, and controlling or avoiding recurrent disease. Finally, consideration must be given to measures that make transplantation unnecessary.

References

1 Evans RW. The National Cooperative Transplantation Study. *Final Report*. Battelle, Seattle, 1991.
2 Annual Report of the US Scientific Registry for Organ Transplantation and the Organ Procurement and Transplantation Network. UNOS, Richmond, VA and the Division of Organ Transplantation, Health Resources and Services Administration, Bethesda, MD, 1990.
3 Scharschmidt B. Human liver transplantation: analysis of data on 540 patients from 4 centers. *Hepatology* 1984; 4: 95S–101S.

10: Immunological complications: rejection late after liver transplantation

GEOFF McCAUGHAN

Background details of the hospital admission

Physicians who are responsible for the management of transplant recipients after discharge from hospital should be provided with adequate information about the admission for transplantation. Details that are crucial in making a subsequent judgement about ensuing or persisting graft dysfunction are shown in Box A. Many patients will have had at least one episode of rejection after the transplant operation, requiring a dose of corticosteroids, and some of these may have received OKT3.

Knowledge about the severity of rejection during the peri-transplantation period will alert the physician to the prospect that the patient is a "high risk rejector". If OKT3 therapy was used for immunosuppression, a relapse may occur in up to 20% of patients during the next 12 months. It is important to realise that the benefit of OKT3 therapy may persist for several weeks after the therapy has finished, despite intercurrent reduction in the doses of standard immunosuppressives, cyclosporin A (cyclosporine), azathioprine, and prednisone. OKT3 therapy may predispose the patient to cytomegalovirus (CMV) disease and repeated courses may predispose to lymphoproliferative disorders. Progressive graft dysfunction in these patients makes uncontrolled rejection a probable cause.

CMV status is important, particularly if the recipient is seronegative and the donor seropositive. In some centres the patient may

176

have received CMV prophylaxis in the form of acyclovir (and/or ganciclovir) in the peri-transplantation period. This may reduce the prevalence of CMV disease but it may still occur. The onset is sometimes delayed, by which time the patient has been discharged and in the care of the referring physician, who should know whether the patient had CMV disease and whether ganciclovir was used. It is uncommon for cytomegalovirus infection to recur following a course of therapeutic ganciclovir.

Although surgical techniques have led to a reduction in the number of early biliary complications post-transplantation, late strictures occur. The likelihood increases in patients who had abnormalities in the biliary tree in the perioperative period. Problems with the hepatic artery, either stenosis or thrombosis, also predispose to late biliary tract strictures.

BOX A   Assessment of graft dysfunction: important background details from the transplant admission

1 *Are there predisposing factors to rejection?*
  (a) Was there postoperative allograft rejection?
  (b) If so, was it severe?
  (c) Did the patient receive OKT3 therapy?

2 *Are there predisposing factors to CMV?*
  (a) What was the cytomegalovirus (CMV) status of the donor and recipient?
  (b) Did the patient have CMV disease during the admission?
  (c) Was anti-CMV prophylactic therapy given?

3 *Are there predisposing factors to biliary tract problems?*
  (a) Were biliary tract abnormalities noted on postoperative cholangiography?
  (b) Did the patient have an end-to-end or Roux-en-Y biliary anastomosis?
  (c) Were there any problems with the hepatic artery post-transplantation?

4 *Are there predisposing factors to recurrent disease?*
  (a) Was the original disease viral hepatitis of type B or type C?
  (b) Was there an associated primary hepatocellular carcinoma?
  (c) Was the original disease autoimmune in origin: Primary biliary cirrhosis? Autoimmune chronic active hepatitis?

The need to be aware of the original diagnosis is important, in particular to know whether the original disease was viral, and whether there was an associated hepatocellular cancer. Furthermore, the possibility of recurrent disease such as primary biliary cirrhosis or autoimmune active hepatitis always needs to be considered in the differential diagnosis of obscure graft dysfunction, and is discussed elsewhere.

The referring physician usually shares responsibility for the care of a patient, when stable graft function and maintenance immunosuppressive therapy have been achieved. The details of maintenance immunosuppressive therapy are given in Chapter 11.

General approach to acute allograft dysfunction in the stable outpatient setting

This section is written on the presumption that the patient has been discharged from hospital within one month of transplantation. Acute allograft rejection is usually the most treatable cause of acute graft dysfunction and this will be discussed in detail later. CMV hepatitis may occur between one and six months post-transplantation and may be part of systemic CMV infection. Recurrence of hepatitis B or C may also occur. Biliary tract problems are a cause of dysfunction during this time, particularly if the record shows that the biliary tree was abnormal at any time post-transplantation.

In the 6–12 month period following discharge from hospital rejection and recurrent viral hepatitis are major causes of graft dysfunction (Table I). Biliary tract problems may begin to manifest themselves even if the biliary tree was normal on earlier studies. In patients who have stable graft function one year post-transplantation, acute rejection may occur, but it is uncommon. Biliary tract problems and chronic viral hepatitis, particularly hepatitis C, begin to emerge as a major cause of graft dysfunction. The possibility of recurrent hepatic malignancy must be considered where appropriate. There is some evidence for histological recurrence of primary biliary cirrhosis late after transplantation, although it does not seem to be a clinical problem. There are a few reports of recurrent autoimmune chronic active hepatitis. It should also be remembered that drug induced liver dysfunction secondary to antibiotics, antihypertensives, or immunosuppressive agents (cyclosporin A and

178

TABLE I—*Aetiology of graft dysfunction more than one month post-transplantation*

Time period post-transplantation*	Diagnosis	Relative importance
1–6 months	Acute cellular rejection	+ + + + +
	CMV hepatitis	+ +
	Recurrent hepatitis B/C/D	+ +
	Biliary tract abnormalities	+ +
6–12 months	Acute cellular rejection	+ + +
	Persisting hepatitis B/C/D	+ +
	Biliary tract abnormalities	+ +
	Chronic ductopenic rejection	+ + +
> 12 months	Persisting hepatitis B/C/D	+ + + +
	Biliary tract abnormalities	+ + +
	Acute cellular rejection	+ +
	Chronic ductopenic rejection	+
	Recurrence of non-viral diseases	+
	Malignancy	
	Autoimmune	

*These time periods are somewhat arbitrary. The list is not exhaustive. Drug induced hepatitis may occur at any time post-transplantation following the introduction of therapies.

azathioprine) may occur at any time post-transplantation. Most drug reactions are idiosyncratic but cyclosporin A may cause dose related hepatotoxicity. Elevated cyclosporin A drug levels, together with rising serum creatinine, may indicate cyclosporin A induced liver dysfunction.

The general diagnostic approach is outlined in Figure 1. Following detection of liver test abnormalities, ultrasonography should be performed to assess hepatic artery and portal vein blood flow, and to detect biliary tract abnormalities. Blood should be taken for CMV early antigen and other markers of CMV, particularly if graft dysfunction occurs within the first six months. Serology for viral hepatitis (hepatitis B surface antigen, HBV DNA, anti-hepatitis C antibody, and HCV RNA) should be performed and cyclosporin A levels estimated. If biliary tract abnormalities are found or if there is a strong history of biliary tract problems, endoscopic retrograde cholangiopancreatography or percutaneous cholangiography should be carried out; otherwise the patient should proceed directly to liver biopsy to assess graft abnormalities.

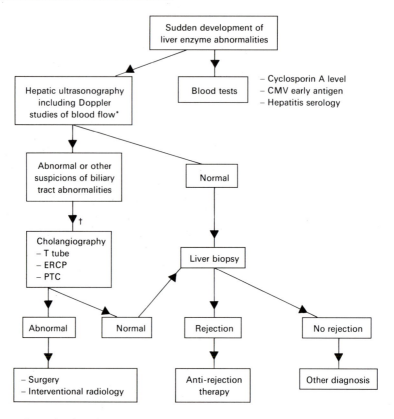

FIG 1—*Investigation of graft dysfunction. *A CT scan of the allograft may be useful at this stage. †Sometimes a hydroxyindoleacetic acid scan may be helpful if ultrasonography is equivocal. ERCP = endoscopic retrograde cholangiopancreatography; PTC = percutaneous transhepatic cholangiogram*

Diagnosis of acute rejection

The diagnosis of acute rejection cannot be made with certainty without the examination of liver biopsy. The pattern of enzyme abnormalities rarely helps in the assessment, although it is uncommon to find aspartate transaminase or alanine transaminase levels greater that 1000 units/litre in acute cellular rejection. The diagnosis may be suspected if the recent cyclosporin A levels have been subtherapeutic. Non-compliance may be a contributing factor, particularly in adolescents or young adults who may have had side effects from drugs such as steroids or cyclosporin A. It must be reiterated that if a patient has had previous episodes of severe rejection or

180

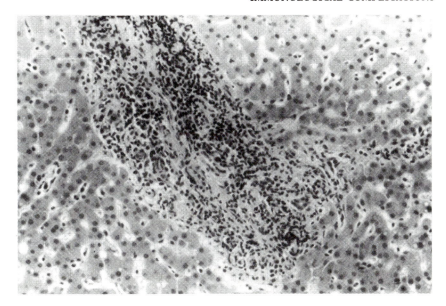

FIG 2—*Acute liver allograft rejection: mixed portal tract infiltrate*

required OKT3 therapy, then the chances of recurrent rejection are increased in the year after discharge from the transplant centre.

Most patients with acute rejection are asymptomatic; at this stage following transplantation it is very unusual for such patients to have impaired synthetic function of the graft. Clotting profiles, serum albumin, and blood glucose should be done, but are nearly always normal during late acute rejection. The key histological features of acute cellular rejection are:

- Portal tract inflammatory infiltrate (mixed)
- Abnormalities of interlobular bile duct epithelium
- Endotheliitis (portal tract and/or central vein).

These are shown in Figures 2–4. The essential abnormality for the diagnosis is a portal tract infiltrate which is predominantly mono-nuclear but contains neutrophils and eosinophils, although it may be a non-specific finding. Other features include changes in the inter-lobular bile ducts, particularly infiltration of the epithelium by lymphocytes, and adherence of mononuclear cells either to the endothelium of the portal vein radicals or sometimes to the central vein. Changes in the hepatic lobule are not particularly prominent but there may be a scattering of lobular lymphocytes. Prominent

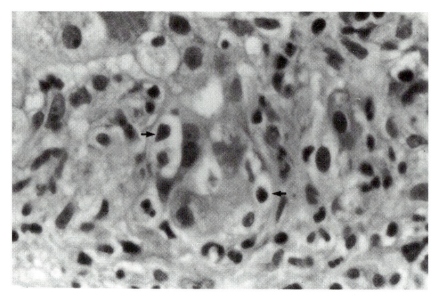

FIG 3—*Acute liver allograft rejection: infiltration of biliary epithelium by mononuclear cells (arrowed)*

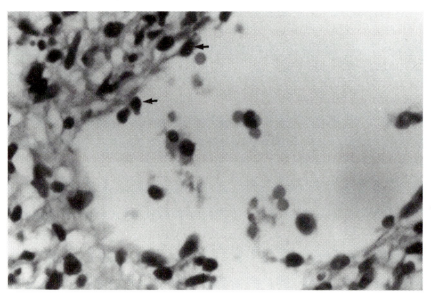

FIG 4—*Acute liver allograft rejection: endotheliitis with adherence of mononuclear cells to venous endothelium (arrowed)*

lobular features such as acidophil bodies should raise the possibility of other diagnoses. Occasionally there may be ballooning of zone 3 hepatocytes. These changes occurring in conjunction with the portal tract changes of acute rejection reflect a degree of ductopenic graft rejection.

Although the above changes are typical of acute cellular rejection, the histology may not be straightforward in a patient who has been recently treated for acute rejection. The biopsy may then show a reduced cellular infiltrate with persisting bile duct damage and little significant endotheliitis. This latter feature disappears quickly after a pulse of corticosteroid therapy. The interpretation of persisting graft dysfunction in the presence of such histological findings is difficult, and the patient is usually best served by referral to the original transplant centre for reassessment.

Therapy for acute rejection

Once rejection has been diagnosed and confirmed histologically, then pulse corticosteroid therapy is the cornerstone of therapy. This can be given either as intravenous methylprednisolone 250 mg to 1 g daily for three days, which can be administered as an outpatient procedure using a butterfly needle over a 30–45 minute period, or as oral prednisolone (200 mg daily for three days). Liver tests are monitored daily during this period. Using the regimen established at Sydney, once the pulse has been given the steroids are tapered according to a sliding scale – for example, 500 mg on day 4, 100 mg on day 5, dropping by 10 mg a day to a maintenance dose of 20 mg/day for a period of one month, although other centres revert to the previous dose of steroids. Following this the steroids are slowly brought back down to a maintenance dose of between 5 mg and 10 mg a day. With such a regimen, 70–80% of patients show rapid improvement in their liver enzyme abnormalities. Side effects of this treatment include water retention, psychosis, hypertension, and glucose intolerance. Pulse therapy increases the rise of opportunist infections, but these are usually not apparent in the short term.

If rejection is not controlled on such therapy, there are two possibilities: first, recycle with another pulse of steroids – this is probably effective in up to 50% of patients if it occurs late during the tapering phase of therapy; second, if there is little response to the

---

BOX B Guidelines for OKT3 rescue therapy

1 Double check to make sure unresolved rejection is the cause of the allograft dysfunction
2 Estimate CD3 and CD2 lymphocyte counts in peripheral blood (percentage and absolute numbers) before and after first dose
3 Careful explanation to patient by medical and nursing staff of the probable side effects
4 Liver enzymes may deteriorate initially, if there are significant systemic side effects
5 Prophylaxis against CMV and Pneumocystis carinii should be instigated (if not already started)
6 Be aware that maximal improvement in liver enzyme abnormalities may not be reached until four weeks after completion of therapy

---

BOX C Side effects of OKT3 therapy*,†

- Fevers, chills, rigors
- Muscle aches and pains
- Vomiting and diarrhoea
- Drowsiness
- Meningism
- Convulsions
- Bronchospasm

* Before the initial dose, methylprednisolone 8 mg/kg, paracetamol 1 g, and an antihistamine – for example, promethazine hydrochloride 25 mg – are given.
† Before each subsequent dose paracetamol 1 g, antihistamines, and methylprednisone 1 mg/kg are given.

---

initial pulse of steroids or early breakthrough, then the use of anti-lymphocyte antibody preparations is indicated. At the hospital in Sydney, the most commonly used agent is the monoclonal antibody OKT3, which is a murine monoclonal antibody raised against human T cells (Box B). The antibody binds to the cell surface CD3 molecular complex and depletes circulating T cells. Before starting OKT3 therapy, a T cell lymphocyte subset count should be done to monitor the effectiveness of T cell depletion from the circulation. A CD3 and CD2 lymphocyte count should be measured before and after the first dose of OKT3. OKT3 therapy has significant side effects (see Box C) and therapy requires a hospital admission. Nearly all patients suffer from fevers, chills, rigors, and general myalgias, but a small percentage (< 10%) have a marked cerebral irritation and aseptic meningitis. A careful explanation of the side effects is helpful to the patient and physician. These symptoms usually resolve after two injections. Amelioration of the symptoms is achieved by the pre-administration of a bolus of corticosteroid therapy, antihistamines, and paracetamol (acetaminophen) according to the manufacturers' instructions (see Box C). The antibody is given as an injection of 5–10 mg daily for 10 days. During this time liver tests are monitored. The initial response to OKT3 therapy may not be seen for 48–72 hours. The side effects described above are due to a cytokine release syndrome which, in itself, may cause a slight deterioration in liver abnormalities after the first injection.

An important aspect of OKT3 therapy is that the maximum benefit may occur after the cessation of treatment. The reason is unknown, but it is possible that OKT3 may shift the balance between rejection and tolerance of the graft in some patients. Significant responses to OKT3 therapy occur in up to 90% of patients.

OKT3 therapy may predispose to CMV and opportunist infections. It is generally advised that, following a course of OKT3 therapy, prophylaxis against CMV reactivation (acyclovir 800 mg four times a day for up to three months) and *Pneumocystis carinii* infection (co-trimoxazole or sulphamethoxazole/trimethoprin 1 tablet (single strength) three times a week for up to six months) be given. Recurrent use of OKT3 therapy is not generally advised as it may predispose to lymphoproliferative disorders.

What happens when anti-rejection fails? (see Figure 5)

Up to 10% of patients may not respond to treatment and develop chronic rejection of the graft. This syndrome is also termed "the vanishing bile duct syndrome", "chronic ductopenic rejection", or "chronic liver allograft rejection". Clinically, the syndrome is characterised by progressive cholestasis with high serum bilirubin levels, and high alkaline phosphatase and γ-glutamyl transferase levels with reasonable preservation of hepatic synthetic function

185

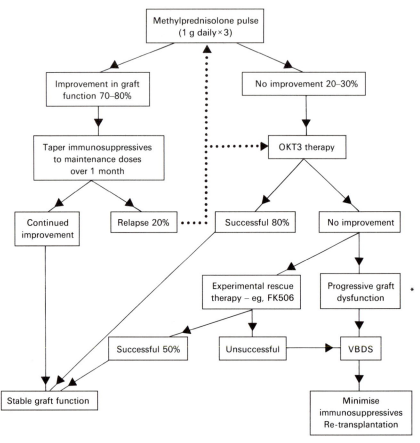

FIG 5—*Therapy and outcomes for acute cellular rejection. *Need for cholangiography should be assessed to look for biliary abnormalities secondary to severe rejection. VBDS = vanishing bile duct syndrome*

(albumin and prothrombin times). The liver is usually large and firm and there may rarely be signs of portal hypertension.

Pathologically the syndrome is associated with destruction of the interlobular bile ducts. There is progressive fibrosis and loss of the cellular infiltrate in the portal tracts. Thus, on biopsy the late features are those of an acellular portal tract with the absence of an interlobular bile duct and sometimes the absence of a portal tract arteriole (Figure 6). Zone 3 (centrilobular) lobular changes usually exist with ballooning and progressive fall out of hepatocytes associated with macrophage and mononuclear cell infiltration. This lobular lesion is probably partly due to ischaemia associated with arterial

186

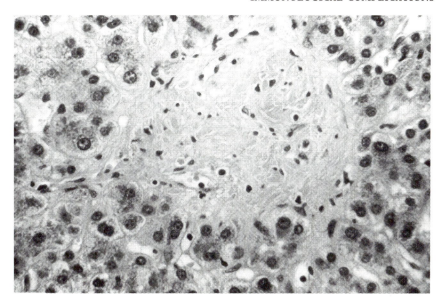

FIG 6—*Chronic liver allograft rejection (vanishing bile duct syndrome): an acellular portal tract without any evidence of an interlobular bile duct*

rejection in the remainder of the allograft. Changes in the larger segmental hepatic arteries are not seen on needle biopsy but are present when the liver is examined at re-transplantation or post-mortem examination. In these cases arterial "cushion" lesions are seen in the lumen. These result from macrophage and lipid accumulation in the wall of the arteries. There is destruction of the internal elastic lamina.

Once significant chronic rejection is established, there are few therapeutic modalities available. It is clear, however, that a small proportion of patients may spontaneously improve over a period of time. In these cases the initial biopsy is not presumably presentative and the lesions may be focal. In most cases, the syndrome is irreversibly progressive and re-transplantation is usually the only therapeutic option, although this need not be done immediately. Often patients prefer to have a break at home away from the transplant centre, while considering the re-transplantation option. Severe ductopenic rejection is usually associated with a progressive downhill course over a 6–18 month period. It is important during this time that excessive immunosuppressive therapy is avoided – for example, there may be little advantage in chasing low cyclosporin A

187

levels and escalating the cyclosporin A dosage as cyclosporin A is poorly absorbed in the presence of cholestasis. Preliminary results have claimed that FK506 may reverse ductopenic rejection, but this remains controversial. These patients may become deficient in fat soluble vitamins, particularly vitamins A, D, and E, and they need to be monitored for such abnormalities. There is an associated renal tubular acidosis, the aetiology of which is unclear, and which may require bicarbonate and potassium supplementation. Steroid therapy should be minimised in an effort to ameliorate progressive metabolic bone disease (osteoporosis).

Patients who fall into an intermediary category, in that they have not completely responded to a course of OKT3 therapy but have not progressed inevitably to severe chronic ductopenic rejection, may respond to immunosuppressive agents such as FK506. This agent is discussed in Chapter 11. If treatment is given before chronic ductopenic rejection has become established, FK506 has been reported to reverse OKT3 resistant rejection in up to 50% of patients. It should be noted that intrahepatic biliary abnormalities may develop secondary to severe rejection. In patients who do not completely respond to OKT3, cholangiography may be required to assess whether interventional endoscopic or radiological procedures can improve graft function.

Re-transplantation for rejection

Re-transplantation may be indicated in patients who have developed chronic ductopenic rejection unresponsive to medical therapy. The results of re-transplantation in such situations are less satisfactory than the initial transplant procedure with only a 50% one year survival (compared with 80% for the initial transplant operation).

Graft versus host disease

Graft versus host disease (GVHD) is a rare complication of liver transplantation. It usually presents between 10 and 100 days after transplantation, with a constellation of features including fever, diarrhoea, pancytopenia, and an exfoliative necrotising skin rash. Although one survivor has been reported, it is usually fatal.[1,2]

Long term outlook

In general, patients surviving for longer than 12 months with completely normal graft function have a very low incidence of acute cellular rejection episodes (less than 5% annually), providing that maintenance immunosuppressive therapy is maintained. The immunosuppressive regimen varies between transplant units – for example, if corticosteroids are not part of the maintenance regimen, then cyclosporin A and azathioprine may have to be used at higher doses than with triple therapy.

References

1 Roberts JP, Ascher NL, Lake J, *et al*. Graft versus host disease after liver transplantation in humans: a report of 4 cases. *Hepatology* 1991; **14:** 274–80.
2 Burdick JF, Vogelsang GB, Smith WJ, *et al*. Severe graft versus host disease in a liver transplant recipient. *N Engl J Med* 1988; **318:** 689–91.

11: Immunosuppressive drugs

MERVYN DAVIES

Introduction

The aim of immunosuppressive therapy[1-11] in liver transplantation is to prevent graft rejection, with the minimum of toxic side effects. Extremely potent immunosuppressive agents are available. Using current immunosuppressive regimens, up to 70% of liver allograft recipients will experience at least one episode of acute cellular rejection. In most cases, this is easily reversed. Chronic ductopenic rejection is usually resistant to immunosuppressive drugs and leads to graft loss.

There are few well designed, controlled, prospective, clinical trials comparing the efficacy of various immunosuppressive drugs. As a result, no single immunosuppressive protocol has been shown to be superior; clinical practice varies widely between centres.

Different centres have different immunosuppressive protocols, involving single, dual, triple, or quadruple therapy. The most commonly prescribed regimens involve corticosteroids and azathioprine combined with either cyclosporin A (cyclosporine) or FK506. Monoclonal antibodies may also be used during the early period post-transplantation either for induction or in response to acute cellular rejection, but are not used long term. Certain diseases may require modification of the standard protocol. Thus, it may be beneficial to minimise steroid therapy in those undergoing transplantation for hepatitis B viral infection; patients with autoimmune chronic active hepatitis may require maintenance therapy with corticosteroids.

It is the policy in some centres to discontinue corticosteroids at three months. Following initial dosage with 20 mg/day, the dose is tapered over the course of three months, except for specific indications such as control of ulcerative colitis. Most other centres continue with the use of low dose steroids indefinitely.

Duration of immunosuppression

For many years, it had been assumed that it was necessary to continue immunosuppression for life. However, there have been anecdotal cases of liver allograft recipients who have discontinued long term immunosuppression with no adverse effect on the graft.[11a] This contrasts with other patients in whom cessation of immunosuppression is followed by rejection and graft loss. It is not clear which factors are responsible for inducing tolerance. Starzl et al.[11a] has proposed that the exchange of migratory leucocytes between the graft and the recipient, with consequent cellular chimerism in both, is the basis for tolerance. There is preliminary evidence to support this hypothesis. However, until those factors that define tolerance and indicate long term graft acceptance have been identified, long term immunosuppression should be withdrawn only under well defined and carefully controlled conditions.

Cyclosporin A

Cyclosporin A is a naturally occurring lipophilic endecapeptide extracted from the fungus *Tolypocladium inflatum Gams*. Following the introduction of cyclosporin A to the field of transplantation in 1978, survival has increased although it is uncertain to what extent this is due to the drug.

Mode of action

Cyclosporin A binds to a ubiquitous cystolic protein, cyclophilin, which acts as a *cis–trans*-peptidylprolyl isomerase (PPIase). The binding of cyclosporin A is associated with loss of the enzyme's activity and it was initially thought that the mode of action was dependent on this effect. It is now clear that the interaction of the cyclosporin–cyclophilin complex with calcineurin is required for an immunosuppressive effect.[9]

191

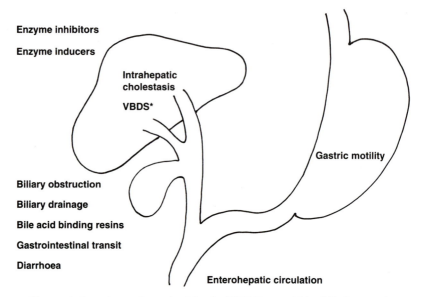

FIG 1—*Factors influencing cyclosporin A levels. VBDS = vanishing bile duct syndrome*

Cyclosporin A exerts its major therapeutic effects by inhibition of T cell activation. At the molecular level, this is achieved by selectively blocking transcriptional activation of genes early in the T cell response. These genes encode cytokines, interleukins 2 and 4 (IL-2 and IL-4), which are the principal T cell growth factors, IL-3, γ-interferon, and the α chain of the IL-2 receptor, required for T cell proliferation.

Pharmacokinetics

Cyclosporin A is highly lipid soluble and partitions extensively into fat; it is approximately 90% protein bound. It crosses the placenta and is distributed into breast milk.

Absorption

There are large inter-individual variations in the bioavailability of cyclosporin A due to slow, incomplete, bile dependent absorption. Cyclosporin A is absorbed with micelles which require bile salts for their formation. Consequently, water soluble vitamin E which forms micelles has been used to increase cyclosporin A absorption.[13]

TABLE I—*Available formulations of oral cyclosporin A*

Form	Concentration	Colour	Comment
Capsules	25 mg	Pale pink	Capsules are bulky
	50 mg	Rusty brown	and patients may find
	100 mg	Dusky pink	difficult to swallow
Liquid	100 mg/ml		

Paradoxically, oral ursodeoxycholic acid, a non-micellar bile salt, may increase cyclosporin A absorption. This is probably due to choloretic effects increasing the amount of bile salts in the gut lumen.[14]

Particular problems may be encountered in liver graft recipients, because disruption of bile flow is common. This may result from external biliary drainage, treatment with bile acid binding resins, such as cholestyramine, or intra- or extrahepatic cholestasis. Achievement of therapeutic blood levels is often a problem in chronic ductopenic rejection. Cyclosporin A absorption is also reduced in patients with diarrhoea, in those with short gut syndrome, and also by drugs that increase gastrointestinal transit. Absorption is reduced in the presence of impaired pancreatic exocrine function and slow gastric emptying. In contrast, metoclopramide enhances absorption because it increases emptying. A new formulation of cyclosporin A, in a microemulsion, is being evaluated and may result in greater absorption.

Cyclosporin A capsules are large and some patients find them difficult to swallow. The bioavailability of the liquid formulation, however, is not greatly different from the oral gelatin capsules. Effective immunosuppression can be achieved by taking a dose once daily, although division of treatment to a twice daily regimen permits dosage reduction of around 40% to achieve a particular trough level. This may benefit patients who are experiencing troublesome side effects.

Storage

It is recommended that cyclosporin A should be stored at less than 30°C. In extremes of temperature, they should be kept in a cool bag, but not refrigerated.

BOX A   Drugs that increase level of cyclosporin A

Aminoglycosides	Ketoconazole
Corticosteroids (high dose)	Lignocaine (lidocaine)
Danazol	Metoclopramide
Diltiazem	Midazolam
Doxycycline	Nicardipine
Erythromycin	Quinidine
Itraconazole	Verapamil

Metabolism

Cyclosporin A is extensively metabolised in the gut and liver by several varieties of cytochrome P450, the dominant of which is P450 IIIA4. More than 30 metabolites are formed, all with their cyclic structure intact. These metabolites are excreted predominantly in the bile. Less than 1% of the dose is excreted unchanged. Most metabolites do not affect the immune system. The metabolite with the greatest imunosuppressive activity is the M1 form, which has around 10% of the activity of the parent compound. M1 is the major metabolite and can achieve significant immunosuppression. A number of the metabolites are nephrotoxic. Because cyclosporin A and its metabolites are excreted in bile, enterohepatic circulation may occur, which accounts for the double peaked concentration/time curve obtained after oral administration.

Urinary elimination of cyclosporin A is of minor importance, contributing less than 5% of the dose; so elimination is not greatly altered in renal failure, although a dosage reduction will often be made under these circumstances, because of the nephrotoxicity of cyclosporin A.

Concomitant medication

Several drugs increase the trough concentrations of cyclosporin A. Some of these are metabolised by the same cytochrome P450 (IIIA4), and therefore competitively inhibit the metabolism of cyclosporin A. These drugs include erythromycin, midazolam, quinidine, lignocaine (lidocaine), nifedipine, and triazolam (see Box A).

BOX B   Calcium antagonists and cyclosporin A levels

Nifedipine   No effect on cyclosporin A levels
Diltiazem \
Verapamil /   Increase cyclosporin A levels

BOX C   Drugs that reduce level of cyclosporin A

Carbamazepine
Isoniazid
Octreotide
Phenobarbitone
Phenytoin
Rifampicin

Of the calcium antagonists, nifedipine appears to be the drug that interferes least with cyclosporin A metabolism (see Box B).

Other drugs which are enzyme inducers may increase the metabolism of cyclosporin A. These include rifampicin, phenytoin, and phenobarbitone (see Box C).

Monitoring

Cyclosporin A exhibits large inter- and intra-individual variation in bioavailability and clearance; the therapeutic window is narrow. It is therefore important that a reliable method of monitoring blood levels is available. Whole blood is the specimen of choice, because whole blood levels are least affected by temperature dependent partitioning. A sample anticoagulated with ethylenediaminetetraacetate (EDTA) should be provided (Box D), and, for the purpose of standardisation, a trough level is taken. Patients on a twice daily regimen have in effect a 12 hour trough level, in contrast to a 24 hour trough level for those on daily therapy.

Several techniques are available for cyclosporin A analysis.

195

> **BOX D   Sample for cyclosporin A assay**
>
> Cyclosporin A dose omitted that morning (trough level)
> Assay of whole blood level
> EDTA sample (same tube as for full blood count)
> Sample can be sent by mail

Radio-immunoassay (RIA), automated RIA (TDX) with polyclonal or monoclonal antibodies, and high performance liquid chromatography (HPLC) are used. Monoclonal antibodies are used to measure parent compounds alone, whereas a polyclonal analysis provides additional information concerning the metabolites, which may be immunosuppressive or toxic. The ratio between metabolites and parent compound varies between approximately 2 and 10 and correlates with renal function and serum bilirubin.

The therapeutic range of cyclosporin A varies between centres; most centres aim for trough whole blood levels of parent compound between 100 µg/l and 200 µg/l. Lower levels should be maintained in the presence of side effects, such as sepsis, opportunist malignancy, neurotoxicity, hypertension, or renal impairment (see later). Where the drug is measured in plasma, therapeutic levels are about 50 µg/ml. For methods measuring parent drug and metabolites, levels are about 2·5 times greater, but in the presence of cholestasis much higher levels of metabolites may make such values difficult to interpret. Whichever method of therapeutic monitoring is used, it is important to consider the whole patient; thus, in the presence of normal liver function but with renal impairment, it may be best to run the whole blood trough levels at below 100 µg/ml.

Side effects (Table II)

Cyclosporin A has a wide range of side effects which can limit the dose used. *Nephrotoxicity* is the most common side effect. Minor abnormalities occur in 80–90% of patients, whereas 40% develop more significant renal dysfunction. During the early stages of cyclosporin A therapy, renal impairment is thought to result from altered renal haemodynamics, with no associated renal morphological change. Subsequently, a combination of tubular atrophy and

TABLE II—*Cyclosporin A side effects and proposed action*

Nephrotoxicity	
Mild/moderate	Avoid concomitant nephrotoxic therapy *
	Check cyclosporin A level
	Divide into twice daily dosage
Severe	Exclude coexistent renal disease
	Consider cyclosporin A withdrawal if severe
Hypertension	Check cyclosporin A level
	First line:
	Calcium channel antagonist
	Thiazide diuretic
	β-Blocker
	Second line:
	ACE inhibitor (check K^+)
Migraine	Check cyclosporin A level
	Divide dose to twice daily
	Introduce pizotifen (patient may gain weight)
	β-Blockers
Severe	Trial of ergotamine
	Sumatriptan
	Consider cyclosporin A withdrawal if extreme
Hyperkalaemia	Check cyclosporin A levels
	Stop potassium sparing diuretics if appropriate
	Stop ACE inhibitors if appropriate
	Sodium bicarbonate 1 g four times daily
Hypertrichosis	Cosmetic assistance, depilation etc.
Fluid retention	Exclude vascular aetiology
	Consider concomitant medication
	Diuretics if persistent and problematic
Arthropathy	
Mild	Check levels and divide dose to twice daily regimen
Moderate/severe	Low dose non-steroidal anti-inflammatory drug only if necessary and if creatinine normal
	Check creatinine level frequently
	Consider corticosteroids as anti-inflammatory if no osteopenia
	Consider cyclosporin A withdrawal if extreme

* See Box E.

interstitial fibrosis may develop, which occasionally leads to renal failure. Biochemical changes that occur include increase in serum uric acid, serum potassium, modest hypomagnesaemia, and decreased serum bicarbonate levels. Concomitant use of other

---

BOX E   Drugs that exacerbate cyclosporin nephrotoxicity

Aminoglycosides
Amphotericin B
Cimetidine
Erythromycin and other macrolides
FK506
Ketoconazole
Melphalan
Non-steriodal anti-inflammatory agents
Ranitidine
Trimethoprim

---

nephrotoxic drugs should be avoided, where possible (drugs that exacerbate cyclosporin A are shown in Box E).

Neurotoxicity is most pronounced during the early period post-transplantation. Tremor is common, but tends to resolve with time. Convulsions are usually associated with high levels of cyclosporin A. Prophylactic phenytoin can be used in the postoperative period in those with a history of epilepsy and in those who develop EEG abnormalities. The dosage of cyclosporin A should be increased following the introduction of this agent, if a therapeutic blood level is to be maintained. Headache can be severe and occasionally warrants withdrawal of treatment, although it often resolves if a reduced dose is prescribed twice daily. The same is true for a peripheral neuropathy which may present with painful dysaesthesiae. Pizotifen, which has antihistamine and anti-serotonin activity, may occasionally be beneficial for the migraine headaches. The drug is started at a dose of 500 µg, prescribed at night, because of sedative side effects. This can be gradually increased to 1500 µg. β-Blockers usually provide ineffective prophylaxis. The newer drug sumatriptan may help, especially for those with a past history of migraine; however, high blood pressure and renal dysfunction are relative contraindications to its use.

Hypertension is present in 60–70% at one year. The incidence increases with duration of follow up. Treatment is with standard hypotensives. Angiotensin converting enzyme (ACE) inhibitors should be used cautiously, because of their tendency to increase serum potassium. The calcium channel blocker nicardipine may be the drug of choice, because it appears to have a beneficial effect on renal haemodynamics, although cyclosporin A levels should be checked following its initiation (see Box B). Others use nifedipine because it has little effect on cyclosporin A levels, but it may be associated with an increased risk of gingival hyperplasia.

Breast fibroadenosis may develop in those on cyclosporin A. It is important to be aware of the possibility of breast carcinoma, especially in those with primary biliary cirrhosis, although in general there has been no increase in this malignancy in the post-transplantation population as a whole.

Pregnancy

There is neither animal nor human evidence to suggest a teratogenic role of cyclosporin A. Ideally a patient should attend for preconception counselling. Close monitoring of cyclosporin A levels is required during pregnancy (see also Chapter 16).

Azathioprine

Azathioprine is an imidazole derivative of 6-mercaptopurine and functions as a structural analogue or "anti-metabolite". It was first used as monotherapy in transplantation in 1961. Subsequently, its synergistic action with corticosteroids and other agents was realised.

Mode of action

Azathioprine is metabolised in the liver to 6-mercaptopurine, which inhibits nucleic acid synthesis, thus interfering with cell division and inhibiting the proliferation and differentiation of T cells in response to antigenic stimulation. Following an oral dose, immunosuppressive activity in the serum peaks at 1–2 hours and declines to baseline over 24 hours, allowing for a once daily dose.

The major toxic side effect of azathioprine therapy is bone marrow suppression, which affects leucopoiesis more than haemopoeisis. Thrombocytopenia may also occur. Bone marrow suppression is dose dependent and reversible, but varies between individuals. In susceptible individuals, azathioprine treatment may

---

BOX F   Recommended monitoring of full blood count while receiving azathioprine

First 8 weeks	monitor weekly
8–26 weeks	monitor 3–4 weekly
Lifelong	monitor 3 monthly

---

result in a normochromic/normocytic anaemia or a megaloblastic anaemia, with macrocytosis. Most units start therapy between 1 and 2 mg/kg per day. It is recommended that full blood count is monitored in patients receiving azathioprine (Box F).

Formulation

Azathioprine is produced by a number of different manufacturers. It is available as 25 mg and 50 mg tablets and in liquid form.

Elimination

Xanthine oxidase is required for azathioprine metabolism, forming 6-thiouric acid prior to excretion in the urine. Concomitant therapy with allopurinol (a xanthine oxidase antagonist) predisposes to azathioprine toxicity, so it should be avoided if possible, or prescribed with a 75% reduction of dose and careful monitoring of the white blood cell count.

Side effects

Other adverse effects associated with azathioprine (Table III) include anorexia, pancreatitis, skin rash, mild alopecia, retinopathy, and gastrointestinal upset, which can be minimised by taking the preparation with food. There have been a number of reports of hepatotoxicity,[8] including elevation of transaminases, cholestasis, veno-occlusive disease, and nodular regenerative hyperplasia; however, these are rare.

Pregnancy

The risks of azathioprine therapy in pregnancy should be considered carefully. It is potentially teratogenic and genotoxic. Animal

TABLE III—*Adverse effects associated with azathioprine therapy*

	Side effect	Action
Bone marrow suppression	Leucopenia Thrombocytopenia Anaemia	Reduce dose Check concomitant drugs Measure haematinics if persists
Gastrointestinal	Nausea, anorexia Dyspepsia Pancreatitis	Take with food Take with food Withdraw drug
Hepatotoxicity	Cholestasis, "Hepatitis"	Withdraw, then rechallenge Withdraw, rechallenge
	Veno-occlusive disease Nodular regenerative hyperplasia	Withdraw Withdraw

experiments have suggested a teratogenic effect, although studies in humans have shown no evidence of an increased risk of congenital malformation. The practice at Birmingham is to continue with azathioprine therapy during pregnancy. Azathioprine is not secreted in breast milk.

Corticosteroids

Corticosteroids continue to play a major role in almost all immunosuppression protocols.

Mode of action

Corticosteroids act at several levels of the immune system, particularly affecting T lymphocytes. They also have a major impact on cytokines and other soluble mediators of the immune system and have anti-inflammatory properties.

Formulation

A number of synthetic corticosteroids are available, which have varying potency. Table IV lists doses required to achieve equivalent anti-inflammatory effects.

TABLE IV—*Equivalent anti-inflammatory doses of various corticosteroids*

Drug	Dose (mg)
Prednisone	5
Prednisolone	5
Methylprednisolone	4
Dexamethasone	0·75
Hydrocortisone	20

TABLE V—*Side effects of corticosteroid therapy*

Gastrointestinal	Dyspepsia	Common
	? Peptic ulcer	
	? Pancreatitis	Rare
Musculoskeletal	Osteoporosis	Duration/dose dependent
	Proximal myopathy	
	Avascular necrosis	Rare
Mineralocorticoid	Mild, fluid retention	
	Potassium loss	
Glucocorticoid	Diabetogenic	
Hypothalmo-pituary axis	Adrenal atrophy	Avoid sudden withdrawal
Skin	Slow healing, bruising, atrophy	
Neuropsychiatric	Depression	
Ocular	Cataract	
	Raised intraocular pressure	

Elimination

Metabolism of corticosteroids occurs through the cytochrome P450 enzyme system. Enzyme inducing agents such as phenytoin and phenobarbitone are likely to reduce the level of corticosteroids, but this is not usually a problem in clinical practice.

Side effects

Side effects of steroid therapy are related to dose and duration of therapy. They are wide ranging (Table V).

Gastrointestinal side effects include dyspepsia, oesophageal candidiasis, and pancreatitis. The link with peptic and oesophageal ulceration is uncertain; however, patients are at risk of such a complication early after transplantation. This period is covered, at Birmingham, with histamine H_2-receptor antagonists, such as ranitidine. A symmetrical proximal myopathy may develop. Other musculoskeletal side effects include osteoporosis, avascular necrosis, and tendon rupture. Mineralocorticoid effects of synthetic corticosteroids are much less marked than their physiological counterparts, but, nevertheless, water retention, hypertension, and potassium loss may occur. Suppression of the hypothalamic–pituitary axis leads to adrenal atrophy after prolonged steroid therapy. A rapid discontinuation of treatment may provoke acute adrenocortical insufficiency. Dermatological side effects include impaired wound healing, easy bruising, skin atrophy, striae, and acne. Neuropsychiatric manifestations tend to be more troublesome during the early period post-transplantation, when the dose of steroids is greatest. These include euphoria, psychological dependence, depression, and insomnia. Ophthalmic side effects may manifest with increased intraocular pressure, glaucoma, papilloedema, or cataract formation.

Pregnancy

The absolute safety of corticosteroids in pregnancy is unproven. There is a suspicion of very slightly increased risk of cleft palate and intrauterine growth retardation. There is no evidence of harmful effects on pregnancy in animals.

Newer agents

Many new agents are entering clinical practice on a trial basis and are discussed briefly below.

FK506

FK506 is a naturally occurring macrolide antibiotic product of the soil fungus *Streptomyces tsukubaensis*.

Mode of action

Studies in vitro and in vivo have shown that the immunosuppressive properties of FK506 and cyclosporin A are similar. It inhibits the proliferative responses of lymphocytes to alloantigen stimulation, expression of the IL-2 receptor and the production of IL-2, IL-3, and γ-interferon. On a molar basis, FK506 is between 50 and 100 times more potent than cyclosporin A. Whether it has advantages in efficacy is still unclear.

The structure of FK506 is different from that of cyclosporin A. It does not bind to cyclophilin, but to a separate protein, FK binding protein (FKBP). Great interest followed the discovery that FKBP also has *cis–trans*-peptidylprolyl isomerase activity, which is inhibited by the binding of FK506. As with cyclosporin A, however, it is not the inhibition of the *cis–trans*-peptidylprolylisomerase activity that is required for its immunosuppressive action, but the effect of the immunophilin–FK506 complex on calcineurin.[9]

Pharmacokinetics

FK506 is well absorbed following oral administration. In contrast to cyclosporin A, absorption is not influenced greatly by bile. This can be of advantage in those requiring prolonged biliary drainage or with prolonged cholestasis following transplantation. Intravenous preparations are available, but their toxicity is greater.

It is uncertain at present how drug levels should be interpreted. The optimum therapeutic range is still unknown, but early results suggest that the therapeutic levels lie between 10 and 20 mg/ml (trough) (TDX). It is unknown whether metabolites accumulate, if they are immunosuppressive, or if they are toxic. The methods of measurement include RIA, TDX, and HPLC.

Metabolism Elimination occurs predominantly by hepatic metabolism with cytochrome P450. Less than 1% of the dose is excreted unchanged in the urine or bile. A number of drugs, however, are thought to interact with FK506 and lead to increased levels (Table VI).

Formulation FK506 is as yet an unlicensed product. It is presently available for intravenous infusion and is also in 1 mg and 5 mg capsules.

TABLE VI—*Drugs thought to interact with FK506*

Potential inhibitors of FK506 metabolism (likely to increase levels)

Cimetidine	Doxycycline	Ketoconazole
Cyclosporin A	Erythromycin	Nicardipine
Danazol	Fluconazole	Troleandomycin
Itraconazole	Verapamil	

Potential inducers of FK506 metabolism (likely to reduce levels)

Carbamazepine	Isoniazid	Phenytoin
Corticosteroids	Phenobarbitone (phenobarbital)	Rifampicin

BOX G   Drugs with potential additive or synergistic nephrotoxicity

Aminoglycosides	Cisplatin	Vancomycin
Amphotericin B	Cyclosporin A	
Non-steroidal anti-inflammatory drugs		

Storage   The manufacturers recommend that FK506 is stored at room temperature. In hot climates it should be refrigerated at 2–8°C.

Side effects

Toxic side effects appear to be at least as common in patients treated with FK506 as with cyclosporin A, despite early experience and anecdotal reports suggesting a toxicity profile that is superior to cyclosporin A. The results of controlled trials in liver transplantation are still awaited. The drug appears to be nephrotoxic, diabetogenic, and neurotoxic, and may induce hyperkalaemia and hypertension. Diabetes appears to occur more commonly than with cyclosporin A and may be quite difficult to stabilise. Boxes G and H list drugs that have the potential to interact with FK506 to exacerbate some of its toxic side effects.

BOX H   Potential additive/synergistic neurotoxicity

Acyclovir	Ganciclovir	Norfloxacin
Ciprofloxacin	Imipenem	

BOX I   Drugs that exacerbate hyperkalaemia

Angiotensin converting enzyme inhibitors
Potassium sparing diuretics

Spironolactone	Amiloride
Most combination diuretics	Triamterene

Pregnancy

Currently, the use of FK506 in the UK and North America is restricted to non-pregnant females who are not planning pregnancy.

Rapamycin

Rapamycin is another macrolide antibiotic. It is produced by *Streptomyces hydroscopicus* and is a potent immunosuppressive agent, both in vitro and in vivo. There are a number of structural similarities with FK506, and yet they possess different immunosuppressive properties. Rapamycin does not inhibit the production of IL-2, but does inhibit cellular proliferation stimulated by IL-2 and IL-4. It binds to FK binding protein and is a potent inhibitor of *cis–trans*-peptidylprolyl isomerase activity. Both FK506 and rapamycin bind to a common receptor, so rapamycin will antagonise the action of FK506, but enhances that of cyclosporin A. Rapamycin is effective in prolonging graft survival in animal studies.

RS-61443

Mycophenolic acid (MPA) is an anti-purine drug, which non-competitively and reversibly inhibits inosine monophosphate dehydrogenase, an enzyme that controls the rate of purine synthesis.[12] It therefore selectively depletes the production of guanosine nucleotides and thus inhibits DNA synthesis. Rapamycin is a morpholinoethyl ester of mycophenolic acid that has a higher bioavailability and is rapidly hydrolysed to MPA. It is unclear whether RS-61443 is more immunosuppressive than MPA, although RS-61443 was more effective in delaying the onset of rejection in the same animal model.[13] RS-61443 is also able to reverse established acute rejection. Although RS-61443 may be effective as monotherapy, combined therapy with low dose cyclosporin A and methylprednisolone was associated with marked prolongation of graft survival in animal studies.

15-Deoxyspergualin

15-Deoxyspergualin (15-DSG) is a synthetic derivative of spergualin, a metabolite of *Bacillus laterosporus*. In vitro and in vivo studies have shown both to be immunosuppressive, although 15-deoxyspergualin is more potent on a weight for weight basis. 15-Deoxyspergualin is effective in animal models of transplantation and more recently has been shown to suppress development of graft versus host disease (GVHD) in a mouse bone marrow transplant model. Its mechanism of action remains unclear, although it appears to suppress the primary humoral response to a variety of exogenous antigens. Because of its effects on B lymphocytes and antibody production, its use has been explored as supportive immunosuppression for renal allografts in which ABO incompatible grafts are performed and in those with transplantation performed in highly sensitised recipients.

Cyclosporin G

This cyclosporin A analogue has similar immunosuppressive properties, but may have a better safety profile. It is currently in phase 3 studies in renal allograft recipients.

Monoclonal antibodies

The mechanisms underlying allograft rejection are becoming increasingly understood. This permits more specific immunomodulatory therapy aimed at particular points in the rejection pathway.

The development of a technique to produce monoclonal antibodies has been used to this end. A number of monoclonal antibodies are already in clinical use and many more are undergoing clinical evaluation.

Those in widespread clinical use include OKT3, targeted to the CD3 receptor on the surface of T cells and anti-thymocyte globulin (ATG), which causes the destruction of T lymphocytes. Others in the development stage include: monoclonal antibodies targeted to the intercellular adhesion molecule ICAM-1; anti-CD4, present on the helper/inducer subset of lymphocytes; anti-cytokines; anti-IL-2 receptor antibodies; and many others. At present, with the exception of OKT3, all are available only on a trial basis.

Conclusions

Immunosuppressive drugs currently used in liver transplantation are highly effective. Unfortunately, toxic side effects are common and therapeutic margins are narrow. There is still a steady rate of allograft attrition due to chronic rejection. Further research is therefore needed to find improved products or combinations of treatment. It is vital that all new agents are formally assessed as part of well designed, controlled, clinical trials to establish whether the product offers definite benefits.

References

1 Marsh JW, Vehe KL, White HM. Immunosuppressants. *Gastroenterol Clin North Am* 1992; **21**: 679–93.
2 Lindholm A. Factors influencing the pharmacokinetics of Cyclosporine in man. *Ther Drug Monit* 1991; **13**: 465–77.
3 Plebani M, Burlina A. Cyclosporin monitoring: Mechanism of action, methods and pharmacokinetics. *Clin Chem Enzym Commun* 1991; **3**: 347–62.
4 Walsh CT, Zydowsky LD, McKeon FD. Cyclosporin A, the cyclophilin class of peptidylprolyl isomerases, and blockade of T cell signal transduction. *J Biol Chem* 1992; **267**: 1315–18.
5 Kahan BD. Cyclosporine. *N Engl J Med* 1989; **321**: 1725–38.
6 Mason J. The pathophysiology of Sandimmune (cyclosporine) in man and animals. Part I. *Pediatr Nephrol* 1990; **4**: 554–74.
7 Mason J. The pathophysiology of Sandimmune (cyclosporine) in man and animals. Part II. *Pediatr Nephrol* 1990; **4**: 686–704.
8 Sterneck M, Wiesner R, Ascher M, *et al*. Azathioprine hepatotoxicity after liver transplantation. *Hepatology* 1991; **14**: 806–10.
9 Schreiber SL, Crabtree GR. The mechanism of action of cyclosporin A and FK506. *Immunol Today* 1992; **13**: 136–42.

10 Morris PJ. Cyclosporine, FK506 and other drugs in organ transplantation. *Curr Opin Immunol* 1991; **3**: 748–51.

11 Thomson AW. The spectrum of action of the new immunosuppressive drugs. *Clin Exp Immunol* 1992; **89**: 170–3.

11a Starzl TE, Demetris AJ. Tiucco M *et al*. Cell migration and chimerism after whole-organ transplantation. *Hepatology* 1993; **17**: 1127–52.

12 Mores RE, Wang J. Comparison of the immunosuppressive effects of mycophenolic acid and morpholinoethyl ester of mycophenolic acid (RS-1443) in recipients of heart allografts. *Transplant Proc* 1991; **23**: 493–6.

13 Sokol R, Johnson K, Karrer FM, *et al*. Improvement of cyclosporin absorption in children after liver transplantation by means of water soluble vitamin E. *Lancet* 1991; **338**: 212–15.

14 Kallinowski B, Theilmann L, Zimmermann R, *et al*. Effective treatment of cyclosporin induced cholestasis in heart-transplant patients treated with ursodeoxycholic acid. *Transplantation* 1991; **52**: 1128.

12: Surgical considerations after liver transplantation

ROBERT M MERION, DAVID MAYER

Vascular complications

Vascular complications of liver transplantation occur uncommonly but are associated with a high level of morbidity, graft failure, and patient mortality. This chapter will focus primarily upon the major vascular complications with consequences for the graft itself and will touch briefly on vascular morbidity unrelated to the transplanted organ. The most widely reported and devastating vascular complications related to the graft are those of the hepatic artery and its reconstruction, but problems related to the portal vein and vena cava have also been reported. Vascular complications of venovenous bypass, invasive haemodynamic monitoring, and miscellaneous unrelated vascular problems will also be discussed.

Hepatic artery

The most commonly reported hepatic artery complication is acute thrombosis. The reported incidence ranges from 10% to 40% of cases, and is usually higher in paediatric recipients. Risk factors reported to be associated with hepatic artery thrombosis include small size of the hepatic artery (< 3 mm), patient weight of less than 7 kg, and use of an anastomotic site without a branch patch or Carrel patch. Donor arterial anomalies, once thought to be an important aetiological factor in the pathogenesis of hepatic arterial thrombosis after transplantation, have more recently been shown to be unassociated with this complication in larger series.[1-3]

Hepatic artery thrombosis may be associated with several dif-

---

BOX A   Presentation of hepatic artery thrombosis

Acute graft failure
Unexplained septicaemia
Biliary tract problems:
  Leaks
  Abscess
  Breakdown of anastomoses
Liver abscess

---

ferent clinical presentations (Box A). The most common presentation is the development of suddenly abnormal liver function tests, dramatic elevations in serum transaminases, cessation of bile production, and marked elevation in prothrombin time. The usual time of presentation of acute hepatic artery thrombosis is from one day to three weeks following transplantation. Thrombosis may be a secondary manifestation of a low flow state associated with intrahepatic oedema seen with severe allograft rejection, and the direct consequences of the immunological attack with associated vasculitis tend to present later.[4]

Initial diagnosis of hepatic artery thrombosis is by duplex sonography (Doppler ultrasonography of the graft vasculature combined with real time scanning). Duplex sonography has been reported to have a sensitivity of 92% for detection of hepatic artery thrombosis.[5] The specificity was not reported in this study, but in another study McDiarmid et al.[6] found a 40% false negative rate among paediatric liver transplant recipients and suggested that patients at high risk for arterial thrombosis should undergo definitive arteriographic examination, even if the duplex sonography suggests an intrahepatic arterial signal. Lomas et al.[7] reported on duplex sonographic findings among 63 patients followed with serial sonographic examinations. The sensitivity was 69% and the specificity 100% in a population with an incidence of hepatic artery thrombosis of 21%.

Complications of hepatic artery thrombosis include haemorrhage associated with uncorrectable coagulopathy, acute hepatic encephalopathy and/or seizures, and the development of progressive multiorgan failure. This fulminant picture requires rapid diagnosis and in most cases urgent re-transplantation is also required. Some authors have advocated thromboembolectomy in selected cases.[8,9] This

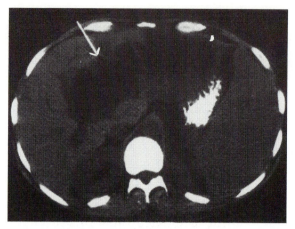

FIG 1—*Computed tomography (CT) scan of a patient following orthotopic liver transplantation. Despite relatively normal liver function tests, this patient harboured a large intrahepatic abscess (arrow) which developed following hepatic artery thrombosis. Percutaneous drainage of the abscess was carried out in preparation for re-transplantation*

approach has not been widely accepted, in part as a result of the high rate of subsequent biliary complications.

Evidence of biliary tract complications should always raise the suspicion of hepatic artery thrombosis. The clinical presentation of biliary leak or obstructive biliary complications associated with intrahepatic strictures and biliary ectasia or bile lakes suggests ischaemia of the biliary tract. Impaired arterial inflow to the grafted liver preferentially affects the biliary tree because of the graft's almost total reliance upon hepatic arterial blood supply.[10] In one study of 31 liver transplant recipients, cholangiograms were found to be abnormal in 84% of patients with complete or partial occlusion of the hepatic artery (thrombosis in 29 and severe stenosis in 2).[11] Leaks from the biliary tree, other than at the surgical anastomosis, were seen in 16 (62%), and 12 of 14 strictures were non-anastomotic. Infection may supervene in areas of necrotic biliary and parenchymal collapse resulting in intrahepatic abscess formation (Figure 1). Patients with this presentation may appear surprisingly well and show little in the way of elevation of standard liver function tests.

Hepatic artery thrombosis may be occult. A clinical picture of relapsing subacute bacterial sepsis may be the only clue and the diagnostic work up must include hepatic arteriography if other investigations for sepsis are not helpful.

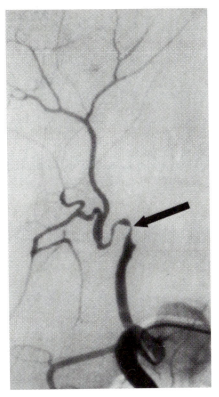

FIG 2—*Arteriographic finding of hepatic artery stenosis over a long segment of redundant donor hepatic artery. This patient underwent resection of the stenotic segment and primary re-anastomosis. Pathological examination of the resected artery revealed intimal atherosclerosis*

Stenosis of the hepatic artery has been recognised more recently as a complication of liver transplantation. The experiences at Ann Arbor with this complication again suggest that a high index of suspicion is necessary when patients present with unexplained abnormalities in liver function tests. Figure 2 shows the arteriographic findings in a patient whose liver tests had gradually deteriorated following an initially uncomplicated course. Doppler examination of the graft vasculature may demonstrate increased velocity in the region of the stenosis and flattened systolic peaks in the post-stenotic area. Such findings should prompt an arteriogram. The patient underwent resection of the stenotic segment of hepatic artery and, after operation, has done extremely well. As an

213

alternative Abad *et al.*[12] have reported successful percutaneous transluminal angioplasty of stenotic hepatic arterial anastomoses in two patients.

Mycotic pseudoaneurysm is a rare but frequently devastating complication of liver transplantation.[13-15] At Ann Arbor only one case has been encountered among over 400 liver transplantations.[16] Fewer than 50 cases have been reported in the literature and the overall incidence is less than 0·5%. Most authors advocate hepatic artery ligation although some have reported encouraging results after resection and reconstruction.[17]

Portal vein

Despite the traditional dogma that large, low resistance veins are prone to thrombotic complications, portal venous thrombosis remains a relatively uncommon occurrence after liver transplantation. This complication is reported in only 2–3% of recipients,[18-19] although the true incidence is almost certainly higher because some patients may have initially silent thrombosis of the transplant organ's portal vein.[20] Subsequent development of variceal haemorrhage or other signs of recurrent portal hypertension may suggest the diagnosis. Endoscopic sclerotherapy should be the initial method of management, but ultimately the patient may require retransplantation, splenorenal shunt, or percutaneous dilatation.[21]

Non-occlusive stenosis can occur at the portal vein anastomotic site. This has been reported most often in paediatric recipients.[22,23] Successful outcomes have been reported with operative revision and percutaneous transhepatic angioplasty.

Hepatic veins and vena cava

Stenosis of the vena cava may occur as a result of technically inadequate construction of either the infrahepatic or suprahepatic vena caval anastomoses. Lerut *et al.*[24] reported three cases of infrahepatic inferior vena caval thrombosis in a series of 336 recipients (<1%). This condition is usually manifested by marked bilateral lower extremity and genital swelling. The diagnosis can be made by physical examination, duplex sonography, and phlebography of the inferior vena cava. Treatment consists of full anticoagulation and long term (3–6 months) administration of warfarin (coumadin). Infrahepatic vena caval stenosis has been successfully treated by transluminal balloon angioplasty.[25]

Patients who receive a liver transplant for Budd–Chiari syndrome are at risk of developing recurrent hepatic vein occlusion. Maintenance of long term anticoagulation with warfarin has been recommended, because recurrence of Budd–Chiari syndrome has been reported in transplant recipients who have discontinued their anticoagulation.[26, 27]

Variceal haemorrhage and aneurysmal rupture

Intra-abdominal portosystemic collaterals present some of the most difficult technical challenges to the surgeon during liver transplantation. Although it is widely believed that portal hypertension is immediately relieved following orthotopic liver transplantation, recent studies suggest that some degree of persistent portosystemic collateralisation remains after successful grafting.[28] Such findings are consistent with clinical observations of persistent, but collapsed, intra-abdominal and gastro-oesophageal varices during the postoperative period. The team at Ann Arbor have had experience with haemorrhage from intra-abdominal and gastro-oesophageal varices in a very small number in the total series of over 450 liver transplantations. Haemorrhage from intra-abdominal varices is usually catastrophic. Gastro-oesophageal variceal haemorrhage has been both rare and easy to control with sclerotherapy.

Visceral arterial aneurysms occur with increased incidence among cirrhotic patients. Reports document the propensity of splenic artery aneurysms to rupture in the postoperative period[29] and operative ligation of the aneurysm during the transplant procedure has been recommended.[30] At Ann Arbor there was success in performing angiographic embolisation of a large splenic artery aneurysm before liver transplantation in a patient with cryptogenic cirrhosis.

Complications of intravascular cannulae

Venovenous bypass has contributed to the ability to perform safe and unhurried liver transplantation.[31] The venovenous bypass circuit entails the placement of cannulae into the lower vena cava via the saphenofemoral venous junction and into the portal vein for systemic and splanchnic decompression, respectively, during the anhepatic phase of the operation. Blood is returned to the systemic circulation via a cannula placed into the axillary vein. Complications related to these cannulation sites have been infrequent, limited primarily to haematomas, seromas, or localised abcesses. No cases of documented upper or lower extremity deep venous thrombosis have been attributed to the use of venovenous bypass in the patient population.

Femoral arterial lines are generally used for haemodynamic monitoring during liver transplantation and have resulted in pseudo-aneurysm formation following their removal in the postoperative period in less than 1% of the recipients at Ann Arbor. Pseudoaneurysm of the femoral artery requires operative repair.

In order to prepare for the need to transfuse large amounts of fluids, blood, and plasma and to provide adequate intraoperative haemodynamic monitoring, multiple central venous access lines are placed percutaneously at the beginning of the operation. Two large bore catheters (8·5 gauge French) and a balloon tipped, flow directed, pulmonary artery catheter are placed. Over 1500 such lines have been placed since the liver transplantation programme was initiated at Ann Arbor. Fewer than 10 serious complications have resulted from the placement of these lines ($<1\%$). Nevertheless, cervical or intrathoracic perforation of a major venous vessel may prove fatal unless the injury is immediately recognised and rapidly treated. In the Ann Arbor programme, two deaths have resulted from such misadventures, but several injuries have been successfully repaired in the neck through a separate cervical incision or in the chest using a median sternotomy or lateral thoracotomy.

Biliary complications

Biliary tract complications remain an important cause of morbidity following liver transplantation. Moreover, they frequently present as a late complication, becoming apparent weeks or months after the transplant operation. Several factors have been implicated in their pathogenesis:

● Biliary epithelium relies upon an adequate arterial blood supply. Thrombosis of the main hepatic artery or its branches is almost always associated with necrosis of the associated bile ducts leading to strictures and leaks

- Bile composition is altered following liver transplantation, predisposing to supersaturation with cholesterol. This may result in sludge and stone formation, particularly if the biliary epithelium has been damaged by ischaemia, rejection, or infection. Prolonged biliary drainage – for example, via a T tube – interrupts the enterohepatic recirculation of bile salts which further promotes supersaturation with cholesterol. Moreover, cyclosporin A (cyclosporine) may inhibit bile salt production
- The transplanted liver is a denervated organ, and it has been suggested that denervation of the biliary tract inhibits bile flow and perhaps alters bile composition
- T tubes are commonly used to protect duct-to-duct biliary anastomosis. The T tube provides a useful conduit to monitor bile production which is a valuable index of liver function in the early postoperative period. The T tube also provides a port to sample bile for microbiology, and to perform cholangiography to assess the biliary tract. However, the T tube stent is a foreign body within the biliary tract, which is prone to bacterial colonisation and forms a focus for the deposition of biliary sludge. Anastomosis of the bile duct to a Roux loop of recipient jejunum is an alternative method of biliary reconstruction, but may promote bacterial colonisation of the bile duct with enteric organisms from the small bowel lumen.

In contrast with the progressive decrease in the incidence of vascular complications at Birmingham over the last few years, the incidence of biliary complications remains stubbornly high at about 15% of the transplanted livers. Other units report similar figures. The biliary complications that have been observed include the following:

- Bile leak
- Bile duct stricture
- Biliary sludge/stones
- Cholangitis
- Cholestasis
- Mucocele of the cystic duct
- Choledochovenous fistula
- Liver abscess.

Presentation

Biliary complications due to technical problems at the time of transplantation are usually apparent in the first few postoperative days. They are recognised by appearance of bile in the surgical drains, cholestatic liver function tests, or on ultrasonography or T tube cholangiography which at Birmingham is performed routinely one week post-transplantation before clamping the T tube. Many biliary complications, however, present later, frequently after the patient has been discharged from hospital. There are two common patterns: first, patients may become acutely septic due to cholangitis, or an infected bile collection, and clearly require immediate admission to hospital for investigation and treatment. Second, increasing jaundice and deteriorating liver function with a high serum alkaline phosphatase may be noted at routine outpatient follow up. Finally, the complication may first be recognised during routine follow up investigations, such as T tube cholangiography performed after three months before removing the T tube, or ultrasonography and liver biopsy which form part of the Birmingham protocol investigations at annual review. Loss of the hepatic artery signal on Doppler ultrasonography is of particular concern. Although hepatocyte function may be unaffected, the biliary tract is liable to ischaemic damage, leading eventually to intrahepatic strictures and bile collections.

Investigations

The septic patient requires urgent investigation and prompt treatment because of the potentially lethal combination of infection and immunosuppression. Occasionally, acute rejection may present in a fulminant fashion with fever and rapid deterioration of liver function which mimics sepsis. Because rejection is treated with increased immunosuppression, whereas infection requires a reduction in immunosuppressive therapy, it is essential to make a rapid and accurate diagnosis.

The "sepsis screen" at Birmingham entails culturing blood, urine, sputum, T tube bile, and, if present, ascites. In addition, urgent chest radiography and ultrasonography of the abdomen are needed, looking for biliary dilatation and intrahepatic and intraperitoneal fluid collections. If a collection is identified, the radiologist is asked to perform a percutaneous aspiration for microbiology. Collections that contain bile or pus are drained with a percutaneous pigtail catheter inserted under ultrasonographic guidance. The T tube (if present) is unclamped and placed on free drainage. A T tube cholangiogram should *not* be performed until the bile culture results are available, the patient has received appropriate antibiotics, and systemic sepsis from cholangitis has resolved. In Birmingham prophylactic antibiotics are given to all patients undergoing either cholangiography or invasive procedures such as liver biopsy.

For the patient presenting with deranged liver function with no evident sepsis, ultrasonography is the initial investigation, looking for biliary dilatation and collections. Until 1987, it was common to use the donor gall bladder as a conduit between the recipient and donor bile ducts, and this will show up on ultrasonography. The gall bladder conduit has now been abandoned because of the very high incidence of biliary sludge and stones which form within it leading to biliary obstruction months or years after the transplant operation. Even though a cholecystectomy is now carried out at Birmingham on the transplanted organ (the recipient's own gall bladder is always removed with the old liver), there may be a remnant of the cystic duct, which can occasionally become obstructed to form a mucocele. This may compress and obstruct the bile duct, and be visualised as an unusual structure on ultrasonography.

Following ultrasonography, a T tube cholangiogram is performed under antibiotic prophylaxis. It is important to ensure that the radiologist does not overfill the biliary system and cause cholangitis. The person making the examination is requested to look for biliary strictures, leaks, and dilatation, *not* to visualise all the small terminal biliary radicals within the liver. For patients without a T tube, endoscopic retrograde cholangiography may be useful in patients with a duct-to-duct biliary anastomosis. For patients with a Roux-en-Y biliary anastomosis, a percutaneous transhepatic cholangiogram is necessary to visualise the biliary tree. This is a potentially hazardous investigation, particularly if there is abnormal clotting or if the biliary tract is dilated. The radiologist should therefore be prepared to drain the biliary tract and dilate or stent strictures visualised at percutaneous transhepatic cholangiography (Figures 3–6).

Cholestatic liver tests (raised bilirubin and alkaline phosphatase) may not be associated with overt biliary pathology. In particular, cholestasis frequently follows severe or protracted rejection episodes

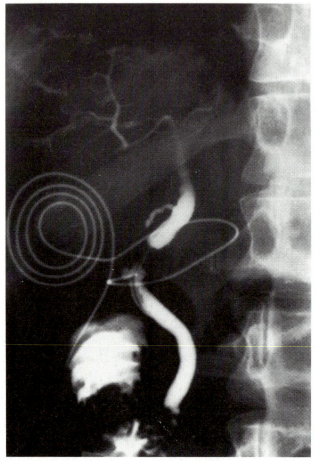

FIG 3— *T tube cholangiogram showing an early stricture at this anastomosis. This settled after endoscopic dilatation*

or preservation injuries to the liver at the time of transplantation. A liver biopsy may show inspissated bile in microscopic bile ducts, and should be performed once bile duct obstruction or infection has been excluded to ensure that there is no active rejection.

Treatment (see Box B)

Any immunosuppressed patient with suspected sepsis should receive broad spectrum antibiotics active against Gram-negative and Gram-positive enteric organisms as soon as specimens have

220

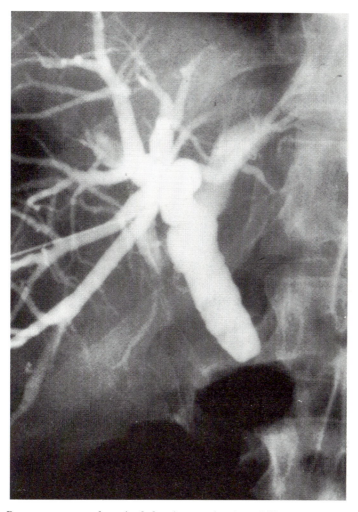

FIG 4—*Percutaneous transhepatic cholangiogram showing a biliary stricture of the bile duct at the anastomosis with a Roux loop. This required surgical intervention*

been taken for microbiological examination. Antibiotic therapy is subsequently modified on the advice of the microbiologist and if necessary, anti-fungal agents are added. If present, the T tube is placed on free biliary drainage. For patients without a T tube, but with biliary dilatation on ultrasonography, percutaneous biliary drainage is usually necessary to treat an associated cholangitis effectively. Similarly, infected bile collections, whether intrahepatic or extrahepatic, require drainage. This can usually be accomplished

221

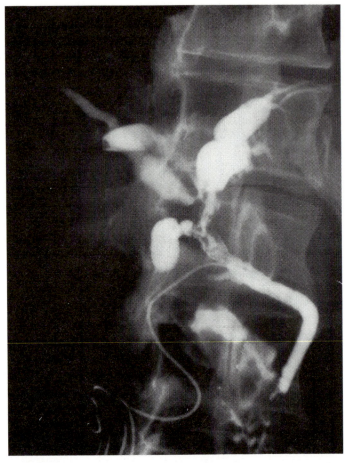

FIG 5—*T tube cholangiogram showing a complex, high, non-anastomotic stricture. Surgery was required*

with a pigtail catheter inserted by the radiologist, but occasionally requires surgical drainage.

Bile may leak from the biliary anastomosis or around the T tube at its insertion into the bile duct, due to faulty surgical technique. This is usually apparent immediately after the operation with bile appearing in the surgical drains. Alternatively, it may be recognised during T tube cholangiography which is routinely performed before clamping T tubes one week postoperatively. Such leaks are initially managed with prolonged T tube drainage and usually heal spontaneously without sequelae. Most bile leaks, however, are probably

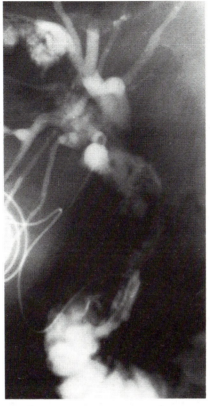

FIG 6—*T tube cholangiogram in a patient with hepatic artery thrombosis. The bile duct has almost totally broken down; there are abscesses in the intrahepatic biliary tree*

BOX B   Biliary problems post-transplantation

- Biliary leaks: treatment by T tube drainage and endoscopic/percutaneous stenting for two weeks
- Early biliary strictures can be treated by endoprosthesis, but often require surgery
- Non-anastomotic strictures (from any cause) do badly and often require surgery or re-transplantation
- Any biliary problem should prompt assessment of the hepatic artery flow

due to ischaemic necrosis at the anastomosis and may only become apparent several days after the operation. They may present with biliary peritonitis or an infected bowel collection. Even if such a leak seals spontaneously, it usually results in a stricture of the anastomosis. Although this can be stented either endoscopically or percutaneously, surgical biliary reconstruction with excision of the stricture and re-anastomosis to a Roux loop of jejunum is the definitive treatment.

Because of the proximity of the biliary anastomosis to the vascular anastomoses of the hepatic artery and portal vein, bile leaks can cause life threatening vascular complications. Hepatic artery thrombosis, portal pyaemia, and ruptured mycotic aneurysms of the hepatic artery and portal vein have been seen at Birmingham as a consequence of infected bile collections at the porta hepatis. Very rarely, a fistula may develop between vascular and biliary anastomoses, resulting in profuse bleeding from the biliary tract. Bile leaks may also occur in the postoperative phase following liver biopsy, but this is almost invariably associated with prior obstruction and dilatation of the biliary tract. Ultrasonography before liver biopsy should ensure against this complication.

Bile duct strictures are classified as anastomotic or non-anastomotic. It has been suggested that non-anastomotic strictures may be caused by long ischaemic times at the time of transplantation. They may also be caused by thrombosis of hepatic artery radicals within the liver. Most bile duct strictures, however, occur at the biliary anastomosis, presumably as a result of local ischaemia. Sludge and debris may collect around the T tube in the bile duct and, radiologically, be difficult to distinguish from a true stricture. Moreover, strictures themselves predispose to sludge deposition because they induce bile stasis and infection. Strictures can be dilated and stented endoscopically or percutaneously. In the experience at Birmingham, dilatation alone provides only a temporary solution and stents, either plastic or metal, may become blocked or chronically infected. Intrahepatic strictures are not usually amenable to surgical correction and re-transplantation may be the only long term solution. For extrahepatic strictures, however, surgical biliary reconstruction is the treatment of choice.

Cholestasis due to the deposition of biliary sludge is the most common late postoperative biliary complication in patients. The pathogenesis is unclear, but contributing factors include chronic rejection, causing ischaemia of the biliary epithelium, prior presence of T tube, and denervation of the biliary tract including the ampulla. Treatment with ursodeoxycholic acid may ameliorate the problem by increasing bile solubility. An endoscopic sphincterotomy is indicated if cholangiography demonstrates stenosis or dysfunction at the ampulla. Sludge and stones can be removed from the biliary tract, either endoscopically or percutaneously by an interventional radiologist. A percutaneous flexible choledochoscope has been successfully employed to clear debris from the bile ducts.

Conclusion

Despite technical modifications to the operation, the biliary tract continues to account for much of the morbidity seen after liver transplantation. Diagnosis is prompted by clinical signs and laboratory abnormalities, and confirmed by radiology. Treatment frequently necessitates a prolonged period of bile drainage. This has important implications for immunosuppression because cyclosporin A is dependent upon bile in the gastrointestinal tract for its absorption. In order to maintain adequate cyclosporin A levels it may be necessary to give the drug intravenously. The preferred alternative at Birmingham, however, is to encourage the patient to drink his bile. The unpleasant taste can be ameliorated by mixing it with orange juice or Guinness!

References

1 Merion RM, Burtch GD, Ham JM, Turcotte JG, Campbell DA. The hepatic artery in liver transplantation. *Transplantation* 1989; **48**: 438–43.
2 Todo S, Makowka L, Tzakis AG, *et al*. Hepatic artery in liver transplantation. *Transplant Proc* 1987; **19**: 2406.
3 Tisone G, Gunson BK, Buckels JAC, McMaster P. Raised hematocrit – a contributing factor to hepatic artery thrombosis following liver transplantation. *Transplantation* 1989; **46**: 162.
4 Samuel D, Gillet D, Castaing D, Reynes M, Bismuth H. Portal and arterial thrombosis in liver transplantation: a frequent event in severe rejection. *Transplant Proc* 1989; **21**: 2225–7.
5 Flint EW, Sumkin JH, Zajko AB, Bowen A. Duplex sonography of hepatic artery thrombosis after liver transplantation. *AJR Am J Roentgenol* 1988; **151**: 481–3.
6 McDiarmid SV, Hall TR, Grant EG, *et al*. Failure of duplex sonography to diagnose hepatic artery thrombosis in a high-risk group of pediatric liver transplant recipients. *J Pediatr Surg* 1991; **26**: 710–13.
7 Lomas DJ, Britton PD, Farman P, *et al*. Duplex doppler ultrasound for the detection of vascular occlusion following liver transplantation in children. *Clin Radiol* 1992; **46**: 38–42.
8 Marujo WC, Langnas AN, Wood RP, Stratta RJ, Li S, Shaw BW. Vascular complications

following orthotopic liver transplantation: outcome and the role of urgent revascularization. *Transplant Proc* 1991; **23**: 1484–6.

9 Yanaga K, Lebeau G, Marsh JW, *et al.* Hepatic artery reconstruction for hepatic artery thrombosis after orthotopic liver transplantation. *Arch Surg* 1990; **125**: 628–31.

10 Northover JMA, Terblanche J. The importance of the blood supply to the bile duct in human liver transplantation. *Transplantation* 1978; **26**: 67.

11 Zajko AB, Campbell WL, Logsdon GA, *et al.* Cholangiographic findings in hepatic artery occlusion after liver transplantation. *AJR Am J Roentgenol* 1987; **149**: 485–9.

12 Abad J, Hidalgo EG, Cantarero JM, *et al.* Hepatic artery anastomotic stenosis after transplantation: treatment with percutaneous transluminal angioplasty. *Radiology* 1989; **171**: 661–2.

13 Houssin D, Ortega D, Richardson A, *et al.* Mycotic aneurysm of the hepatic artery complicating human liver transplantation. *Transplantation* 1988; **46**: 469–72.

14 Zajko AB, Tobben PJ, Esquivel CO, Starzl TE. Pseudoaneurysms following orthotopic liver transplantation: clinical and radiologic manifestations. *Transplant Proc* 1989; **21**: 2457–9.

15 Madariaga J, Tzakis A, Zajko AB, *et al.* Hepatic artery pseudoaneurysm ligation after orthotopic liver transplantation – a report of 7 cases. *Transplantation* 1992; **54**: 824–8.

16 Merion RM, Burtch GD, Ham JM, Turcotte JG, Campbell DA. The hepatic artery in liver transplantation. *Transplantation* 1989; **48**: 438–443.

17 Langnas AN, Marujo W, Stratta RJ, Wood RP, Shaw BW. Vascular complications after orthotopic liver transplantation. *Am J Surg* 1991; **161**: 76–83.

18 Calne RY, McMaster P, Portman B, *et al.* Observations on preservation, bile drainage, and rejection in 64 orthotopic liver allografts. *Ann Surg* 1977; **186**: 282.

19 Starzl TE, Porter KA, Putnam CW, *et al.* Orthotopic liver transplantation in ninety-three patients. *Surg Gynecol Obstet* 1976; **142**: 49.

20 Helling TS. Thrombosis and recanalization of the portal vein in liver transplantation. *Transplantation* 1985; **40**: 446–8.

21 Rouch DA, Emond JC, Ferrari M, Yousefzadeh D, Whitington P, Broelsch CE. The successful management of portal vein thrombosis after hepatic transplantation with a splenorenal shunt. *Surg Gynecol Obstet* 1988; **166**: 311–16.

22 Scantlebury VP, Zajko AB, Esquivel CO, Marino IR, Starzl TE. Successful reconstruction of late portal vein stenosis after hepatic transplantation. *Arch Surg* 1989; **124**: 503–5.

23 Rollins NK, Sheffield EG, Andrews WS. Portal vein stenosis complicatiing liver transplantation in children: percutaneous transhepatic angioplasty. *Radiology* 1992; **182**: 731–4.

24 Lerut J, Tzakis AG, Bron K, *et al.* Complications of venous reconstruction in human orthotopic liver transplantation. *Ann Surg* 1987; **205**: 404–14.

25 Rose BS, Van Aman ME, Simon DC, Sommer BG, Ferguson RM, Henry ML. Transluminal balloon angioplasty of infrahepatic caval anastomotic stenosis following liver transplantation: case report. *Cardiovasc Intervent Radiol* 1988; **11**: 79–81.

26 Halff G, Todo S, Tzakis A, Gordon R. Liver transplantation for the Budd–Chiari syndrome. *Ann Surg* 1990; **211**: 43–9.

27 Campbell DA, Rolles K, Jamieson N, *et al.* Hepatic transplantation with perioperative and long term anticoagulation as treatment. *Ann Surg* 1992;

28 Navasa M, Feu F, Garcia-Pagan JC, *et al.* Hemodynamic and humoral changes after liver transplantation in patients with cirrhosis. *Hepatology* 1993; **17**: 355–60.

29 Brems JJ, Hiatt JR, Klein AS, Colonna JO, Busuttil RW. Splenic artery aneurysm rupture following orthotopic liver transplantation. *Transplantation* 1988; **45**: 1136–7.

30 Ayalon A, Wiesner RH, Perkins JD, Tominaga S, Hayes DH, Krom RA. Splenic artery aneurysms in liver transplant patients. *Transplantation* 1988; **45**: 386–9.

31 Griffith BP, Shaw BW, Hardesty RL, Iwatsuki S, Bahnson HT, Starzl TE. Veno-venous bypass without systemic anticoagulation for transplantation of the liver. *Surg Gynecol Obstet* 1985; **160**: 271.

13: Medical complications

DANIEL K BRAUN, MERVYN DAVIES,
JOHN R LOWES, DAVID MUTIMER

Infections in the liver transplant recipient

Postoperative infections are a serious problem, contributing to the morbidity and mortality following orthotopic liver transplantation. Between 66% and 83% of all transplant recipients experience at least one episode of infection post-transplantation and many patients experience multiple occurrences of infection.[1-5] Up to 88% of deaths following liver transplantation have been attributed to infectious complications.[2-6] The greatest period of risk of infection seems to be in the first two months following orthotopic liver transplantation.[4] After six months, many infections caused by opportunist organisms are only observed infrequently.[4]

Evaluation for infection pre-transplantation

Before surgery, the liver transplant candidate should be evaluated for previous exposure to infectious agents which might pose significant problems with the institution of immunosuppression.[7-10] Blood may be taken for evidence of past viral infection, including herpes simplex viruses (HSV) types I and II, varicella-zoster virus, cytomegalovirus, and Epstein–Barr virus. In those with antibodies, a significant rise in titre after transplantation may indicate reactivated infection, whereas seroconversion usually denotes primary infection. Other blood tests routinely obtained pre-transplantation may include those for hepatitis B, C, and D, and HIV, syphilis (Venereal Disease Reference Laboratory (VDRL) slide test and fluorescent treponemal antibody test – absorbed (FTA-Abs)),

Legionella sp., and *Toxoplasma gondii*. Skin testing for tuberculosis is also done in some centres; those candidates who are PPD (purified protein derivative) positive, but without evidence of active disease, may be given prophylaxis with isoniazid. Patients from tropical or subtropical regions should have their stools examined for ova and parasites, and appropriate therapy given before surgery. Transplant candidates from south-eastern USA should be evaluated for infection with the nematoid *Strongyloides stercoralis*. Those with positive stool specimens should be treated with thiabendazole before transplantation.

Liver donors are also routinely screened for various infectious agents, and some donations are precluded by evidence of HBV, HCV, or HIV seropositivity. Many transplant programmes will not accept a liver from a donor who is anti-HCV antibody positive or who has either HBsAg or anti-HBc antibody. It is uncertain whether donor livers from those who are HCV positive or with past or active HBV infection should be transplanted into recipients already infected with the viruses. Donors who are anti-HBs antibody positive are acceptable if they are known to have received anti-hepatitis B vaccine. In the case of cytomegalovirus, it is preferable to choose a cytomegalovirus-seronegative donor for a seronegative recipient to limit transfer of latent virus. Given the short supply of available donors, however, such limitations are frequently not possible.

Diagnosis of infection post-transplantation

The evaluation for possible infection in the liver transplant recipient can present a considerable challenge to the physician:

- Rejection of the allograft may present similarly to acute infection
- Potentially toxic drugs may cause fever, which may be mistakenly attributed to infection
- The technical complexity of the operation predisposes the patient to infections at a higher rate than in some other types of transplantation
- Many infections are due to opportunist pathogens which do not usually cause serious disease.

In the immunocompromised transplant recipient, illness may

develop slowly with only subtle manifestations present until the process becomes life threatening.

In the month after liver transplantation, infection may occur due to many different pathogens, including bacteria, viruses, fungi, and parasites.[4] During this period, abdominal infections associated with the surgical procedure are common, including liver and other abdominal abscesses, cholangitis, and peritonitis. Common organisms responsible for such infections include enterococci, Gram-negative aerobes, anaerobes, Candida sp.,[4,8,11] Staphylococcus aureus and coagulase negative staphylococci.[11] Abdominal infections in the peri-transplantation period usually manifest with fever and abdominal pain, abdominal distension, ascites, and, in cases of liver abscess and cholangitis, jaundice. The evaluation of such signs and symptoms is often helped by abdominal ultrasonography or computed tomography, showing fluid collections, organomegaly, or biliary dilatation. More invasive investigations which may help include T tube cholangiography, endoscopic retrograde cholangiopancreatico-graphy (ERCP), and liver biopsy. Culture of the blood or aspirated fluid will frequently identify the micro-organisms responsible for the abdominal infection and help in guiding specific therapy. In the absence of other localising signs and symptoms, positive blood cultures for bacteria and fungi may indicate colonisation of indwelling intravenous catheters.

Other sites commonly infected in the peri-transplantation period include the lungs and the urinary tract. The former may be involved as a consequence of tracheal intubation, whereas the latter may become infected secondary to the effects of catheterisation or of bacteraemia.

As the time for transplantation extends beyond a month, the spectrum of infection changes as opportunist pathogens become relatively more common aetiological agents.[4,8,10] The physician may encounter a post-transplant recipient with a fever but no other localising signs or symptoms. Organ systems that are not frequently sites of infection immediately after transplantation must be considered (ie, the central nervous system) in the differential diagnosis of fever in this patient. Infections commonly observed in non-immunocompromised hosts should not be overlooked.

Some transplant recipients with low grade fever do not always receive intensive therapy. This includes those grafted more than six months earlier and who appear only mildly ill. For the transplant

229

recipient with no obvious source of infection, diagnostic evaluation should include:

- Complete blood count with differential
- Liver function tests
- Urinalysis
- Chest radiograph
- Abdominal ultrasonography
- Stains and cultures of blood and other bodily fluids such as sputum, cerebrospinal fluid, and urine obtained in the course of the work up
- Head computed tomography (CT) and possible lumbar puncture if there is headache, mental status change, or localising neurological signs (lumbar puncture should be performed if there are no contraindications such as a mass with midline shifts)
- Possible chest CT scan to allow further definition of any abnormalities noted
- Abdominal CT scan including the allograft and biliary tree
- Evidence for a liver abscess should always lead to investigation of the patency of the hepatic artery.

Such cultures should be held by the microbiology laboratory for sufficient time to allow slow growing pathogens, such as fungi, viruses, such as cytomegalovirus, and various other slow growing organisms, such as *Nocardia* sp. and *Mycobacterium tuberculosis* to be identified. Examination of the chest radiograph may disclose an infiltrate or other significant abnormality such as a mass, but sputum may be unobtainable. In this case bronchoscopy may be performed to obtain specimens for staining and cultures, because infections, such as *Pneumocystis carinii* pneumonia or aspergillosis, may be missed. Shell-vial cultures for cytomegalovirus may be most helpful in identifying the presence of this organism as a potential pathogen. (The shell-vial technique uses a monoclonal antibody to a protein of CMV to yield fluorescence of infected cells on a specially prepared slide. Results may be obtained in 24 hours.) Even without localising signs or symptoms, the abdomen and pelvis may harbour an infectious process identifiable by computed tomography. Additionally, immunological evaluation for seroconversion from negative to positive or for a significant rise in titre may be useful in assessment of viral or parasitic infection.

If the initial evaluation does not disclose a probable source of infection, further studies may be useful. Radionuclide scanning with gallium, or with indium-labelled leucocytes, is highly sensitive and may provide information that is not available from any other technique for identification of a site of infection. Bone marrow biopsy with culture may identify infection with agents such as *M. tuberculosis* or fungi. Biopsy of the transplanted liver may be needed to differentiate between direct infection, cholestasis secondary to disease in the biliary tree, drug induced hepatitis, or rejection. Similarly, biopsy of masses found on imaging studies may be necessary for identification of the aetiology of fever. Microscopic examination and culture of biopsied material are essential to establish the diagnosis.

Although the liver transplant recipient provides a wider spectrum of potential infections than many non-compromised hosts, it is usually possible to establish the aetiology for fever in such patients with a careful and thorough diagnostic search. Most infections in liver transplant recipients, even those caused by unusual pathogens, can be identified with sufficient consideration given to the types and specific kinds of micro-organisms involved with illness in the compromised host.

Specific infections and associated pathogens

Infections early post-transplantation

Infections within the first month of liver transplantation include those that have existed before surgery, such as those due to viral hepatitis, and those that result from the operation. Some viral and fungal infections are common within the first month following transplantation.

Bacterial infections Surgically related infections are frequently associated with the vascular or biliary anastomoses. Thrombosis or occlusion of the hepatic or portal veins and the hepatic artery have been associated with bacteraemia and clinical deterioration in the first few days following surgery.[8] A particular problem is hepatic artery occlusion with development of hepatic infarcts and subsequent gangrene or abscess development.[1,8,12] Unexplained fever should always indicate the need for assessment of hepatic artery patency. Fever, ascites, and biochemical dysfunction of the allograft are commonly seen.[12] Inadequate vascular supply to the biliary anastomosis may result in breakdown of the anastomosis with a bile leak and development of abscesses, deep soft tissue infections, cholangitis, and systemic spread.[8] Microbial organisms responsible for such infections include enterococci, Gram-negative coliform bacilli, anaerobes, and *Candida* spp.[4, 8, 11]

The biliary anastomosis is a common source of infection in the early period post-transplantation even with an intact vascular supply. Although the optimal biliary anastomosis is a choledocho-choledocostomy with retention of the sphincter of Oddi, this is not always feasible.[8, 12] An alternative is choledochojejunostomy with Roux-en-Y, which has less tendency than other procedures for development of biliary contamination from flora of the gastrointestinal tract.[8, 12] However, reflux of gut contents may give rise to infection of the biliary tree. With either of these anastomoses, biliary leaks with secondary infection are possible.[8, 12] The choledocho-choledocostomy is also prone to obstruction with development of infection.[8, 12] Most liver transplant recipients will have colonisation of the bile by normal gut flora, but in most cases this does not present a problem unless bile leaks or obstruction of the ducts occurs.[8, 10]

Because of the technical complexity of the liver transplantation procedure, postoperative infections are more likely than with transplantation involving other organs. In the early post-transplantation period, development of fever, dysfunction of the allograft, or bacteraemia should be evaluated aggressively. The diagnostic evaluation should include ultrasonography and/or computed tomography of the allograft and related anatomy, and may also include cholangiography and hepatic angiography if necessary.[8]

Abdominal infection not directly related to vascular or biliary anastomoses may also be observed in the first month after transplantation. These include cholangitis after radiological examination such as cholangiography or ERCP, infected intra-abdominal haematoma, abdominal abscesses remote from the allograft, and peritonitis associated with abscesses, cholangitis, or disruption of bowel integrity.[4, 8, 11] Cholangitis may require liver biopsy to distinguish it from rejection. The presence of an accompanying bacteraemia may be suggestive. Because of the tendency for significant bleeding during surgery and the transfusion of large quantities of blood both during and after operation, there is a possibility of intra-abdominal haematoma, which may become secondarily infected.[8] Abdominal

abscesses occur most frequently in those who have multiple operations or surgery of extended duration.[11] Ultrasonography and CT of
the abdomen and pelvis are diagnostic methods of choice for
location of abscesses and guided aspiration will frequently yield
material for microbiological culture. Bile peritonitis may often occur
after removal of a T tube and secondary infection may develop.[11]

Cholangitis, abscesses, soft tissue infections, and peritonitis occur
commonly following transplantation. In the series of 101 transplant
recipients of Kusne et al.,[4] there were 16 cases of intra-abdominal
abscess, 10 cases of soft tissue infection, 9 cases of cholangitis, and 7
cases of peritonitis. Many of these occurred in the early period after
transplantation, exemplified by 7 of 9 abdominal abscesses diagnosed within 30 days of surgery.

Other infections occurring in the early period post-transplantation include nosocomial pneumonias, skin and superficial wound
infections, urinary tract infections, and infections related to intravenous catheters. Post-surgical pneumonia is a common problem
following any extensive operative procedure and is related to aspiration of pharyngeal flora and atelectasis. In the hospitalised patient,
the most common micro-organisms are anaerobic Gram-positive
cocci, *Staphylococcus aureus*, and Gram-negative bacilli. Other
potential causes of pneumonia in the first month following surgery
include *Legionella* sp., *Aspergillus* sp., herpes simplex virus, and
Toxoplasma gondii.[11] The clinical presentation of postoperative
pneumonia typically includes fever, leucocytosis (frequently with
left shift), respiratory insufficiency, physical findings of consolida-
tion or other lung abnormalities, and evidence of pulmonary infiltrates on chest radiograph. Identification of the pulmonary
pathogens(s) may require bronchoscopy with lavage or transbronchial biopsy if sputum specimens are not diagnostic. Rarely, open
lung biopsy may be required for diagnosis. Infections of the skin and
superficial wounds are quite common following liver transplantation, but are not usually life threatening. *S. aureus*, various viruses
(discussed below), dermatophytes, and *Candida* spp. are common
skin pathogens.[11] The most common micro-organism infecting
wounds is *S. aureus*, but other staphylococci, Gram-negative bacilli,
and *Candida* spp. may also be responsible.[11] Urinary tract infections
are often observed and may be related to Foley catheterisation or
seeding during bacteraemia from another source.

The widespread use of intravenous catheters in hospitalised

patients of all types has led to the common occurrence of catheter-related infections, both at the site of insertion and with development of bacteraemia. Peripheral catheters should be changed frequently, and sterile technique practised rigorously in manipulation of indwelling central lines to avoid colonisation of micro-organisms. Staphylococci and *Candida* spp. are the most common colonisers of catheters. Local inflammation at the site of access, and comparison of quantitative cultures drawn both peripherally and through a central line may suggest line-related infection.

Infection in the first month and beyond

After the first postoperative month, incidence of infections decreases steadily with time.[4] Bacteria continue to be significant pathogens at this time, even though infectious complications directly related to the surgical procedure decline in numbers, whereas proportionally more opportunist infections related to chronic immunosuppression occur. Among bacterial pathogens, organisms such as *Mycobacterium tuberculosis*, atypical mycobacteria, and higher bacteria such as *Nocardia asteroides* should be considered, although the last named have not been commonly observed in liver transplant recipients.[4,5] This contrasts with the relatively frequent occurrence of nocardiosis in heart transplant recipients.[13] Community acquired pneumonia due to *Streptococcus pneumoniae*, *H. influenzae*, and other agents may be seen in patients with liver allografts. *Listeria* sp. is the most common cause of meningitis in the immunocompromised host.[19] Other bacteria causing acute meningitis in the imunocompromised host include *Streptococcus pneumoniae*, *S. aureus*, and Gram-negative bacilli. Although fungal infections decline in incidence after the first month post-transplantation, viral and parasitic infections show an increased incidence[4] which may peak in the second month (viral) or continue for several months (protozoal). Beyond the first 6 months post-transplantation, some bacterial and fungal infections may still be observed (though with significantly decreased frequency), but viral and protozoal infections become very uncommon.[4]

Fungal infection The vast majority of fungal infections in liver transplant recipients occur in the first 2 months after transplantation. Earlier series compiled during the era of immunosuppression with azathioprine and prednisone,[14] as well as during the first years of cyclosporin A (cyclosporine) use,[15] demonstrated a high incidence of significant fungal infections. In the latter series, up to 42% of liver transplant recipients developed fungal infections. More recently, the incidence of such infections has declined to 16–25% of transplant recipients, and yet the mortality due to invasive fungal disease remains high. In the series of Kusne et al., death occurred in 81% of those with severe fungal infections.[4]

The most common fungal infections in transplant recipients are those due to Candida spp., with over three-quarters of cases of fungal disease resulting from this yeast.[4,5,14,16] C. albicans has been found in most cases, although other species including C. glabrata, C. tropicalis, and C. kruzei have been observed.[4,14] Candida spp. are small, yeast-like organisms which reproduce by budding. Pseudo-hyphae and hyphae may also be found in infected tissue and bodily fluids. Candida spp. are normal inhabitants of the bowel in 10–50% of the general population,[17] and yeast from this reservoir is believed to be the source of most of the infections observed with this pathogen. Disruption of bowel integrity, secondary to the surgical procedure, appears to be a major factor in the predisposition of liver transplant recipients to develop infections with Candida spp. Other factors that have been reported to increase the risk of infection by fungi in general are increased use of antibiotics and prolonged time of surgery.[4]

Invasive candidiasis is diagnosed by candidaemia, isolation of Candida spp. from the abdomen, in association with peritonitis or an abdominal abscess, and by histologically documented candida invasion of tissue. Sites of invasive disease other than the abdomen may include the eye, oesophagus, lungs, heart, kidneys, thyroid, central nervous system, bladder, subcutaneous tissues, and wounds (Figure 1).[14,18] Disseminated candidiasis, defined as infection at two or more anatomically distinct sites, is common and is associated with a very high mortality. Despite the serious nature of invasive candidiasis, clinical manifestations may be subtle and the diagnosis difficult. In one series, 4 of 10 cases of invasive disease due to Candida spp. were diagnosed only at postmortem examination.[4]

Candida infections in liver transplant recipients are often seen in conjunction with concurrent bacterial and viral infections. The high mortality rates observed probably do not result from fungal infection alone but are believed to be caused by the combined effects of

235

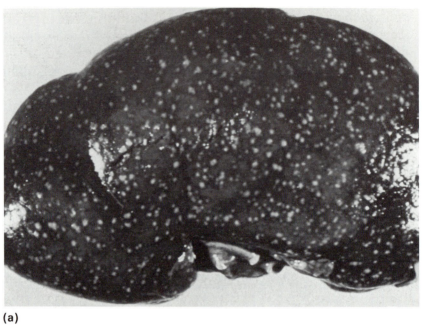

(a)

(b)

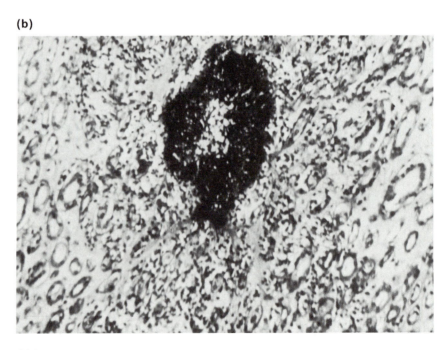

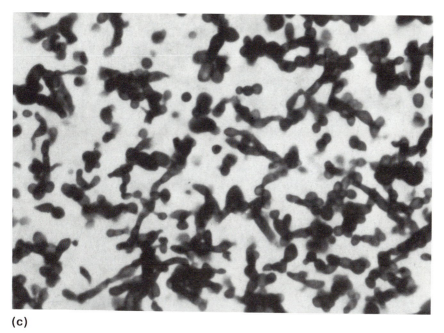

(c)

FIG 1—*(a) Kidney from a case of disseminated candidiasis demonstrating multiple microabscesses. (b) Histopathological section of a renal microabscess. (c) Microscopic appearance of biopsied liver from a patient with hepatic candidiasis demonstrating budding yeast and pseudohyphae*

multiple pathogens and other non-infectious factors, such as graft rejection and haemorrhage.

Infection with *Aspergillus* sp. is observed less often than with *Candida* spp., but aspergillosis has been associated with a fatal outcome in 75% or more of cases in various series.[4, 14–16] *Aspergillus* sp. is a ubiquitous fungus which is present in many environments and which frequently acts as an opportunist pathogen in immunocompromised hosts. Microscopically, *Aspergillus* sp. appears as dichotomously branching hyphae which are usually septate. Commonly the lungs are involved, although disseminated disease involving multiple organs is also observed (Figure 2). Infection is thought to occur by inhalation of spores from the air. Of particular concern in the immunocompromised host is the propensity for tissue erosion and invasion of blood vessels by *Aspergillus* sp., leading to localised necrosis, infarction, and haemorrhage, and permitting dissemination to other sites. As with *Candida* spp., specific indications of infection by this organism are frequently lacking. In one series, only

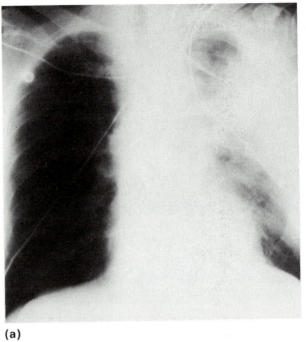

(a)

(b)

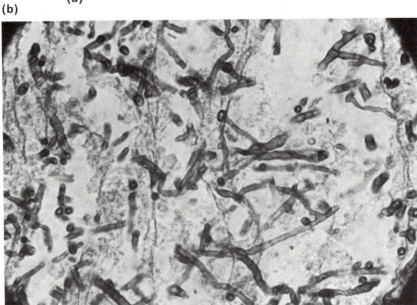

FIG 2—*(a) Chest radiograph showing wedge-shaped infiltrate characteristic of invasive pulmonary aspergillosis. (b) Silver stained histopathology of lung demonstrating acutely branching, septate hyphae of Aspergillus* sp.

238

3 of 10 liver transplant recipients developing invasive aspergillosis were suspected of having the disease before death.[14] Unlike *Candida* spp., which are frequently cultured from blood, urine, wounds, and drains, *Aspergillus* sp. is rarely found in these sites. This contributes to the difficulty in early diagnosis, which probably plays an important role in the exceedingly poor prognosis.

Infections due to other fungi have been recognised in liver transplant recipients, although these appear to be uncommon. Mucormycosis has been reported to occur in conjunction with a candida infection in one patient, and an additional case involving obstruction of the hepatic artery by a fungal abscess has been observed. Both patients died.

The encapsulated yeast *Cryptococcus neoformans* is an opportunist pathogen which may infect the immunocompromised host. The most common sites of infection are the central nervous system and the lungs. However, infection with *Cryptococcus* sp. may be associated with a better outcome than is noted with other fungi in liver transplant recipients. The most common infection observed is cryptococcal meningitis, which may present in a subacute fashion with minimal symptoms of headache, visual changes, and low grade fever. Thus, a high degree of suspicion is necessary in order to recognise the often subtle findings of cryptococcal meningitis. The diagnosis may be established by finding encapsulated yeast or cryptococcal antigen in the CSF. Pulmonary disease accompanies meningitis in many cases of cryptococcal infection. Cutaneous lesions caused by *Cryptococcus* sp. may also be observed.

Infections caused by endemic fungi such as *Histoplasma capsulatum* and *Coccidioides immitis* are occasionally observed in liver transplant recipients. *H. capsulatum*, commonly found in central USA, most often causes pneumonitis, but disseminated disease involving the liver, spleen, bone marrow, and lymph nodes is often seen in the immunocompromised host. *Coccidioides immitis* is endemic in south-western USA. Pneumonitis is the illness caused most commonly by this agent, but cutaneous, musculoskeletal, and central nervous system disease may also be observed. Histopathological identification of the organism using stains specific for fungi is the most helpful test for diagnosis of infection caused by endemic fungi.

Viral infection Viral infection is a significant cause of morbidity and mortality following liver transplantation, with most episodes

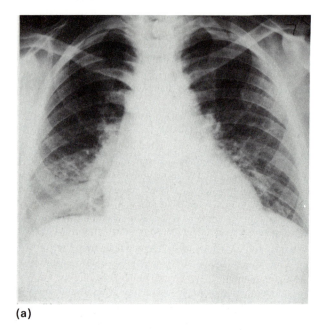

(a)

(b)

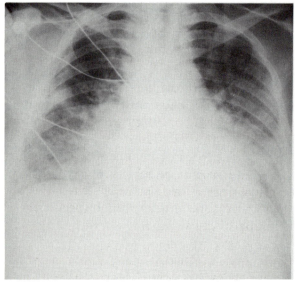

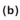

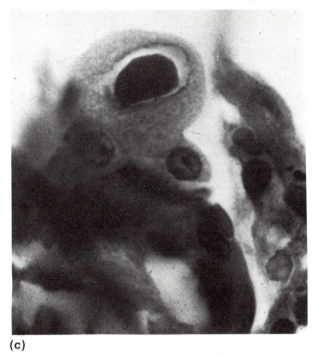

(c)

FIG 3—*(a) Chest radiograph illustrating typical bilateral, interstitial pattern of cytomegalovirus pneumonitis. (b) After this progression to confluent air–space disease in 3 days. (c) Histopathological appearance of biopsied lung from a patient with cytomegalovirus pneumonitis demonstrating characteristic intranuclear inclusion. (With permission of C. Kauffman)*

occurring in the first few months post-transplantation. The single most common agent responsible for viral infection is cytomegalovirus, a member of the herpes virus family. In one study of 136 severe infections in liver transplant recipients, 22 (16%) were due to cytomegalovirus, more than any other single pathogen of any type, and death occurred in 5 (5%) of these patients, all from disseminated disease.[4] Another report from the same institution examined 93 adult liver transplant recipients and found that 55 (59%) developed cytomegalovirus infections, ranging from a viral syndrome to a disseminated disease.[20] Five of 27 patients (18%) with symptomatic infection died. A study of 211 paediatric and adult liver transplant recipients at another medical centre reported that 73 (35%) experienced cytomegalovirus pneumonitis, hepatitis, enteritis, or infection at multiple sites.[21] Four of these patients (5%) died with evidence of cytomegalovirus-related disease. Cytomegalovirus may

241

cause disease due to primary infection in the previously seronegative recipient or secondary to reactivation of latent virus in the host with prior exposure.[21] Seronegative recipients receiving livers from seropositive donors are at greatest risk of developing cytomegalovirus infection.

Several syndromes may be observed with cytomegalovirus-related illness. The most common is a mononucleosis-like syndrome with malaise, fever, neutropenia, and atypical lymphocytosis.[4, 11] Thrombocytopenia may also be seen. Mild to moderate elevations of serum transaminase may occur but jaundice is uncommon. This presentation may be associated with viraemia and/or viruria, which may be found with shell-vial or more traditional viral culture. Fever may be prolonged but many episodes of this syndrome are often self-limiting and do not require treatment.

Of greater concern are cytomegalovirus infections involving the lungs, transplanted liver, or disseminated disease. Cytomegalovirus pneumonitis is usually manifested as a bilateral, interstitial process, and may progress to the appearance of adult respiratory distress syndrome on chest radiograph (Figure 3). Many of the deaths associated with cytomegalovirus in liver transplant recipients occur with viral infection of the lungs, either alone or as one component of disseminated disease. Bronchoalveolar lavage or tissue biopsy may be required for diagnosis but an appearance on chest radiograph typical of cytomegalovirus pneumonitis in conjunction with viraemia is suggestive of the diagnosis. Cytomegalovirus may be obtained by lavage without being associated with disease, so care must be exercised in interpretation of bronchoalveolar lavage results. Demonstration of intranuclear inclusions on biopsy is strong evidence for cytomegalovirus pneumonia (Figure 3). Cytomegalovirus pneumonitis may be seen in conjunction with *Pneumocystis carinii* pneumonia.[4]

Cytomegalovirus hepatitis is another common opportunist viral infection following liver transplantation. In the study of Stratta *et al.*,[21] the liver was the most frequent site of disease. Risk factors include primary cytomegalovirus infection, previous OKT3 therapy, and re-transplantation.[22] Cytomegalovirus hepatitis frequently presents similarly to allograft rejection with fever, malaise, anorexia, abdominal discomfort, hepatomegaly, and biochemical evidence of liver dysfunction.[12] Although non-invasive testing may help in diagnosis, the most definitive procedure to distinguish cytomegalovirus hepatitis from rejection or other causes of hepatitis is liver biopsy, with appropriate histopathological and culture studies (Figure 4). Even with biopsy, however, some instances of cytomegalovirus hepatitis may be difficult to distinguish from rejection. Cytomegalovirus may cause ulcerative disease in the gastrointestinal tract, from the oesophagus to the rectum.

Disseminated cytomegalovirus disease involving multiple organs may also be observed in the liver transplant recipient and carries a high mortality. Previous treatment for rejection with OKT3 appears to predispose to this widespread viral disease in those with primary cytomegalovirus infection.[20] Death in liver transplant recipients with such disseminated disease may be multifactorial, because concurrent infection with other pathogens frequently occurs. In addition to directly causing significant disease at single or multiple sites in the transplant recipient, cytomegalovirus is also thought to contribute to immunosuppression which predisposes to other opportunist infections.[23-25] Cytomegalovirus hepatitis may be diagnosed by culture, seroconversion, an increase in cytomegalovirus IgG titre, or demonstration of cytomegalovirus on histological examination of liver, duodenum, or colon.

Herpes simplex virus (HSV) is another common viral pathogen in the liver transplant recipient, 34% of patients experiencing HSV infections in one study.[4] Approximately half of all HSV-related illness in the liver transplant recipient occurs within the first three weeks after surgery.[4] Mucocutaneous oral or genital infections are most common and are usually due to reactivation of latent HSV in the immunocompromised host. Lesions are usually vesicular or ulcerated. Most HSV infections are not severe and diagnosis can be readily accomplished with the Tzanck test and viral culture of fluid from the typical vesicular lesions. Occasionally, HSV will cause more serious disease in the liver transplant recipient and cases of HSV oesophagitis, colitis, hepatitis, and disseminated disease have been described.[4,19] Oesophagoscopy, colonoscopy, or liver biopsy is required to diagnose such disease. As with cytomegalovirus, visceral HSV infection in the liver transplant recipient is associated with high mortality.

Varicella-zoster virus also causes cutaneous lesions in the liver transplant recipient, but these are less common than those due to HSV.[4] Children may contract primary varicella (chickenpox), whereas in adults reactivated herpes zoster is observed more often.

243

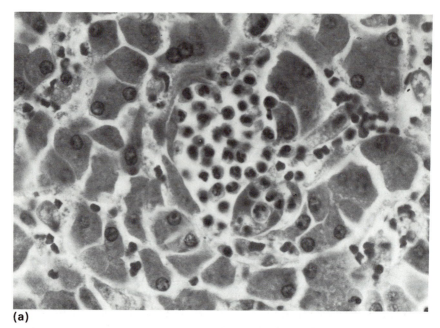

(a)

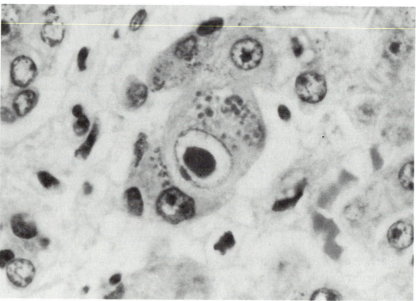

(b)

FIG 4—(a) *Microscopic appearance of biopsied liver from a patient with cytomegalovirus hepatitis showing a microabscess with lymphocytic infiltrate. (b) Hepatocyte with intranuclear inclusion from another patient with cytomegalovirus hepatitis. (Both micrographs used with permission of Charles Slack and Company)*

244

Lesions in the former case are more widespread than those of HSV, whereas in the latter they are most often confined to one or more dermatomes. Varicella-zoster virus infections, including herpes zoster, are most common in the first six months after transplantation.[11] As with HSV, the Tzanck test and culture of the lesions are useful for diagnosis. Illness due to varicella-zoster virus in the transplant recipient is usually self-limiting, although it may be more severe than in the non-immunocompromised host. Occasionally, disseminated disease involving visceral organs may occur.

Epstein–Barr virus is commonly associated with infectious mononucleosis in the normal host. Primary infection is most common in paediatric transplant recipients, whereas reactivated or secondary infection occurs more often in adults.[11] Most commonly, transplant infections with Epstein–Barr infections develop no specific signs or symptoms. However, lymphoproliferative disorders or syndromes related to Epstein–Barr virus, of several types, may be observed,[11, 26–29] especially in those in whom primary infection occurs within three months of transplantation.[11, 26, 27] One large study found that 4% of paediatric and 0.8% of adult transplant recipients developed such a lymphoproliferative syndrome.[26] The first type observed consists of an infectious mononucleosis syndrome with fever, tonsillitis, and lymphadenopathy, and is usually self-limiting. The second type of lymphoproliferative syndrome frequently begins with a mononucleosis-like syndrome which develops into a polymorphous B cell infiltrative process involving many organs. This syndrome has been associated with high mortality. The third type of lymphoproliferative disorder consists of localised, solid tumour in which Epstein–Barr DNA and/or antigens are found. These tumours are lymphomas that may occur in diverse anatomical sites. Diagnosis of such disorders relies on serological evidence of viral infection and on biopsy of involved tissue with special staining for viral antigens.[26–28] The presence of Epstein–Barr virus genomes may be indicated by DNA hybridisation studies.[26–28]

Systemic infections with adenovirus or enterovirus do not appear to be common in the liver transplant recipient.[5, 22] Cutaneous warts, caused by a papilloma virus, may enlarge and sometimes become malignant cancers of the cervix, vagina, and anus in the immunosuppressed transplant recipient. Warts that demonstrate a change in appearance should be evaluated by a dermatologist. Infections due to hepatitis viruses B, C, and D are discussed elsewhere in the book.

Other infections Infections with parasites have been encountered less frequently in the liver transplant recipient than infections due to other types of pathogens such as bacteria, viruses, or fungi. Additionally, such infections occur less often in the liver transplant recipient than in some other immunocompromised hosts, such as people with AIDS. The two protozoans most likely to be seen are *Pneumocystis carinii* and *Toxoplasma gondii*. Although traditionally considered to be a protozoan, there is evidence that *Pneumocystis carinii* may really be a fungus, based on studies of ribosomal RNA.[30] This organism has been associated with serious and often life threatening pneumonia in the compromised host. In one study of 101 liver transplant recipients, *Pneumocystis carinii* pneumonia (PCP) was observed in 11 transplant recipients.[4] Presenting symptoms included fever (100%), cough (45%), and shortness of breath (30%), whereas 80% had diffuse interstitial infiltrates on chest radiography. Most cases occurred several months after transplantation. There were three deaths in this series, and all had coexistent cytomegalovirus pneumonia. In another series of 35 liver transplant recipients, no cases of PCP were observed.[5] Diagnosis may sometimes be made by examination of induced sputum. However, bronchoalveolar lavage or transbronchial biopsy provides increased sensitivity. Specimens should be stained with Gomori's methenamine silver stain to detect the organism. Widespread use of prophylactic trimethoprim-sulphamethoxazole for 1–3 months has largely eradicated infection with this organism.

Toxoplasma gondii has been an uncommon cause of infection in the liver transplant recipient. This protozoan most often causes meningoencephalitis or single or multiple mass lesions of the brain. One case of toxoplasma infection of the central nervous system was reported in the series of Kusne *et al.*[4] Infection with this pathogen may be primary or reactivated. The clinical presentation usually includes fever, mental status changes, and focal neurological findings. Seizures and visual disturbances are common. Cerebrospinal fluid may show a mild pleocytosis. Contrast CT of the brain most frequently shows multiple, nodular, or ring-enhanced lesions. Definitive diagnosis usually requires biopsy.

Although not commonly observed in the liver transplant recipient, infection with *Strongyloides* sp. poses a significant risk to immunocompromised hosts because of the tendency for autoinfection and disseminated disease (hyperinfection syndrome), which may be lethal. Organ systems involved may include the skin, lungs, gastrointestinal tract, and central nervous system (meningitis). Secondary sepsis with Gram-negative bacilli frequently accompanies this syndrome. Eosinophilia is commonly seen with strongyloidiasis, but may be absent in the immunocompromised host, especially those on corticosteroids. The diagnosis of infection with *Strongyloides* sp. depends on the demonstration of larvae in a stool sample or body fluid such as duodenal aspirate.[31]

Treatment of infection

Bacterial infection

As bacteria constitute the most common pathogens observed in the early period post-transplantation, therapy directed against these micro-organisms will be frequently employed during this time. Intra-abdominal infections are frequently associated with fluid collections (eg, abscesses) demonstrated by imaging techniques, which may require drainage. Drainage may be accomplished by ultrasonography or CT-guided aspiration, but surgical drainage and tissue débridement may be necessary in cases of large or complex collections. Surgical corrections of predisposing factors (eg, bile leak in a biliary anastomosis, hepatic artery thrombosis) may also be required. In addition, appropriate antibiotic therapy is very important for optimal treatment.

Ideally, the choice of antibiotics should be directed by culture and sensitivity results from the microbiology laboratory. Often it is necessary to begin antibiotic treatment before the results of, or without the availability of, definitive staining, cultures, and sensitivity tests. In these cases, choice of antibiotic is largely empirical. Treatment of skin and superficial wound infections should be directed against Gram-positive cocci, especially *Staphylococcus aureus*. Penicillinase resistant penicillins such as nafcillin or oxacillin, or a first generation cephalosporin such as cefazolin, is appropriate for this use unless the possibility of methicillin resistant organisms is high, in which case vancomycin is a better choice. Local wound débridement may also be beneficial. In patients who develop nosocomial pneumonia, antibiotics should be chosen that have activity against Gram-negative micro-organisms such as *Eschericia coli*, *Enterobacter* sp., or *Pseudomonas* sp. Broad spectrum penicillins (eg, pipericillin or ticarcillin) and second and third generation cephalosporins (eg, cefoxitin, cefotetan, cefotaxime, ceftriaxone, ceftazidime) should be considered for treatment of such pneumonias. Community acquired pneumonias may be due to such pathogens as *Streptococcus pneumoniae* or *Staphylococcus aureus* and antibiotics should be chosen accordingly. Intra-abdominal infections are frequently due to enterococci, Gram-negative aerobic bacilli, and anaerobes. Ampicillin or vancomycin, together with an aminoglycoside such as gentamicin, is usually optimal for enterococci. Broad spectrum penicillins or second or third generation cephalosporins have activity against many Gram-negative bacilli, with the choice guided by culture and sensitivity results if possible. Anaerobes are usually sensitive to agents such as pipericillin, cefoxitin, cefotetan, clindamycin, and metronidazole. Combinations of penicillin with β-lactamase inhibitors such as sulbactam and clavulanic acid have broad activity against many Gram-positive cocci, Gram-negative bacilli, and anaerobes, as does imipenem, which is among the most broadly acting antimicrobials available. Drugs of choice for meningitis caused by *L. monocytogenes* include ampicillin and penicillin. The use of an aminoglycoside for synergy may also be beneficial for treatment of listeria meningitis.[32] Third generation cephalosporins are useful for many instances of bacterial meningitis caused by other organisms, because they penetrate inflamed meninges. In most cases, liver transplant recipients require initial therapy with intravenous antibiotics. Consultation with the appropriate specialist is recommended for assistance in making therapeutic decisions, including the choice of antibiotics.

Fungal infection

Treatment of invasive fungal disease in the liver transplant recipient has generally relied upon the polyene amphotericin B given intravenously. This agent has a very broad spectrum of activity against both endemic mycoses, such as histoplasmosis, blastomycosis, and coccidioidiomycosis, as well as the opportunist fungal infections most likely to be encountered in those who have undergone liver transplantation, such as candidiasis or aspergillosis.[33] Therapy with amphotericin B is associated with a number of problems, including the relatively frequent occurrence of fever, nausea, and rigors during administration, the need to provide intravenous therapy over many hours on a daily basis, and the

248

significant nephrotoxicity with most therapeutic courses. Despite the drawbacks of amphotericin B, there is more experience using the drug than with any other antifungal agent, and most of the associated problems are manageable.

Acute reactions during administration with amphotericin B can be minimised in most cases by premedicating the patient with aspirin, paracetamol (acetominophen), compazine, or diphenhydramine. Hydrocortisone 25–50 mg may be added to the infusion if necessary. Phlebitis at the site of infusion can be avoided by use of a central venous catheter. The dose of amphotericin B is usually started at 5–10 mg and escalated by between 5 and 15 mg/day for cryptococcal and less severe candida infections (eg, candida peritonitis without abscess or evidence of dissemination), to a dose usually not exceeding 1·0 mg/kg per day. However, for systemic infections caused by *Aspergillus* or *Mucor* spp., or for life threatening candida infections (eg, candidaemia with hypotension), the dose of amphotericin B should be increased rapidly to achieve a value of 0·7–1·0 mg/kg per day within two days of starting therapy. A common mistake made by physicians unfamiliar with the use of amphotericin B is the failure of aggressive escalation of the dose when treating critically ill patients who have fungal infections. During a typical therapeutic course with amphotericin B, the serum creatinine rises to 2·0–3·0 mg/dl. The dose of the drug should be regulated to keep the serum creatinine below 3·0 mg/dl. In order to do this, some patients may require alternate day dosing.

Amphotericin B may be used for treatment of invasive fungal infections with *Candida* sp., *Cryptococcus* sp., *Aspergillus* sp., and Zygomycetes (*Mucor* sp.) seen in the liver transplant recipient. Duration of therapy is dependent upon the site as well as the organism causing the infection. Long term maintenance therapy may be required with fungal infections in the compromised host. Some alternatives to amphotericin B are discussed later. In general, candida infections usually require at least 0·5–1 g amphotericin B and higher total doses may be necessary for infection of the eye, liver, or heart valves. Candida endocarditis is usually not curable with medical therapy alone. Cryptococcal meningitis is usually treated using a combination of amphotericin B and the oral antifungal 5-fluorocytosine, because the combination appears to be at least as effective as amphotericin B alone and lower doses of this agent may be employed, thus reducing nephrotoxicity. The usual regimen uses amphotericin B 0·3 mg/kg per day and 5-fluorocytosine at 150 mg/kg per day in four divided doses.[34] Monitoring of 5-fluorocytosine levels is essential to avoid bone marrow toxicity. 5-Fluorocytosine levels should be less than 100 µg/ml when obtained 1·5–2 hours after the dose. Amphotericin B is also the standard therapeutic agent for invasive aspergillosis or mucormycosis. These fungal infections are difficult to treat and high mortality has been observed both in patients who have undergone liver transplantation as well as in other hosts. High doses of amphotericin B over long durations may be required for adequate treatment. Infections in the immunocompromised host caused by *Histoplasma* or *Coccidioides* spp. should be treated with amphotericin B. Effective treatment of life threatening infections in the liver transplant recipient, caused by fungi or other pathogens, may require significant induction or discontinuation of immunosuppressive agents despite the attendant risk of allograft rejection. Liposomal preparations may be less nephrotoxic but are much more expensive.

The oral azole agents fluconazole and itraconazole may have a role in treatment of certain fungal infections in the liver transplant recipient. For those with cryptococcal meningitis, long term therapy with oral fluconazole may be beneficial following initial treatment with amphotericin B and 5-fluorocytosine – this initial therapy with antifungals is usually for 6–10 weeks. If the clinical status and results of serial lumbar punctures show improvement and clearing of intrathecal organisms with significant reduction of cryptococcal antigen titre in the cerebrospinal fluid, maintenance therapy with oral fluconazole may be considered (C. Kauffman, personal communication). Treatment may consist of 400 mg/day for 6 months, with discontinuation if there is no evidence of continued infection. Fluconazole may also be employed for treatment of superficial infections with *Candida* sp. The role of fluconazole in the treatment of deep seated candida infection in the transplant patient is in evolution. Itraconazole is another oral imidazole which may be useful in treatment of fungal infections in the liver transplant recipient. Given the poor outcome typically seen in systemic aspergillosis in liver transplant recipients, there is no good alternative at present to therapeutic courses of amphotericin B for treatment of this infection. However, should significant improvement occur with amphotericin B, long term treatment with oral itraconazole may provide similar efficacy with less toxicity than amphotericin B. For now, it cannot be recommended as primary therapy because data regarding response are limited. Both fluconazole and itraconazole affect cyclosporin A levels and adjustments in the dosage of cyclosporin A may be necessary with concomitant use of these imidazoles. Consultation about infectious diseases is advised for treatment of fungal infection in the liver transplant recipient.

Viral infection

There has been considerable improvement in the ability to treat opportunist viral infections since the earliest orthotopic liver transplantations. The most important advances have included the introduction of the antiviral agents acyclovir and ganciclovir, useful against various herpes viruses.[35, 36] Ganciclovir is the most commonly employed drug for treatment of cytomegalovirus infections. This agent is an analogue of the natural nucleoside guanosine and has in vitro activity against all of the clinically significant herpes viruses. It acts by inhibiting viral DNA polymerase after the drug has been activated by triphosphorylation within the infected cell. Ganciclovir is currently only available for intravenous use and is excreted almost exclusively by the kidneys, necessitating dose reduction in renal insufficiency. The most prominent toxicity of ganciclovir is a reversible neutropenia which has been observed in 25–67% of recipients in various studies.[37–41] Other toxicities observed have been skin rashes, anaemia, thrombocytopenia, liver dysfunction, and mild to severe effects on the central nervous system. Overall, however, most patients can tolerate a course of ganciclovir with appropriate monitoring for side effects and dosing adjustments as necessary.

Studies of ganciclovir treatment of cytomegalovirus infection in the liver transplant recipient have generally been small and in most cases uncontrolled. Dosages have varied, typically being 7·5–10 mg/kg per day in divided doses, and duration of therapy varies for less than one week to three weeks or more. A dose of 5 mg/kg every 12 hours for two weeks is recommended for those with normal renal function with dose reduction necessary for those who have renal insufficiency as advised in the package insert by the manufacturer. A longer duration of therapy may be required in some patients, depending on clinical response. Some of these studies will now be described.

One of the largest series of cytomegalovirus infections in liver transplant recipients was reported by Stratta et al.[21] They described the response to treatment with ganciclovir in 69 liver transplant recipients with cytomegalovirus infection of lungs, liver, gastrointestinal tract, or multiple anatomical sites. Of these patients, 51 (74%) showed significant clinical improvement and negative viral cultures after therapy, whereas another 18 (27%) required retreatment. Fourteen of the latter group responded to retreatment such that successful resolution of disease was ultimately observed in 94% of those treated. Therapy also included a variable reduction in immunosuppression, but the authors believed this alone was insufficient to account for resolution of viral disease. Some patients who developed rapidly progressive disease despite antiviral therapy were also treated with immune globulin. A later study from the same transplant centre found similar results in treatment of cytomegalovirus infection with ganciclovir.[41] Despite the limitations of data interpretation imposed by such factors as changes in immunosuppression and use of immune globulin, it appears that ganciclovir offers significant benefit in the treatment of cytomegalovirus-associated disease in liver transplant recipients. Several studies of bone marrow transplant recipients with cytomegalovirus pneumonitis have suggested improved outcome when ganciclovir is combined with either pooled human immune globulin or cytomegalovirus immune globulin.[42, 43] Whether this information can be applied to recipients of liver transplants is unclear. Foscarnet is another antiviral agent with activity against cytomegalovirus and may be useful for treatment of cytomegalovirus resistant to ganciclovir. However, this agent has considerable nephrotoxicity and has not been well studied in the treatment of visceral disease in organ transplant recipients. Cytomegalovirus immunoglobulin is used in addition to ganciclovir in some centres, although its value has yet to be proved conclusively.

There has been considerable interest in prophylaxis to prevent disease caused by cytomegalovirus in solid organ transplant recipients. Recent studies have indicated that prophylactic ganciclovir may prevent cytomegalovirus-associated disease among heart and liver transplant patients, although no benefit was shown for cytomegalovirus donor-positive, recipient-negative organ recipients – the patients at the highest risk.[44, 45] Another recent investigation found that prophylactic cytomegalovirus immune globulin reduced the rate of severe, cytomegalovirus-related disease by 40% in liver transplant recipients, but no protection was found for the donor-positive, recipient-negative subgroup.[46] No studies have examined the potential benefit of prophylaxis using a combination of an antiviral agent with cytomegalovirus immune globulin.

Acyclovir is the drug of choice for therapy of HSV and varicella-zoster virus in liver infection transplant recipients.[36] This agent is another guanosine analogue and inhibits viral DNA polymerase. However, it has no proven efficacy for treatment of cytomegalovirus or Epstein–Barr virus infections in the liver transplant recipient. Acyclovir is available in topical, oral, and intravenous forms. Most of the drug is excreted unmetabolised in the urine, necessitating dose reduction in those with significant renal insufficiency. Acyclovir is relatively non-toxic, with the most common significant side effect being a reversible renal toxicity observed at high doses.[36] This is seen most often with bolus administration of the intravenous preparation in a patient who is not well hydrated or has underlying renal insufficiency. Central nervous system side effects may include delirium, tremors, or EEG changes, and are occasionally seen with high doses. Overall, this drug has an excellent safety record.

Infections due to HSV or varicella-zoster virus may be treated with acyclovir. Mucocutaneous HSV lesions generally respond to intravenous acyclovir given at a dose of 5 mg/kg every 8 hours and, though not as well studied, daily oral treatment with 2 g/day in divided doses for 10 days may also provide safe and effective therapy for such lesions.[36] Treatment of visceral disease requires intravenous therapy at high doses, usually 10 mg/kg every 8 hours. Acyclovir is also of value for prophylaxis of HSV infections in immunocompromised hosts.[36] Acyclovir can be given prophylactically at an oral dose of 200 mg daily in adults for 30 days after the transplantation. Varicella-zoster virus infection may also be effectively treated with acyclovir.[36] Treatment of primary varicella or reactivated herpes zoster uses intravenous acyclovir in the organ transplant recipient. In children, acyclovir may be administered at 500 mg/m^2 every 8 hours, and adults may be treated with 10–15 mg/kg every 8 hours for 7–10 days. Visceral disease may be treated similarly. Although high dose oral therapy may be beneficial, definitive studies of its use in immunocompromised hosts are lacking. As varicella-zoster virus is less responsive than HSV to acyclovir, intravenous therapy is preferred for serious illness. Transplant recipients who are varicella-zoster seronegative may benefit from prophylactic administration of varicella-zoster immune globulin (VZIG) if exposed to people with varicella-zoster associated disease.

The therapeutic options for Epstein–Barr related lymphoproliferative disorders are limited, because treatment with acyclovir has in general not been effective,[36] and ganciclovir has not been well studied for use against the virus. One small study showed progressive improvement of Epstein–Barr virus hepatitis, with or without lymphoproliferative disease, in four of five patients treated with ganciclovir.[47] All patients had discontinued cyclosporin A so that evaluation of any antiviral effects of ganciclovir is difficult. Reduction in dose or discontinuation of immunosuppressive agents appears to constitute the best therapy currently available for Epstein–Barr virus related lymphoproliferative disorders in the liver transplant recipient (Figure 5).

The treatment of choice for PCP is co-trimoxazole (trimethoprim–sulphamethoxazole), in which there is a combination dose of between 15 and 20 mg/kg per day of the trimethoprim component.[48] Therapy is usually provided in four divided doses per day and given for 2–3 weeks. Initial therapy is intravenous, but may be changed to oral with significant improvement or mild disease. Some patients are unable to tolerate co-trimoxazole therapy; fever, rash, and neutropenia may occur. For these patients, intravenous pentamidine isethionate is an alternative.[48] This drug is given at 4 mg/kg per day as a single dose administered over 1–2 hours. Adverse effects are common with pentamidine and necessitate careful monitoring of the patient. Common toxicities noted include hypotension, hyper- or hypoglycaemia, nephrotoxicity, and neutropenia. Prophylaxis with trimethoprim–sulphamethoxazole is often employed after the surgical procedure at many transplant centres to reduce the likelihood of subsequent development of PCP. One double-strength tablet (containing 160 mg trimethoprim and 800 mg sulphamethoxazole) per day is commonly used for prophylaxis in adults.

Toxoplasma infections are most often treated with a combination of pyrimethamine and sulphadiazine (sulfadiazine).[49] Pyrimethamine is given orally with a 100–200 mg loading dose, followed by 25–50 mg/day. Folinic acid 5–10 mg/day is usually provided as a supplement to reduce bone marrow toxicity. Sulphadiazine is provided orally at 100 mg/kg per day up to 8 g/day in divided doses. Recommended dosages are for adults. Treatment is provided for at

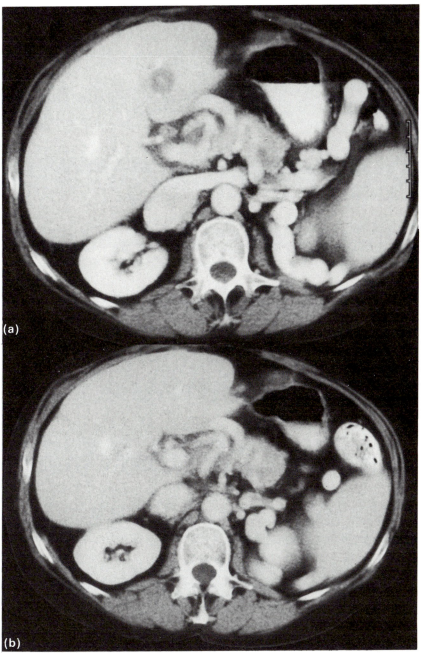

FIG 5—*(a) Abdominal CT scan showing intrahepatic lymphoma which developed in a liver transplant patient. (b) The tumour resolved with reduction of immunosuppressives.*

TABLE I—*Treatment of infections in the liver transplant recipient*

Site	Probable pathogens	Therapy
Skin and superficial wounds	Bacteria: staphylococci, anaerobic Gram-positive cocci, Gram-negative bacilli	Débridement of wounds, removal of intravenous catheter if present at site Antibiotics for bacteria*
	Fungi: dermatophytes, *Candida* sp., *Cryptococcus* sp.	Local therapy for dermatophytes Consider fluconazole for *Candida* sp., *Cryptococcus* sp.
	Viral: herpes simplex virus, varicella-zoster	Acyclovir for HSV, VZV
Oral cavity, oesophagus (mucosal disease, ulceration)	Fungi: *Candida* sp.	Oral nystatin or clotrimazole, fluconazole for more severe cases and ulcerative disease due to *Candida* sp.
	Viral: herpes simplex virus	Acyclovir for HSV mucosal disease
Lungs (pneumonitis)	Bacteria: anaerobic Gram-positive cocci, *S. aureus*, Gram-negative bacilli most common in early period *S. pneumoniae* common for community acquired pneumonia *Legionella* sp. occasionally	Antibiotics for bacteria*
	Protozoa: *Pneumocystis* sp.	Trimethoprim–sulphamethoxazole for *Pneumocystis* sp.
	Fungi: *Candida*, *Aspergillus*, possibly *Cryptococcus* spp.	Amphotericin B for *Candida*, *Aspergillus*, *Cryptococcus* spp.
	Viral: Cytomegalovirus most often; occasionally herpes simplex virus	Ganciclovir for CMV Acyclovir for HSV

Site	Organisms	Treatment
Abdomen (abscess, cholangitis, peritonitis)	Bacteria: Gram-positive cocci, Gram-negative bacilli, anaerobes	Drainage of fluid collections; antibiotics for bacteria*
	Fungi: Candida sp.	Amphotericin B for Candida sp.
Allograft	Viral: cytomegalovirus most often; occasionally herpes simplex virus	Ganciclovir for CMV Acyclovir for HSV
Blood (associated with intravenous catheter colonization)	Bacteria: staphylococci, Gram-positive cocci, Gram-negative bacilli	Removal of peripheral catheter Removal of central catheter frequently required (Candida sp. and many bacterial species; sepsis syndrome) Antibiotics for bacteria*
	Fungi: Candida sp.	Amphotericin B for Candida sp.
Central nervous system	Bacteria: Listeria sp.	Antibiotics for bacteria*
	Fungi: Cryptococcus sp. Protozoa: Toxoplasma sp.	Amphotericin B + 5-fluorocytosine for Cryptococcus sp. Pyrimethamine + sulphadiazine for Toxoplasma sp.
Urinary tract	Bacteria: Gram-positive cocci, Gram-negative bacilli	Removal of indwelling catheter if present Antibiotics for bacteria*
	Fungi: Candida sp.	Amphotericin B or fluconazole for upper tract fungal infection; amphotericin B bladder washes or fluconazole for lower tract infection.
Lymphoproliferative disorder (diverse sites)	Viral: Epstein–Barr virus	Reduction of immunosuppression for severe infectious mononucleosis and other lymphoproliferative syndromes

* See text for antibiotic suggestions.

least 4–6 weeks. Clindamycin, 600 mg every 6 hours, may be an alternative for those unable to tolerate sulphadiazine.

Treatment of strongyloides infections employs thiabendazole. For eradication of carriage before surgery, the dose is 22 mg/kg twice daily for 2 days (up to 1.5 g/dose). Patients with the hyperinfection syndrome have a high mortality rate, but may recover with several weeks of therapy.[31] Thiabendazole is only available in oral form. Side effects occur often and most commonly include anorexia, nausea, vomiting, and dizziness.[50]

A summary of the recommended treatment of various infections in the liver transplant recipient is provided in Table I.

De novo malignancy post-transplantation

Immunodeficiency is associated with an increased incidence of a number of malignant tumours, whether the deficiency is congenital, or due to the HIV virus or immunosuppressive therapy. It is assumed that impaired immune surveillance may result in the uncontrolled growth of a neoplastic cell arising from somatic mutation or oncogenic viral infection.

The clearest evidence for a viral aetiology of de novo malignancy in solid organ graft recipients relates to Epstein–Barr viral infection and lymphoproliferative conditions, and will be discussed later. Another probable causal association is between subtypes of human papilloma virus and the development of cervical, vaginal, and anal cancer. Less clear association exists between de novo hepatoma and recurrent viral hepatitis infection, especially HBV.

Since the first reports of an increased incidence of lymphomas were noted in renal transplant recipients in 1968, data have accumulated concerning the incidence of neoplasia in the post-transplantation setting, the spectrum of disease that may develop, and factors that influence the likelihood of such a complication arising.[51–56]

In addition to the effects of drug therapy on the immunological control mechanisms of neoplasia, the possibility of a direct effect of the drug on DNA replication (genetic mechanisms) must be considered. Steroids, anti-lymphocyte antibodies and cyclosporin A (cyclosporine) appear to have no direct effect on DNA and thus do not belong to the group of genotoxic drugs. Azathioprine, on the other hand, is metabolised to mercaptopurine, and has the potential to be genotoxic.

The earliest reports of de novo malignancy were derived from small groups of patients with short follow up. Since this time, a large amount of information has been gathered, with follow up exceeding 20 years in the case of liver transplantation and longer for renal grafts. This, together with the introduction of new immunosuppressive agents, has resulted in the recognition of changing patterns of malignancy.

The tumours that are most over-represented in the post-transplantation population are non-Hodgkin's lymphoma, Kaposi's sarcoma, carcinoma of the vulva, vagina, and anus, and squamous carcinoma of the skin. Numerous other tumours occur with greater than expected rates, and behave more aggressively than otherwise similar tumours in a normal population.

Lymphoproliferative disease

The most closely studied group of post-transplantation malignancies are the lymphomas.[57,58] These are almost invariably B cell in origin. They give rise to a wide spectrum of disease, collectively described as post-transplantation lymphoproliferative disease (PTLD). This should be considered in a number of different categories:

- A variety of mononuclear cell abnormalities similar to those seen in infectious mononucleosis.
- Polyclonal B cell proliferation, occurring frequently in young patients soon after transplantation. This often resolves following a reduction of immunosuppression, but may progress to malignant lymphoma.
- The monoclonal malignant lymphoma, which may be rapidly fatal.

The malignant lymphomas typically behave in a very aggressive fashion, with a far greater incidence of extranodal presentation and invasion of the central nervous system, when compared with a population who have not undergone transplantation. They may occur at a very early stage post-transplantation and some cases have masqueraded as acute rejection on liver histology.[59] A particularly close association has been noted following therapy with the monoclonal antibody OKT3. In one series of heart transplants, 9 of the 79 patients treated with this agent developed PTLD (fatal in 6 of these) with a median time of onset of 1·75 months.[60] The incidence was highest in those with a cumulative dose of OKT3 exceeding 75 mg. There is evidence to suggest that the widespread use of cyclosporin A has coincided with a small, but significant, increase in the incidence of lymphoma, which has an earlier onset,[61] and Kaposi's sarcoma.

The data must be interpreted cautiously, because follow up is incomplete, the dosage schedule for cyclosporin A has decreased greatly since its early use, and the comparison between the use of "conventional immunosuppression" and cyclosporin A involves interpreting data from very different historical cohorts.

The role of the Epstein–Barr virus

The Epstein–Barr virus is thought to play an important aetiological role in the development of PTLD. Frequently Epstein–Barr virus nuclear antigen is present in lymphomatous tissue and Epstein–Barr virus specific DNA sequences have been incorporated into the genome of some of these tumours. It is postulated that immunosuppressive agents inhibit certain T cell functions, permitting unrestricted B cell proliferation in response to primary viral infections or reactivation of latent virus. The initial polyclonal response may progress to oligoclonality and finally monoclonality.

Statistics from the Australia and New Zealand Combined Dialysis and Transplant Registry

Data from this registry have been compiled by Sheil.[56] It relates to renal transplant recipients. This database is referred to, because it is larger than published data on liver transplantation, and the registry has been diligently maintained, with almost complete detail on all 6067 renal allograft operations performed in these countries since the initiation of the programme in 1963. Mean follow up is 7 years (maximum 28 years). The incidence of almost all tumours is increased (Tables II, III, and IV).

Time of tumour onset (Table V)

The relative contribution of lymphoma to post-transplantation malignancy has declined, since the first reports. Previously,

260

TABLE II—*Non-skin cancer occurring in 362 (6%) of 6067 renal allograft recipients*

Tumour type	Observed*		Expected	Risk ratio
	No.	(%)		
Genitourinary	130	(33)	30·6	4·2
Digestive organs	77	(20)	30·0	2·6
Lymphoma	48	(12)		
Diffuse non-Hodgkin's	32		4·3	7·4
CNS	16		0	+ + +
Respiratory system	39	(10)	16·6	2·1
Leukaemia	21	(5)	3·3	6·4
Breast	20	(5)	17·6	1·1
Kaposi's sarcoma	12	(3)	0	+ + +
Endocrine	9	(2)	0	+ + +
Miscellaneous	36	(9)	11·1	3·2
Totals	389		113·5	3·4

*The percentages have been rounded up or down; + + + greatly increased incidence. Reproduced with permission from Sheil.[41]

TABLE III—*Genitourinary malignancies*

Tumour type	Observed	Expected	Risk ratio
Vulva and vagina	18	0·5	35·5
Cervix			
In situ	28	7·7	3·6
Invasive	11	2·4	4·5
Uterus	6	2·7	2·2
Prostate	5	4·9	1·0
Testis	3	1·3	2·2
Bladder	26	5·3	4·9
Kidney	26	2·8	9·2
Ureter	7	0	+ + +
Totals	130	(33%)	

+ + + Greatly increased incidence. Reproduced with permission from Sheil.[41]

lymphoma was reported to represent around 40% of cases, but more recent data show this figure to be about 10% of the total. This is mainly because the duration of follow up has increased, and a disproportionate number of lymphomas occur in the first year.

TABLE IV—*Malignancies of the digestive organs*

Tumour type	Observed	Expected	Risk ratio
Buccal cavity	10	4·8	2·1
Pharynx	2	1·0	2·0
Oesophagus	8	1·0	8·0
Stomach	5	3·7	1·4
Small intestine	1	0·3	3·2
Colon	25	9·2	2·7
Rectum and anus	13	6·1	2·1
Liver	6	0·7	9·2
Biliary	2	1·1	1·9
Pancreas	5	2·1	2·3
Totals	77		

Reproduced with permission from Sheil.[41]

TABLE V—*Timing of onset of post-transplantation tumours*

Time post-transplantation	Tumour	Management
First 3 months	Polyclonal PTLD	↓Immunosuppression (Ix) Usually resolves
	Malignant lymphoma	↓Immunosuppression Intravenous acyclovir Cytoxic chemotherapy Frequently fatal
3–12 months	Malignant lymphoma	As above
	Kaposi's sarcoma	↓Ix – may regress Chemotherapy ± DXR
Beyond 1 year	Basal cell carcinoma Squamous cell carcinoma Malignant melanoma Others	All may behave highly malignantly: excise + DXR and close follow up Maintain high index of suspicion. Consider ↓ Ix Frequently more aggressive than non-immunosuppressed cohort

Ix = immunosuppression. DXR = deep radiotherapy.

TABLE VI—*Screening for post-transplantation malignancy*

Tumour	Screening	Additional tests
PTLD	? Lymphadenopathy	Excision biopsy
		Lymphocyte surface markers
Colorectal	Surveillance colonoscopy	Carcinoembryonic antigen
Cancer in PSC		
Cervix	Cervical smear annually to	
	detect in situ lesion	
Others	High index of suspicion	

Skin cancer

Skin cancer is the most common malignancy occurring post-transplantation. These tumours are frequently omitted from overall cancer statistics. Skin cancers, however, may behave in a highly malignant fashion in the immunosuppressed individual; they are not only locally invasive, but frequently multiple, locally recurrent, and have a tendency to both lymphatic and haematogenous spread. Squamous cell carcinomas outnumber basal cell carcinomas in the post-transplantation group, in contrast to a normal population. The incidence in countries such as Australia is likely to be greater than in the UK, because of the intensity of sunshine there. Patients on immunosuppressive agents should be warned against excessive exposure to the sun. Sunscreen should be applied to exposed skin in sunny weather.

Caution is required when interpreting data on tumour prevalence and incidence. Some tumours may be associated with the underlying disease, and occur in excess even in the absence of any immunosuppressive therapy – for example, primary biliary cirrhosis has a slightly increased incidence of breast carcinoma; some chronic renal diseases are associated with urogenital malignancy and non-Hodgkin's lymphoma. Also, patients post-transplantation have a close level of surveillance, so that the diagnosis and reporting of tumours may be more complete than in a non-transplant recipient population.

Surveillance (Table VI)

The high incidence of neoplasia and the altered behaviour of tumours when they arise dictate that post-transplantation patients require close surveillance for evidence of early tumour formation.

TABLE VII—*Prognosis in some post-transplantation related malignancies*

Tumour	Metastases (%)	Survival rate* (%)
Lymphoma	50	20–40
Kaposi's sarcoma	41	66
Skin squamous cell carcinoma	8	96
Malignant melanoma	30	80

* Survival is at the time of data collection, not five year survival. These figures do not relate to cure.

Outcome and treatment

The outcome of patients with lymphoma following liver transplantation is shown in Table VII. In general, tumours are managed according to the usual treatment protocols, but in all cases it should be asked whether the level of immunosuppression can be reduced. This is particularly important in the setting of PTLD, and Kaposi's sarcoma,[62] because reduction of immunosuppression is associated with regression of the disease. This policy, however, is not without significant risk, as complete withdrawal of immunosuppression is likely to be accompanied by rejection of the allograft, which may be an acceptable price in renal transplantation, because of dialysis facilities, but is not acceptable with a liver allograft. A compromise has to be reached, which usually involves corticosteroids as the dominant immunosuppressive.

There is some evidence to support the use of acyclovir in PTLD, especially if it is associated with Epstein–Barr virus. Disseminated lymphoma, however, often requires more aggressive treatment in the form of cytotoxic chemotherapy. Results are frequently disappointing, due to disease recurrence following partial remission. Such recurrence is often in the form of CNS invasion, which is usually incurable. Promising results have been achieved by treating lymphoma with a murine monoclonal anti-B cell preparation (anti-CD24 and anti-CD21), but further studies are awaited.

In summary, de novo malignancy is a complication of immunosuppressive therapy. Its frequency will be reduced by adopting less aggressive treatment regimens, but this may be at the cost of increasing rejection. Any case of suspected neoplasia should be investigated urgently, because early reduction of immunosuppression may result in regression of the neoplastic process.

Recurrent disease

As the results of liver transplantation improve and patient survival increases, it is becoming apparent that certain diseases may occur. In some cases, the rate and severity of recurrence are such that grafting may not be indicated. In other circumstances, there may be recurrences but the patient remains well and has an excellent quality of life.

Metabolic diseases

Transplantation for those metabolic diseases where the liver is the locus of the abnormality will result in "cure" of the patient. These conditions include the following:

- α_1-Anti-trypsin deficiency
- Anti-thrombin III deficiency
- Protein C deficiency
- Protein S deficiency
- Wilson's disease
- Tyrosinosis
- Byler's disease
- Galactosaemia
- Crigler–Najjar syndrome
- Haemophilia A and B.

In some of these conditions, there will be a beneficial effect on extrahepatic disease. Thus, transplantation for galactosaemia or the Crigler–Najjar syndrome will avert further neurological damage; grafting for tyrosinosis or primary oxaluria will prevent further renal damage.

In some cases, metabolic disease may be associated with severe damage to other organs, so that although the liver function is well maintained, liver replacement is indicated. Indications in this category include the following:

- Primary oxaluria

- Primary hypercholesterolaemia
- Haemophilia A and B.

Patients with primary oxaluria may also require a renal graft and those with hypercholesterolaemia may, in addition, need a heart transplant. Although a liver graft is not required just for cure of haemophilia, these patients may have cirrhosis due to viral hepatitis acquired from contaminated blood products, and end stage liver disease, as the indication for grafting.

There are some diseases where the metabolic defect is generalised and the disease recurs. Such diseases include the following:

- Genetic (hereditary) haemochromatosis
- Niemann–Pick disease
- Gaucher's disease
- Sea blue histiocyte syndrome
- Congenital protoporphyria
- Cystic fibrosis.

In some cases, the disease recurrence may be such that grafting is inappropriate, such as sea blue histiocyte syndrome. However, in the case of genetic haemochromatosis, where it is believed that the metabolic defect lies, in part, in the enterocyte, there may be a slow reaccumulation of iron. Early detection and treatment will prevent progression of the disease. Furthermore, the rate of iron accumulation is slow so that it is likely to be years before this becomes a clinical problem. In protoporphyria, the porphyrins accumulate; institution of treatment with cholestyramine may delay any symptomatic disease.

Primary biliary cirrhosis

Recurrence of primary biliary cirrhosis (PBC) is the subject of controversy although most agree that, if recurrence does happen, it is unlikely to have a detrimental effect on the patient, at least for the first decade.

The reason for the uncertainty lies in the means of diagnosis. There is general agreement that the serological features of PBC persist after grafting – patients remain with an elevated serum IgM and anti-mitochondrial antibodies (of the PBC specific variety – anti-E2) – and that patients are still at risk of developing the extrahepatic manifestations of the syndrome, such as sicca syndrome, Raynaud's phenomenon, and thyroid disorders. The diagnosis of recurrence, however, rests on the interpretation of histological features. Although PBC and allograft rejection share some features, there are differences. In de novo PBC, diagnostic features include granulomatous bile duct damage, bile duct proliferation, and the deposition of copper associated protein, initially in the absence of cholestatis.[63] Chronic ductopenic rejection is associated with arterial lesions, not seen in PBC.

Many patients, however, have a minor degree of bile duct damage after transplantation, which may give rise to some of the histological features associated with PBC (see chapter 15). Some of the features may be attenuated by immunosuppression. It has been suggested that, in patients receiving FK506, PBC recurrence is accelerated.

Although the controversy remains unresolved, there are broad areas of agreement: not all patients grafted for PBC will develop recurrence; if disease does recur, it does so slowly so that patients remain well for at least a decade. The possibility of late disease should not be considered as a contraindication to grafting.

Autoimmune chronic active hepatitis

There have been isolated reports of autoimmune chronic active hepatitis recurring after transplantation. In the initial stages, the diagnosis was made on the basis of a systemic illness, development of spider naevi, and increases in serum aminotransferases, autoantibodies, and immunoglobulins, after corticosteroids had been withdrawn. After reinstitution of steroids, patients improved clinically, serologically, and histologically, and they have remained well. Other reports are less clear cut. Histological differentiation of autoimmune chronic active hepatitis from other causes, such as hepatitis C or drugs, may be difficult (see chapter 15). Thus, the potential for disease recurrence must be considered especially in those not receiving corticosteroids.

Primary sclerosing cholangitis

As with PBC, it is difficult to confirm recurrence of primary sclerosing cholangitis (PSC). In patients who are not transplant recipients, PSC is diagnosed by a combination of features, including cholestatic liver tests, hyperglobulinaemia, anti-neutrophil cytoplasmic antibodies, characteristic biliary radiology, and suggestive histological features. The characteristic histological features include "onion-skin" fibrosis around bile ducts, but is not always present in needle biopsies. Recurrence of the serological features does not necessarily mean that the disease will recur. Most surgeons will fashion a Roux loop, rather than a duct-to-duct anastomosis; this precludes subsequent ERCP. Radiological features of intrahepatic PSC (ductal strictures, dilatation, and beading) are not pathognomonic for disease in the graft because similar changes can be observed in biliary sepsis.

Although there has, as yet, been no systematic evaluation of the livers in patients grafted for PSC, there are a small number of case reports suggesting PSC recurrence. Preliminary studies (Hubscher and Harrison, personal communication) suggest that the characteristic "onion-skin" lesions of PSC can be found some patients. As with PBC, patients with recurrence, if that is indeed what it is, have remained asymptomatic. Thus, the possibility of PSC recurrence should be remembered but not considered as a contraindication to transplantation, or even to re-transplantation.

Alcoholic liver disease

As alcoholism is a life-long disease, it is to be expected that it should persist after liver transplantation. Current estimates suggest that up to 30% of alcoholics who survive liver transplantation will resume drinking within the first three years. Pathological drinking will occur in a smaller proportion, perhaps 10%. It is not clear why the incidence of pathological drinking after transplantation is so low. Careful selection policies and fear of the consequences probably contribute to the relatively low rate of recidivism. Longer follow up is needed to determine if the rate of recidivism increases after three years.

The incidence of alcoholic liver disease after liver transplantation is low and has not been well documented. This reflects the infrequency of abuse in the early post-transplantation period and the short duration of follow up in published studies. Similarly, the frequency of non-compliance with medication does not differ in alcoholic and non-alcoholic recipients. Nevertheless, there are anecdotal reports of allograft dysfunction in alcoholics which has been attributed to alcoholic relapse with or without an associated non-compliance with immunosuppressive medications.

Viral hepatitis

Hepatitis A viral infection

Two patients have been described who have had recurrent hepatitis A viral infection.[64] Both were grafted for fulminant hepatic failure. One patient, who died seven months after a re-graft for chronic rejection, persisted with high titre anti-HAV and had viral infection, but no hepatitis documented on the resected liver; the other patient developed a self-limiting hepatitis 58 days after transplantation. The authors state that in both cases the re-infection was clinically, biochemically, and histologically mild, although a carrier state was suggested in the patient who died.

Hepatitis B viral infection

As hepatitis B virus (HBV) is not confined to the liver, but may infect lymphocytes, pancreas, bone marrow, and other cells, it is perhaps to be expected that HBV re-infection may occur after transplantation. In North America, most HBV infected patients referred for transplantation have evidence of active viral replication.

Recurrence of disease is associated with reduced graft survival; thus the Pittsburgh group reported one and five year survival rates of 57% and 40%, respectively, in HBsAg positive patients, compared with 78% and 71% in those with cryptogenic cirrhosis.[65]

The cumulative experience of a number of transplant centres can be summarised as follows:

- The major prognostic factor for prediction of HBV recurrence is the pre-transplantation HBV DNA level. Thus, according to the Paris group, HBV re-infection rates, which correlate inversely with patient and graft survival, were 37% in HBV DNA negative recipients, compared with 92% in the HBV DNA positive group.[66]
- Recurrence is less common in those grafted for fulminant hepatitis B, possibly because many of these patients have cleared the virus by the time of transplantation.
- HBV DNA may be a better predictor of recurrence than HBeAg, because some pre-core mutant viruses are associated with absent serum HBe antigen despite active replication.
- Immunosuppressive therapy may be modified in patients grafted

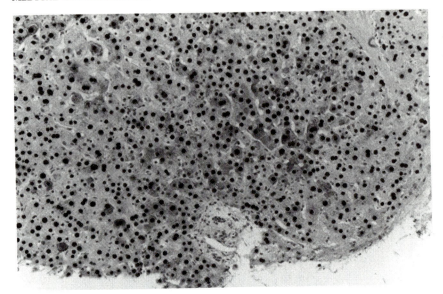

FIG 6—*Recurrent hepatitis B in liver allograft. Biopsy taken 12 months after grafting from an asymptomatic patient. There is diffuse nuclear immunostaining for hepatitis B core antigens. Focal cytoplasmic staining is also positive. Immunoperoxidase stain. (Courtesy of Dr S Hubscher)*

for HBV related disease, because there is preliminary evidence that corticosteroids enhance viral replication.[67]

- In the presence of coexisting delta infection, re-infection rates are lower, possibly because HBV replication rates are reduced. Patients who are re-infected by both hepatitis B and D viruses after transplantation have a more benign clinical course than those affected by hepatitis B virus alone.[68, 69]
- A variety of clinicopathological patterns of HBV re-infection of the graft exist:
  acute, resolving hepatitis
  fibrosing cholestatic hepatitis
  chronic persistent hepatitis
  lobular hepatitis
  chronic active hepatitis
  cirrhosis
  late onset hepatic failure.

These represent a spectrum of abnormalities. The earliest histological feature of re-infection is expression of HBcAg in hepatocyte nuclei (Figure 6). This is often followed by large forms of HBsAg

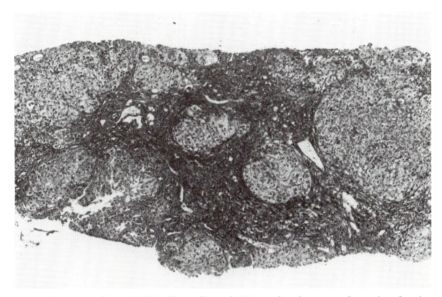

FIG 7—*Recurrent hepatitis B in liver allograft 12 months after transplantation showing an established cirrhosis. Haematoxylin and eosin stain. (Courtesy of Dr S Hubscher)*

which are transported inefficiently by hepatocytes and result in the formation of abundant, large, "ground-glass" hepatocytes. The development of post-transplantation patterns of HBV thereafter is variable[54] (Figure 7).

Another pattern is that of fibrosing cholestatic hepatitis (FCH), which occurs in up to one quarter of patients, and is characterised by rapidly progressive liver failure; this may lead to death.[55] Histologically, there is extensive periportal and pericellular fibrosis, and cellular and canalicular cholestasis in the presence of a mild inflammatory infiltrate and extensive HBV antigen expression (Figure 8). The course of the cirrhosis may be rapid and evident with the first year (Figure 7). One case of de novo hepatoma has been reported in a graft infected by HBV.[71]

Because of the poor results, attempts have been made to modify the patterns of graft re-infection. Immunisation has proved of little value: passive immunisation, giving high titre anti-HBs immunoglobulin (HBIg) during the anhepatic phases and maintaining levels of anti-HBs above 100 units/ml, has been attempted. In practice, this has been difficult to achieve – the supply of immunoglobulin is limited and not always reliable. The immunoglobulin is often given intravenously, but at present in both the USA and the UK it is

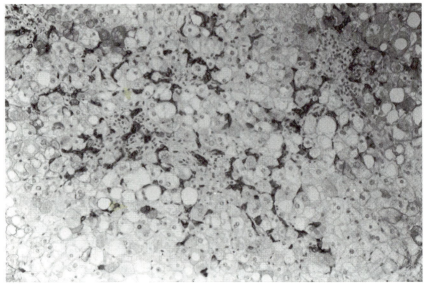

FIG 8—*Fibrosing cholestatis hepatitis: immunostaining for bile duct cytokeratin (AE1) shows numerous small dutules which extend from a portal tract into the parenchyma. (Courtesy of Dr R Harrison)*

unlicensed for intravenous use: anaphylactic reactions may occur. Whether the maintenance of high levels of anti-HBs is associated with improved graft survival is uncertain. Other approaches include giving interferon and other anti-virals. These remain, at present, research projects and should, in the view held at Birmingham, be carried out only in controlled studies.

A radical approach has been to use a baboon graft because the baboon liver appears to be resistant to HBV infection.[72] Xenografting remains a highly specialised approach.

Hepatitis C viral infection

Infection of the graft with HVC may occur as a result of re-infection or de novo infection, because of the use of contaminated blood or donor organs.

The incidence of HCV graft re-infection will be under-estimated if the standard antibody tests are used, without measurement of HCV RNA (using the polymerised chain reaction or PCR). Recurrent HCV infection occurs in nearly all recipients who are serum HCV RNA positive at the time of transplantation. Furthermore, anti-HCV positive patients, who are HCV RNA negative prior to transplantation, may become viraemic after grafting.[73]

HCV recurrence is rarely apparent for the first month after grafting, but thereafter patterns of re-infection are variable, ranging from a mild, self-limiting hepatitis, to a mild chronic hepatitis, and to an active hepatitis progressing to cirrhosis. HCV type II may be associated with a more rapid recurrence and poor response to therapy. Liver tests do not parallel the histological activity.

Both the natural history of recurrent HCV and any effect of therapy with interferon, or other anti-virals, have not yet been well defined. Use of interferon may predispose to graft rejection. Although graft re-infection appears to be common, patient survival remains good.

Hepatitis D viral co-infection

Recurrence of HDV in the graft is well recognised. Although many patients with both HBV and HDV before transplantation will not re-infect the grafts in some patients, recurrence of HDV appears to be a transplant phenomenon when HBV infection is not acquired simultaneously. When patients are infected with both hepatitis B and D viruses, there is a more benign clinical course after transplantation, often with long survival.

Non-A, non-B hepatitis

Despite the increasing sensitivity of tests for the presence of viruses, there remains a significant number of patients who present with a fulminant hepatitis, and in whom all virological tests are negative. As the presence of this putative virus cannot be detected, it is impossible to document whether recurrence occurs. Although it is the clinical impression at Birmingham that such patients may have more inflammatory activity in the graft than control subjects, the possibility of recurrence can only be surmised (see Chapter 15).

Malignancy

The poor survival of patients with unresectable primary hepatic malignancy treated with chemotherapy encouraged the use of transplantation. Although most of these patients survive the operation, they remain at risk of recurrence.

Primary hepatocellular carcinoma

The recurrence rates depend on the size of the tumour. Those tumours that are small (<5 cm diameter) and found incidentally during routine screening carry the best prognosis, with two and five year survival figures ranging from 60% to 75%. The other factors that predict poor survival are discussed earlier in this chapter. There is no convincing evidence that survival of patients grafted for the fibrolamellar variant is much greater than for other types of hepatoma.

Recurrence is most commonly observed in the liver and less commonly in the lungs. Recurrence has been observed at the site of a previous liver biopsy, suggesting seeding of tumour along the biopsy tract. For patients grafted for hepatoblastomas, two year survival rates lie between 50% and 60% with a five year survival rate of around 50%.

Other primary hepatic tumours such as epithelioid haemangio-endotheliomas, haemangiosarcomas, and others do recur, but numbers of patients grafted for these indications are too few to draw useful conclusions on recurrence rates.

As discussed earlier, cholangiocarcinomas have a high recurrence rate, with predominantly local recurrence. The two year survival rates of patients grafted with a known cholangiocarcinoma (as distinct from that diagnosed incidentally at surgery) of 25% makes such patients poor candidates.

Conclusions

Although many diseases recur after transplantation, the possibility of recurrence does not necessarily constitute a contraindication to transplantation. The survival of patients with primary liver cancer who receive medical treatment is so poor that grafting may be indicated even when the chances of cure are low. As with transplantation for viral hepatitis, there is an urgent need to consider additional strategies to lessen the risk of graft failure due to recurrent disease. Such therapeutic interventions should be undertaken in controlled studies. The shortage of donor livers makes it necessary for careful consideration to be given to which patient will stand to benefit most from the surgery.

References

1 Schröter GPJ, Hoelscher M, Putnam CW, Porter KA, Hansbrough JF, Starzl TE. Infections complicating orthotopic liver transplantation. *Arch Surg* 1976; **111**: 1337–47.
2 Dummar JS, Hardy A, Poorsatter A, Ho M. Early infections in kidney, heart, and liver transplant recipients on cyclosporine. *Transplantation* 1983; **36**: 259–67.
3 Ho M, Wajszczuk CP, Hardy A, *et al*. Infections in kidney, heart, and liver transplant recipients on cyclosporine. *Transplant Proc* 1983; **15**: 2768–72.
4 Kusne S, Dummer JS, Singh N, *et al*. Infections after liver transplantation. *Medicine* 1988; **67**: 132–43.
5 Colonna JO II, Winston DJ, Brill JE, *et al*. Infectious complications in liver transplantation. *Arch Surg* 1988; **123**: 360–4.
6 Fulginiti VA, Scribner R, Groth CG. Infections in recipients of liver homografts. *N Engl J Med* 1968; **279**: 619–26.
7 Ho M, Dummer JS. Risk factors and approaches to infections in transplant recipients. In: Mandell GL, Douglas RG Jr, Bennett JE, eds. *Principles and Practice of Infectious Diseases*, 3rd Ed. New York: Churchill Livingstone, 1990: 2284–91.
8 Rubin RH. Infection in the renal and liver transplant patient. In: Rubin RH, Young LS, eds. *Clinical Approach to Infection in the Compromised Host*, 2nd Ed. New York: Plenum, 1988: 557–609.
9 Perloth MG. The role of organ transplantation in medical therapy. In: Rubenstein E, Federman DD, eds. *Scientific American Medicine*. New York: Scientific American, 1989: CTM V, 1–16.
10 Sinnott JT IV, Rubin RH. Infections in transplantation. In Reese RE, Betts RF, eds. *A Practical Guide to Infectious Diseases*, 3rd ed. Chicago: Little Brown & Co, 1991: 619–42.
11 Ho M, Dummer JS, Peterson PK, Simmons RL. Infections in solid organ transplant recipients. In: Mandell GL, Douglas RG Jr, Bennett JE, eds. *Principles and Practice of Infectious Diseases*, 3rd Ed. New York: Churchill Livingstone, 1990: 2294–303.
12 Busuttil RW, Goldstein LI, Danovitch G, Ament ME, Memsic LDF. Liver transplantation today. *Ann Intern Med* 1986; **104**: 377–89.
13 Simpson GL, Stinson EB, Eggar MJ. Nocardial infections in the immunocompromised host: A detailed study in a defined population. *Rev Infect Dis* 1981; **3**: 492–507.
14 Schröter GPJ, Hoelscher M, Putnam CW, Porter KA, Starzl TE. Fungus infections after liver transplantation. *Ann Surg* 1976; **186**: 115–22.
15 Wajszczuk CP, Dummer JS, Ho M, *et al*. Fungal infections in liver transplant recipients. *Transplantation* 1985; **40**: 347–53.
16 Castaldo P, Stratta RJ, Wood RP, *et al*. Fungal infections in liver allograft recipients. *Transplant Proc* 1991; **23**: 1967.
17 Odds FC. *Candida and Candidosis. A Review and Bibliography*, 2nd Ed. London: Baillière Tindall, 1988.
18 Edwards JE Jr. *Candida* species. In: Mandell GL, Douglas RG Jr, Bennett JE, eds. *Principles and Practice of Infectious Diseases*, 3rd Ed. New York: Churchill Livingstone, 1990: 1943–58.
19 Rubin RH, Hooper DC. Central nervous system infection in the compromised host. *Med Clin North Am* 1985; **69**: 281–96.
20 Singh N, Dummer JS, Kusne S, *et al*. Infections with cytomegalovirus and other herpesviruses in 121 liver transplant recipients: Transmission by donated organ and the effect of OKT3 antibodies. *J Infect Dis* 1988; **158**: 124–31.
21 Stratta RJ, Shaefer MS, Markin RS, *et al*. Clinical patterns of cytomegalovirus disease after liver transplantation. *Arch Surg* 1989; **124**: 1443–50.

22 Markin RS, Langnas AN, Donovan JP, Zetterman RK, Stratta RJ. Opportunistic viral hepatitis in liver transplant recipients. *Transplant Proc* 1991; **23**: 1520–1.
23 Rand KH, Pollard RB, Merigan TC. Increased pulmonary superinfections in cardiac-transplant patients undergoing primary cytomegalovirus infection. *N Engl J Med* 1978; **298**: 951–3.
24 Chatterjee SN, Fial M, Weiner J, Stewart JA, Stacey B, Warner N. Primary cytomegalovirus and opportunistic infections. *JAMA* 1978; **240**: 2446–9.
25 Rubin RH. The indirect effects of cytomegalovirus infection on the outcome of organ transplantation (Editorial). *JAMA* 1989; **261**: 3607–9.
26 Ho M, Jaffe R, Miller G. The frequency of Epstein–Barr virus infection and associated lymphoproliferative syndrome after transplantation and its manifestations in children. *Transplantation* 1988; **45**: 719–27.
27 Ho M, Miller A, Atchinson RW. Epstein–Barr virus infections and DNA hybridization studies in post-transplantation lymphoma and lymphoproliferative lesions: role of primary infection. *J Infect Dis* 1985; 876–86.
28 Starzl TE, Porter KA, Iwatsuki S, *et al*. Reversibility of lymphomas and lymproliferative lesions developing under cyclosporin-steroid therapy. *Lancet* 1984; **I**: 583–7.
29 Hanto D, Frizzera G, Gajl-Peczalska K, Simmons RL. Epstein–Barr virus, immunodeficiency, and B cell lymphoproliferation. *Transplantation* 1985; **39**: 461–72.
30 Edman JC, Kovacs JA, Masur H. Ribosomal RNA sequence shows *Pneumocystis carinii* to be a member of the fungi. *Nature* 1988; **334**: 519–22.
31 Mahmoud AAF. Intestinal nematodes (roundworms). In Mandell GL, Douglas, RG Jr, Bennett JE, eds, *Principals and Practice of Infectious Diseases*, 3rd ed. New York: Churchill Livingstone, 1990: 135–40.
32 Armstrong D. *Listeria monocytogenes*. In Mandell GL, Douglas RG Jr, Bennett JE, eds, *Principles and Practice of Infectious Diseases*, 3rd ed. New York: Churchill Livingstone, 1990: 1587–93.
33 Bennett JE. Antifungal agents. In Mandell GL, Douglas RG Jr, Bennett JE, eds. *Principles and Practice of Infectious Diseases*, 3rd Ed. New York: Churchill Livingstone, 1990: 361–70.
34 Bennett JE, Dismukes WE, Duma RJ. A comparison of amphotericin B alone and combined with flucytosine in the treatment of cryptococcal meningitis. *N Engl J Med* 1979; **301**: 126–31.
35 Laskin OL, Douglas RG Jr. Antiviral agents. In: Reese RE, Betts RF, eds. *A Practical Guide to Infectious Diseases*, 3rd Ed. Boston: Little Brown and Co, 1991: 764–800.
36 Whitley RJ, Gann JW Jr. Acyclovir: a decade later. *N Engl J Med* 1992; **327**: 782–9.
37 Collaborative DHPG Treatment Study Group. Treatment of serious cytomegalovirus infections with 9-(1,3-dihydroxy-2-propoxymethyl) guanine in patients with AIDS and other immunodeficiences. *N Engl J Med* 1986; **314**: 801–5.
38 Laskin OL. Ganciclovir for the treatment and suppression of serious infections caused by cytomegalovirus. *Am J Med* 1987; **83**: 201.
39 Buhles WC Jr. Ganciclovir treatment of life- or sight-threatening cytomegalovirus infection: experience in 314 immunocompromised patients. *Rev Infect Dis* 1988; **10**(Suppl 3): S495–506.
40 Harbison M, DeGirolami PC, Jenkins RL, Hammer JM. Ganciclovir therapy of severe cytomegalovirus infections in solid-organ transplant recipients. *Transplantation* 1988; **46**: 82–8.
41 Shaefer MS, Stratta RJ, Markin RS, *et al*. Ganciclovir therapy for cytomegalovirus disease in liver transplant recipients. *Transplant Proc* 1991; **23**: 1515–16.
42 Emanuel D. Cytomegalovirus pneumonia after bone marrow transplantation successfully treated with the combination of ganciclovir and high-dose intravenous immunoglobulin. *Ann Intern Med* 1988; **109**: 777–82.
43 Reed EC, Bowden RA, Dandliker PS, Lilleby KE, Meyers JD. Treatment of cytomegalovirus pneumonia with ganciclovir and intravenous cytomegalovirus immunoglobulin in patients with bone marrow transplants. *Ann Intern Med* 1988; **109**: 783–8.
44 Merigan TC, Renlund DC, Keay S, *et al*. A controlled trial of ganciclovir to prevent cytomegalovirus disease after heart transplantation. *N Engl J Med* 1992; **326**: 1182–6.

45 Martin FM, Martin M, Manez R, *et al.* A randomized controlled trial comparing high-dose oral acyclovir to ganciclovir for the prevention of cytomegalovirus infection in adult liver transplant recipients. Abstract 113. Presented at the XIV International Congress of the Transplantation Society. Paris, France, August 1992.

46 Snydman DR, Werner BG, Dougherty NN, *et al.* and The Boston Center for Liver Transplantation CMVIG-Study Group. A randomized, double-blind, placebo controlled trial of cytomegalovirus immune globulin prophylaxis in liver transplantation. *Ann Intern Med* (in press).

47 Langnas AN, Castaldo P, Markin RS, Stratta RJ, Wood RP, Shaw BW Jr. The spectrum of Epstein–Barr virus infection with hepatitis following liver transplantation. *Transplant Proc* 1991; **23**: 1513–14.

48 Masur H. Prevention and treatment of pneumocystis pneumonia. *N Engl J Med* 1992; **327**: 1853–60.

49 McCabe RE, Remington JS. *Toxoplasma gondii.* In: Mandell GL, Douglas RG Jr, Bennett JE, eds. *Principles and Practice of Infectious Diseases,* 3rd Ed. New York: Churchill Livingstone, 1990: 2090–103.

50 Webster LT Jr. Drugs used in the chemotherapy of helminthiasis. In Gilman AG, Goodman LS, Rall TW, Murad F, eds, *The Pharmacologic Basis of Therapeutics,* 7th ed. New York: Macmillan. 1985: 1009–28.

51 Penn I. Cancers complicating organ transplantation. *N Engl J Med* 1990; **323**: 1767–9.

52 Penn I. The changing pattern of posttransplant malignancies. *Transplant Proc* 1991; **23**: 1101–3.

53 Penn I. Cancer in the immunosuppressed organ recipient. *Transplant Proc* 1991; **23**: 1771–2.

54 Penn I. Lymphomas complicating organ transplantation. *Transplant Proc* 1983; **15**: 2790–7.

55 Sheil AGR, Disney APS, Matthew TH, Amiss N, Excell L. Cancer development in cadaveric donor renal allograft recipients treated with azathioprine (AZA) or cyclosporine (CyA) or AZA/CyA. *Transplant Proc* 1991; **23**: 1111–12.

56 Sheil AGR. Development of malignancy following renal transplantation in Australia and New Zealand. *Transplant Proc* 1992; **24**: 1275–9.

57 Nalesnik MA, Jaffe R, Starzl TE, *et al.* The pathology of posttransplant lymphoproliferative disorders occurring in the setting of cyclosporine A–prednisone immunosuppression. *Am J Pathol* 1988; **133**: 173–92.

58 Hanto DW, Frizzera G, Gajl-Peczalska KJ, Simmons RL. Epstein–Barr virus, immunodeficiency, and B cell lymphoproliferation. *Transplantation* 1985; **39**: 461–72.

59 Howard TK, Klintmalm GBG, Stone MJ, *et al.* Lymphoproliferative disorder masquerading as rejection in liver transplant recipients – an early aggressive tumor with atypical presentation. *Transplantation* 1992; **53**: 1145–7.

60 Swinnen LJ, Costanzo-Nordin MR, Fisher SG, *et al.* Increased incidence of lymphoproliferative disorder after immunosuppression with the monoclonal antibody OKT3 in cardiac-transplant recipients. *N Engl J Med* 1990; **323**: 1723–8.

61 Alfrey EJ, Friedman AL, Grossman RA, *et al.* A recent decrease in the time of development of monomorphous and polymorphous posttransplant lymphoproliferative disorders. *Transplantation* 1992; **54**: 250–3.

62 Starzl TE, Nalesnik MA, Porter KA, *et al.* Reversibility of lymphomas and lymphoproliferative lesions developing under cyclosporin–steroid therapy. *Lancet* 1984; **i**: 583–7.

63 Hubscher S, Elias E, Buckels J, Mayer A, McMaster P, Neuberger J. Primary biliary cirrhosis: histological evidence of disease recurrence after liver transplantation. *J Hepatol* 1993; in press.

64 Fagan E, Yousef G, Brahm J, *et al.* Persistence of hepatitis A virus in fulminant hepatitis and after liver transplantation. *J Med Virol* 1990; **30**: 131–6.

65 Iwatsuki S, Starzl T, Todo S, *et al.* Experience in 1000 liver transplants under cyclosporine–steroid therapy: a survival report. *Transplant Proc* 1988; **20**: 498–504.

66 Rizzetto M, Recchia S, Salizzoni M. Liver transplantation in carriers of the HBsAg. *J Hepatol* 1991; **13**: 5–7.

67 Lau J, Bain V, Smith H, Alexander G, Williams R. Modulation of Hepatitis B viral

antigen expression by immunosuppressive drugs in primary hepatocyte culture. *Transplantation* 1992; **53**: 894–8.

68 Samuel D, David M, Gigou M, *et al*. Liver transplantation for post-hepatitis C cirrhosis. *Hepatology* 1991; **14**: 23.

69 Lucey MR, Graham DM, Martin D, *et al*. Recurrence of hepatitis B and delta hepatitis after orthotopic liver transplantation. *Gut* 1992; **33**: 1390–6.

70 O'Grady J, Smith H, Davies S, *et al*. Hepatitis B virus reinfection after orthotopic liver transplantation, *J Hepatol* 1992; **14**: 104–11

71 Luketic VA, Shiffman ML, McCall J, *et al*. Primary hepatocellular carcinoma after orthotopic liver transplantation for chronic hepatitis B infection. *Ann Intern Med* 1991; **114**: 212–13.

72 Starzl T, Fung J, Tzakis A, *et al*. Baboon-to-human liver transplantation. *Lancet* 1993; **341**: 65–71.

73 Wright TL, Donegan E, Hsu HH, *et al*. Recurrent and acquired hepatitis C viral infection in liver transplant recipients. *Gastroenterology* 1992; **103**: 317–22.

14: Rehabilitation

QUALITY OF LIFE

JANET BELLAMY, ELWYN ELIAS, JAMES NEUBERGER

Introduction

There is little doubt that liver transplantation is associated with a significant improvement not only in the quality of the patient's life but also in the life expectancy. It must be remembered, however, that liver transplantation does not represent a cure for patients. Indeed, in some respects, patients are doing no more than swopping one disease that is leading to either an intolerable quality of life or very poor life expentancy for another that would allow them to lead normal lives. Patients will remain on immunosuppressive therapy with the consequent need for monitoring and possible complications; these are related not only to possible recurrence of disease but also to the side effects of the drugs themselves. Many patients, because of their poor quality of life, enter into the transplant procedure with an unrealistic expectation. In many units it is the practice to ensure that potential transplant recipients and their families meet other patients and families who have already gone through the procedure; in the experience at Birmingham, the option of a significant improvement in lifestyle obscures the possible down side of the procedure. Although the quality of life achieved by many patients is excellent overall, it can in no way be considered that transplant recipients have a completely normal life.

In this section the longer term physical and psychological sequelae of liver transplantation are discussed. Although many of the problems are outlined in detail, it must be remembered that the great majority of patients return to a normal and fulfilled way of life.

Quality of life after transplantation

Quality of life remains an elusive concept, difficult to define and therefore difficult to assess, but, nevertheless, of fundamental importance to the patient. When seen in terms of restoration of overall functional capacity with unrestricted options for employment or activity, it can be assessed with objective quantitative measures. However, the extent of restoration and the definition of "unrestricted" remain within the subjective context of the patient's own evaluation and perception of life.

A helpful definition has been provided by Kuchler et al.[1]: "the quality of life is determined by subjective experience and as well as by objective factors in the following main dimensions: somatic, psychological, interpersonal, socio-economic and spiritual." These dimensions overlap and interact; it is essential, however, to appreciate their significance for each individual patient who presents problems after discharge.

Psychological adjustment on discharge will depend partly on the extent of adjustment before and during surgery. This in turn will be influenced by the psychopathology of the patient, by the experience of illness and treatment, and by the interaction of these two factors. It must be remembered that transplant recipients have been exposed not only to the experience and trauma of terminal illness, major surgery, and long periods of hospitalisation, but also to the implications of organ donation and the death of another person. Dependency issues, high anxiety levels, impaired confidence, and diminished self-esteem are therefore common, particularly in the first year, but generalisation is always dangerous. What follows is an attempt to outline some of the problems that some patients face after transplantation. The experience of those with chronic liver disease differs in some ways from that of patients with fulminant liver failure; they will therefore be considered separately.

Following chronic liver disease

Patients who have been ill for a considerable period of time before the operative may find it difficult to relinquish the sick role. Reduced activities, permanent or temporary cessation of employment, special diets, periods of hospitalisation, and a permanent preoccupation with physical symptoms may have become so much part of their identity that the possibilities and expectations afforded by the transplantation are seen as threatening. Where family dynamics have been changed considerably (for example, by a partner leaving work or changing lifestyle to care for the patient) both may collude with the sick role. The patient may feel too insecure to adjust to the possibility of a return to "normal" life and the end of being the centre of attention. The partner may have vested interests in maintaining the dependency of the patient. In such relationships, there is likely to be a very slow rehabilitation, a high level of anxiety about physical symptoms, and an unhealthy willingness to return to hospital.

For other patients, however, transplantation may enable such a rapid return to normal life that the partner experiences adjustment problems. Relationships can be very vulnerable in these circumstances; it is significant that frequently the patient's partner becomes ill, as if demanding the attention from the patient and others that has been denied for so long. Dependent children in the family may also find adjustment difficult and in themselves add to the complexity of family dynamics and stress.

Where there are relationship tensions, there are also likely to be sexual difficulties. Although there are no restrictions on sexual activities, patients may continue to experience a loss of libido. There may also be significant concerns about body image: there is a large scar to adjust to, there may have been considerable weight gain or loss, and the unwelcome effects of steroids can cause additional problems. Some patients feel "inferior" and lack the self-confidence to make new relationships. Some fear pregnancy or fatherhood in case the child inherits liver disease or because of anxiety about their own life expectancy. For older women, psychosexual problems associated with the menopause may need to be acknowledged and addressed.

The effect of transplantation on relationships is therefore profound, and provides a key factor in subjective assessments of the quality of life. For some people, the experience is enriching; for others it is damaging; for all it involves significant change. Some patients, however, have no close relationships. It is significant that there is an increased incidence of death within the first year for this group of patients. It is therefore important to facilitate alternative support in order to minimise social isolation and lack of self-esteem.

Quality of life is dependent upon the patient's perception of its value. Those who believe that they have much to live for are likely to make better progress. Some patients, however, may undergo transplantation because it seems the lesser of two evils; they may see possible death on the operating table as infinitely preferable to the continuing agonies of intractable pruritus, the demoralising effects of recurrent ascites or variceal bleeds, or the inevitability of a slow and certain death. Others may seek transplantation as an attempt to help their families; they see themselves as an intolerable burden on others. After transplantation, such patients may feel a sense of emptiness and find life meaningless.

At the opposite end of the spectrum, many have pinned unrealistic hopes on the efficacy of transplantation; they feel disillusioned when they discover that it does not solve pre-existing non-liver related problems whether psychological, social, or physical. In such instances, there may be a failure to achieve a quality of life acceptable to them or commensurate with their physical recovery.

Some patients may experience feelings of guilt and unworthiness, and these may remain with them or resurface occasionally during the post-transplantation period of rehabilitation. It can be difficult to accept that one's own life is dependent on the death of another person. Patients who have had two transplants sometimes identify with the relatives of the first donor and feel responsible for the second "bereavement". Others feel unworthy of their families or friends. Failure to meet perceived expectations or an awareness of continuing to contribute to the stress of others can be intolerable. Sometimes this feeling is extended to medical staff – for example, the patient feels that to produce symptoms, particularly puzzling ones, is a sign of ingratitude and thus efforts may be made to disguise them. Some patients feel the injustice of their continued survival when other patients they have known have died. A minority of families may continue to struggle with moral and ethical issues regarding the cost of treatment or the concept of transplantation itself. A Jehovah's Witness who has accepted a transplant may have been ostracised by his or her community; in addition to the considerable psychosocial problems caused by this, post-transplantation complications may be interpreted as punishment. Similarly, a minority of fundamentalist Christians may respond in this way. It is obviously essential that patients be encouraged to express and work through their feelings and to refer them for specialised counselling as appropriate.

Anxiety levels are high both pre- and post-transplantation and these do not readily disappear. The pre-transplantation period is marked by rapid swings of mood between hope and despair, and this is echoed in the post-transplantation period. Every biopsy, blood test, or unexplained physical symptom carries with it thoughts of the risk of complications, hospitalisation, rejection, re-graft, or even death. Research has shown that there are no significant changes in anxiety indices: there is a latent but constant anxiety for years which rises immediately in any crisis or situation.[1]

Anxiety is particularly evident when recurrence of the original liver disease is a known possibility or when the transplantation or its aftermath has led to economic hardships or relationship problems. The effect of anxiety on quality of life is clearly determined by the patient's ability to tolerate it, his or her coping strategies and the external factors that may provoke a crisis.

Levels of depression, however, seem to decrease after transplantation, although there may be considerable loss of confidence, especially if levels of expectation from family, employers, or doctors are perceived as inappropriate. A large number of patients with primary biliary cirrhosis have been found to have experienced a significant loss (usually death or divorce) within the 5–10 year period before diagnosis. If the grief remains unacknowledged during their pre-transplantation period, their quality of life after transplantation may well be diminished by further illness or signs of stress. The loss of their health and the possible loss of their life may have activated some of the unresolved issues from the past and bereavement counselling may be helpful. Many of these patients are "type C" personalities; it is helpful to recognise their tendency to subordinate their own needs, and their own needs to "bottle" feelings or to comply with perceived expectations. Where pre-transplantation counselling can begin this process, recovery post-transplantation is enhanced.

Following fulminant hepatic failure

It is noticeable that patients who have little opportunity to prepare for transplantation, and thus to work through the implications of organ donation and terminal illness, have more difficulties with psychological adjustment during the postoperative period. This may or may not be reflected in physical problems. In addition, these patients are more likely to experience a psychotic episode immediately after the transplantation; some of them continue to suffer nightmares or flash-backs for several months afterwards. It is therefore very important to give them opportunities to acknowledge and work through their feelings – for example, anxieties about organ donation, feelings of unworthiness, identification with the grief of the death of the donor's family, disbelief that death could have been so near, confusion and anxiety about "lost days", mortification about reported or remembered behaviour while confused, insecurity about relationships, or anxiety about the future. Lack of preparation also means that, unlike the chronically ill patients, there has been no opportunity to build up trusting relationships with hospital staff. If physical recovery is without complication, the period of hospitalisation may be comparatively short; there is thus an even greater need for such patients to have appropriate help.

Patients whose liver failure arose as a result of paracetamol (aceteminophen) overdose will need particular care. Not only is it necessary for them to adjust to transplantation and its aftermath, but also to adjust to the feelings of guilt, inadequacy, or depression. If the precipitating crisis remains unresolved, it is important to help the patient to discover more appropriate resources, both internal and external.

Similarly, the families and friends of patients with acute liver failure need special help. They have no preparation, they are likely to have undergone trauma and to be exhausted, and thus the task of caring for a discharged patient can arouse extra anxieties. If they are also coming to terms with an attempted overdose, there is an added pressure. These relatives may need as much help as the patient in coming to terms with a mixture of guilt, shame, fear, anger, and anxiety for the future.

Conclusions

The return to an acceptable quality of life will be a different process based on different criteria for each patient. It is therefore misleading to attempt to define its nature, or the stages by which it may be reached, too closely. It is the patient's own evaluation that is significant; it is thus essential that patients are given sufficient opportunity to express their anxieties and acknowledge their feelings so that confidence and self-esteem can be restored. They have received a new life through their liver transplant; it is a new life which carries no guarantees and which will have had significant and permanent implications not only for them but for all who are close to them. If medical staff and others caring for them are aware of these wider dimensions, they are more likely to contribute to the enhancement of its quality.

Follow up

The follow up arrangements will vary from centre to centre. The frequency of follow up appointments will depend on a number of factors including the time after transplantation, the normality of liver function and geographical factors. Because of the need for centralisation of liver transplant services, many patients will live some distance away from transplant centres and, therefore, shared care will be necessary. The crux of good patient management is close liaison between the transplant centre and the attending physician.

When complications develop, it is crucial that the transplant team is contacted; although allograft recipients are always at risk of general infections, and other ailments that affect the normal population, there may be additional problems consequent on the procedure itself or its treatment. Furthermore, the normal patterns of illnesses and especially infections may be masked by immunosuppressive treatment. Whether or not patients need to be referred back to the transplant centre will depend on the local prevailing conditions.

Diet

Patients should be encouraged to eat a normal and well balanced diet. Although some are reluctant to change ingrained habits of avoiding fat, salt, or protein, it must be emphasised that, with normal liver function, they should maintain a normal diet.

However, obesity represents a significant problem in patients post-transplantation, with weight gain of over 10 kg being reported by up to 30% of patients. The reasons for this weight gain are probably multi-factorial and relate to the increased nutrition after receipt of the transplant, increased absorption, lack of dietary restrictions, and the use of corticosteroids. In general, the weight tends to fall after two years, but in the interim only dietary advice is indicated.

Alcohol

Few data exist on which to base sound advice about the resumption of alcohol consumption. It is our practice to advise patients that they can return to alcohol consumption when liver tests have returned to normal, but the conventional guidelines should be adopted in that men should consume less than 21 units per week and women less than 14 units. It is important that excess alcohol intake be avoided, not only to protect the graft but also to avoid fluctuations in cyclosporin A (cyclosporine) levels, affected by the enzyme inducing effects of alcohol.

For patients who undergo transplantation for alcoholic liver disease, most centres advise complete abstinence. However, in rare circumstances, if the patient can control alcohol intake and has no history of abusive dependence, it may be possible to advise a limited intake. The effect of alcohol use on the post-transplantation period by a previously alcohol dependent patient who is on subsequent re-transplantation for graft failure remains controversial, even when graft failure is unrelated to alcohol. In many programmes, these patients will be denied a second transplant. (See the section at the end of the chapter on psychiatric evaluation post-transplantation.)

Sexual activity

In general, there should be no restrictions placed on when the patient resumes normal sexual activity. It is suggested that the women avoid pregnancy until after the first year; contraceptive advice is given elsewhere (p 307–8, 322–3).

Sport

A return to sporting activity should be encouraged once the patient has made a good physical recovery and the scar is well healed. Resumption of sporting activity should be gradual. Contact sports, such as boxing, should be avoided.

Work patterns

The date of return to work will depend on many factors including the nature of the work involved and the motivation of patients. Patients themselves will normally be aware when they are fit enough to return to work. In general, in the Birmingham experience, patients return to work between 3 and 12 months after transplantation. There are no specific contraindications to any particular types of work although clearly commonsense must be used.

Travel

Many patients wish, after transplantation, to take a well deserved holiday and this should be encouraged. In the first year, travel too far from a recognised transplant centre is probably inadvisable but, thereafter, the need to allow patients to run their lives as they wish must be balanced against the problems of complications when they are remote from sophisticated medical help. In general, commonsense should prevail.

Advice must be given to the patient about arranging adequate insurance cover and it should be emphasised that it is necessary to make sure the insurance company is informed that the patient has received a liver transplant.

Advice to patients

- The patient must take adequate amounts of immunosuppressive agents with him or her
- Details of storage of cyclosporin A and other drugs are given in the relevant sections
- In general patients should ensure that the medication is carried in hand luggage. A medical letter will often ease any problems at Customs
- Advice on diarrhoea and vomiting: patients should be advised that if they develop diarrhoea or vomiting, the dose of immunosuppressive agent should be doubled until the symptom settles. If vomiting persists for more than 24 hours then medical help should be sought urgently

---

PSYCHIATRIC EVALUATION OF LIVER TRANSPLANT RECIPIENTS

THOMAS BERESFORD, ROBERT HOUSE

Psychiatric disorders

Delirium post-transplantation has been reported as the most common psychiatric complication in transplant recipients.[2,3] Usually it is self-limiting and can be traced to metabolic disturbances such as infection, cytomegalovirus, rejection, or adverse drug reaction (Table I). Sleep deprivation and cerebral oedema secondary to hepatic insufficiency must also be considered.[4] Correction of the underlying problem will bring about resolution of the delirium. Haloperidol or other anti-psychotic medicines may be used to treat the agitation that often accompanies delirium. These agents are specific for the disturbances of thought and perception characteristic of delirium, and offer patients considerable relief from hallucinations, delusions, and other such symptoms. Advantages include few side effects and multiple routes of administration. In addition to the use of medication, the patient must be protected from harm to self or others. This may require the use of restraints and one-to-one nursing care.

Depression is not uncommon soon after transplantaton. Often this occurs as the dose of steroids is decreased and may be short-lived. Survivor guilt, difficulty assimilating someone else's liver, and the advent of postoperative complications may lead to episodes of depression. Weight gain, hirsutism, acne, and cushingnoid facies (moon faces) which are common side effects of cyclosporin A (cyclosporine) and steroids may also cause depression. When use of an antidepressant is indicated, dosages should start low and be increased every 3–5 days to reach a therapeutic level. With a healthy liver, patients generally tolerate standard therapeutic doses, so serum levels should be followed to prevent toxicity. The use of psychostimulants offers a safe, short term alternative when the traditional antidepressants are contraindicated. Stimulants usually act rapidly and may improve motivation, energy, appetite, sense of well-being, and mood. Treatment may be initiated with 5–10 mg methylphenidate each morning and increased by 5 mg daily up to 30–60 mg. The principal drawback in stimulant use is the acquisition of tolerance, thereby limiting effectiveness. At this time, no long

TABLE I—*Drugs used in transplantation*

Drug	Neuropsychiatric effects	Comments
Cyclosporin A (cyclosporine)	Anxiety, delirium, hallucinations, seizures, tremor, paraesthesiae, hirsutism	Nephrotoxic, hepatotoxic Cimetidine, ketaconazole, erythromycin, metoclopramide increase serum level Phenobarbitone (phenobarbital), phenytoin, rifampicin (rifampin), lower serum level Verapamil may potentiate Methods of assay controversial Intramuscular injection erratically absorbed
FK506	Anxiety, delirium, insomnia, tremor, paraesthesiae	Experimental; used mainly in liver transplantation
OKT3 (Muromonab-CD3)	Aseptic meningitis, seizures, tremors, malaise, photophobia	Monoclonal antibody Treatment of rejection eisodes Blocks T cell functions Serum levels available
Steroids	Delirium, euphoria, depression, mania, insomnia, tremors, irritability	Phenobarbitone may decrease serum level May increase metabolism of drugs by liver
Azathioprine	Meningitis type syndrome (rare)	May cause bone barrow suppression Use in transplantation less common
Antibiotic	Delirium, hallucinations, fear of impending death (usually at high doses)	Half-life depends on excretion mode
Antiviral	Delirium, irritability, topical hallucinations	
Antifungal	Depression, hallucinations	

term, placebo controlled studies offer guidance on the point and time limited use is probably the best course.

Anxiety is often seen in response to medications, as shown in Table I. In addition, anxiety often accompanies fears of rejection, liver biopsies, and any change in the patient's health. As the patient nears discharge, anxiety may again occur as the patient worries about leaving the security of the hospital and the immediate availability of medical help. For mild anxiety, relaxation techniques, imaging, or biofeedback may be helpful. For those with more severe anxiety, benzodiazepines or low dose neuroleptics may be useful.

Postoperative adjustment can be a complicated process. Following discharge most patients do well. However, during this period several problems may arise. Fears of rejection and infection may last for a long time. Sexual concerns include issues of attractiveness, fear of damage to the transplanted organ, and performance anxiety. Sexual functioning must be specifically asked about during follow up visits. Changes in family dynamics may also be problematic. Before transplantation, the patient's family is often preparing for death and now must reintegrate the patient into the family. Re-establishing a new equilibrium may be difficult and may require couples of family psychotherapy.

Outcome for alcohol dependent allograft recipients

To date, survival studies from different centres providing liver transplantation to people with alcohol dependence have noted identical survival rates among alcoholic and non-alcoholic liver allograft recipients.[5-7] The more serious question has been to assess the occurrence of abstinence in the alcholic group post-transplantation. Recently a one year follow up was reported at Colorado, comparing alcoholic and non-alcoholic subjects; it was found that the rate of alcohol use was identical between the two.[8] The overall rate of return to any drinking among the alcoholic subjects was about 90%. Preliminary data of a sample of 38 alcohol dependent patients followed for three years suggest that Beresford's rate is likely to drop to approximately 74% in the second and third years. In this series, approximately 10% returned to drinking that required further hospitalisation either for graft rejection or for some intercurrent illness caused by drinking, such as pancreatitis or alcohol withdrawal. In the two cases in which graft rejection was a factor, both patients had returned to drinking and had not taken their immunosuppressive regimen properly. One of the patients died and the second suffered irreparable liver damage.

In the main, however, these preliminary data suggest that there is a high probability of continued abstinence in this highly selected group of transplant recipients. Outcome studies of alcoholism treatment suggest that a 50% one year abstinence rate is a remarkable feat, with the average more often being in the 30–40% range. Studies proceeding beyond two years suggest that a 30% abstinence rate is a very optimistic result.[9] If the preliminary data from Colorado for alcohol dependent, liver allograft recipients can be corroborated by other studies, it may transpire that highly selected cases in this setting can double the characteristic abstinence rates. A definitive study on this topic must be carried out to verify and improve upon both selection procedures pre-transplantation and continued surveillance and support of the abstinent patient post-transplantation.

References

1 Kuchler T, Kober B, Broelsch C, Henne-Bruns D, Kremer B. Quality of life after liver transplantation: can a psychosocial support program help? *Transplant Proc* 1991; **23**: 1541–4.
2 Freeman AM, Watts D, Karp R. Evaluation of cardiac transplant candidates: preliminary observations. *Psychosomatics* 1984; **25**: 197–207.
3 Freeman AM, Folks DG, Sokol RS, *et al*. Cardiac transplantation: clinical correlates of psychiatric outcome. *Psychosomatics* 1988; **29**: 47–54.
4 Surman O. Liver transplantation. In: Craven J, Rodin GM, eds. *Psychiatric Aspects of Organ Transplantation*. New York: Oxford Medical Publications, 1992: 177–88.
5 Kumar S, Stauber RE, Gavaler JS, *et al*. Orthotopic liver transplantation for alcoholic liver disease. *Hepatology* 1990; **11**: 159–64.
6 Lucey MR, Merion RM, Henley KS, *et al*. Selection for and outcome of liver transplantation in alcoholic liver disease. *Gastroenterology* 1992; **102**: 1736–41.
7 Bird GL, O'Grady JG, Harvey FA, Calne RY, Williams R. Liver transplantation in patients with alcoholic cirrhosis: selection criteria and rates of survival and relapse. *BMJ* 1990; **301**: 15–17.
8 Beresford TP, Schwartz J, Wilson D, Merion M, Lucey MR. The short-term psychological health of alcoholic and non-alcoholic liver transplant recipients. *Alcoholism: Clinical and Experimental Research* 1992; **16**: 996–1000.
9 Vaillant GE. *The Natural History of Alcoholism*. Cambridge, MA: Harvard University Press.

15: Histological findings in long term survivors following liver transplantation

S G HUBSCHER

With improved survival following liver transplantation, there is increased interest in long term histological changes occurring in the liver allograft. Policies vary regarding histological monitoring of grafts after the early postoperative period. In centres where this is done routinely, histological abnormalities are frequently detected.[1-3] The aetiology, clinical significance, and natural history of the often minor histological abnormalities that are seen in long term survivors following transplantation are largely unknown.

In the Birmingham programme, liver biopsy is obtained as part of an annual review, the main components of which are summarised in Table I. In a recent review of 353 biopsies obtained from 188 patients more than 12 months post-transplantation, only 7% were considered to be completely normal (Table II).[3] The remainder can be divided into seven main categories which are described further below. Subdivisions between the individual categories are sometimes blurred and some cases have overlapping features. It should be emphasised that the majority of these long term biopsies are obtained from patients who are clinically well with normal or near normal biochemistry.

Non-specific inflammation

Histology

There is mild, patchy portal and/or parenchymal inflammation (Figure 1). Portal inflammation is not associated with inflammatory

292

TABLE I—*Clinical assessments, laboratory investigations, and radiology carried out at annual review on patients surviving long term following liver transplantation**

Assessment	Test
Clinical	History and physical examination
Haematology	Full blood count, clotting profile
Biochemistry	Liver function tests (aspartate transaminase, alkaline phosphatase, bilirubin), albumin, globulin, creatinine clearance
Serology	Autoantibodies, serum immunoglobulins viral hepatitis screening
Radiology	Ultrasonography of liver and biliary tree
Histology	Liver biopsy

* Individual tests vary according to the clinical status at the time of assessment and the original disease for which transplantation was carried out.

TABLE II—*Histological diagnoses in 353 biopsies obtained from 188 patients more than 12 months post-transplantation*

Histological diagnosis	Biopsies		Patients	
	No.	(%)	No.	(%)
Normal	25	(7)	22	(12)
Non-specific inflammation	140	(40)	97	(51)
Chronic hepatitis	97	(28)	73	(39)
Biliary obstruction	37	(10)	22	(12)
Recurrent primary biliary cirrhosis	16	(5)	13	(16)*
Rejection ("acute" – 3, "chronic" – 9)	12	(3)	8	(4)
Recurrent hepatitis B	11	(3)	4	(2)
Other	15	(4)	14	(7)
Total	353	(100)	188†	(100)

In cases where more than one of the above patterns was present, only the main histological diagnosis is included.

* 13 out of 83 patients receiving transplants for primary biliary cirrhosis = 16%.

† A total of 253 diagnoses was made in the 188 patients. Several patients had more than one biopsy, in which different histological changes were observed.

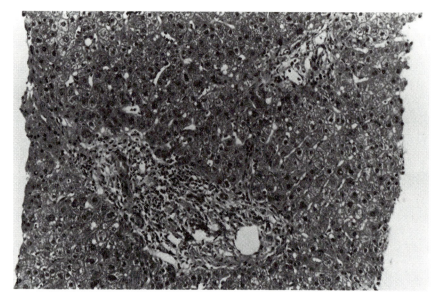

FIG 1—*Mild non-specific inflammation in liver allograft: needle biopsy, 12 months post-transplantation. One portal tract contains a light infiltrate of mononuclear inflammatory cells. Another portal tract (top right) appears normal. (Haematoxylin and eosin; magnification × 120.) (In this figure and all the figures, the original magnification is stated, but there has been a reduction to two-thirds the size in reproduction)*

spillover or fibrosis; parenchymal inflammation is not accompanied by conspicuous hepatocyte damage. Histological changes may resemble those otherwise described as non-specific "reactive" hepatitis or, when portal inflammation predominates, chronic persistent hepatitis.

Aetiology

The aetiology is unknown.

Clinical/biochemical changes

Almost all of these patients are clinically well, and most have normal or near normal biochemistry. Minor elevations of transaminases are sometimes found.

Chronic hepatitis

Histology

This is characterised by predominantly portal inflammation, which is more dense and diffuse than in non-specific inflammation,

294

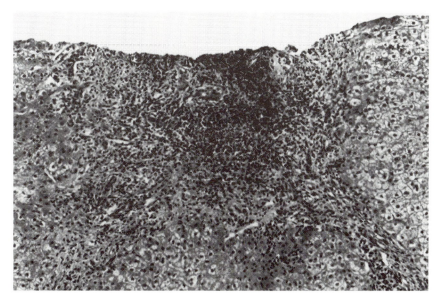

FIG 2—*Chronic hepatitis in liver allograft: needle biopsy, 2 years post-transplantation. Portal tract shows fibrous expansion and contains a dense lymphocytic infiltrate. There are several foci of inflammatory spillover into periportal regions. (Haematoxylin and eosin; magnification × 120)*

with periportal spillover also present. Piecemeal necrosis may be conspicuous in more severe cases (Figure 2).

Parenchymal inflammation is also frequently present. This tends to be most marked in perivenular areas and is often associated with small areas of confluent necrosis (Figure 3). In more severe cases there may be bridging necrosis and, rarely, areas of panacinar necrosis.

Minor degrees of fibrosis are common but severe fibrosis is rare, even in cases where chronic hepatitis has been present on several occasions over a period of years. Occasional cases have developed progressive fibrosis with features suggestive of macronodular cirrhosis (Figure 4).

Most cases of chronic hepatitis are graded as "mild" in terms of inflammatory activity. Distinction between milder forms of chronic hepatitis and non-specific inflammation is difficult. This is in keeping with recent concepts about the classification of chronic hepatitis in a liver that has not undergone transplantation.[4]

Fluctuating levels of inflammatory activity are often seen in serial biopsies from individual patients. Thus, for example, a biopsy 12

295

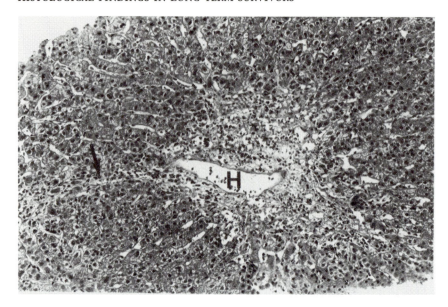

FIG 3—*Chronic hepatitis in liver allograft: needle biopsy, 3 years post-transplantation. Parenchymal inflammation and lytic necrosis are present in a perivenular area. There is a narrow zone of early bridging necrosis (arrowed) extending to an adjacent perivenular region. H = hepatic venule. (Haematoxylin and eosin; magnification × 120)*

months post-transplantation, graded as chronic hepatitis (mild), may be followed by another 24 month post-transplantation biopsy classified as non-specific inflammation; a third, 36 month post-transplantation biopsy could show features of chronic hepatitis (moderate).

Aetiology

Many factors may be implicated in the syndrome of chronic hepatitis, following liver transplantation. A detailed discussion of these is beyond the scope of this chapter. However, some of the main possible causes are listed below.

Hepatitis C

Hepatitis C is increasingly implicated as a cause of chronic hepatitis, either as recurrent disease (see Chapter 13) or de novo

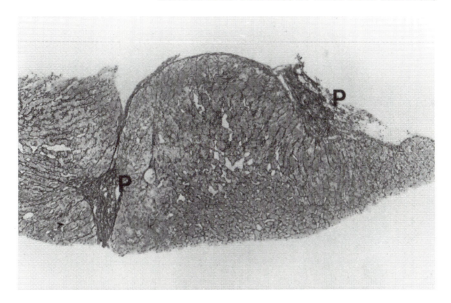

FIG 4—*Chronic hepatitis (quiescent) in liver allograft with probable macronodular cirrhosis: needle biopsy, 4 years post-transplantation. Portal tracts (P) contain a light infiltrate of inflammatory cells without spillover into the liver parenchyma. The presence of septum formation along the top edge of the biopsy is suggestive of cirrhosis. (Reticulin; magnification ×60)*

infection. The latter could be related to transmission by blood products or latent infection in the donor liver.

Hepatitis B

Hepatitis B virus (HBV) infection may also be associated with acute and chronic hepatitis (see Chapter 4). Recurrent HBV infection is associated with characteristic histological and immunohistochemical findings, as well as serological changes, which enable a diagnosis to be readily made. Rapid progression to a distinctive form of "post-necrotic" cirrhosis occurs in some cases.[5]

"Non-A, non-B, non-C" hepatitis

A higher incidence of chronic hepatitis has been observed in patients initially receiving a transplant for fulminant "non-A, non-B, non-C" hepatitis than in those receiving a transplant for other diseases.[2] In the absence of a demonstrable infective agent the mechanism for chronic hepatitis in these patients is uncertain.

297

Autoimmune chronic hepatitis

A small number of patients receiving a transplant for autoimmune chronic active hepatitis have developed histological features of chronic hepatitis in the liver allograft, with serological changes suggesting recurrent disease (see Chapter 13).

Unknown

For the great majority of patients in the programme at Birmingham with chronic hepatitis post-transplantation, none of the above factors can be implicated.

Clinical/biochemical changes

Most patients are clinically well, even those with quite marked histological abnormalities, and most have normal or near normal biochemistry. Elevated serum transaminases, usually no more than twice the upper limit of normal, are present in approximately 40% of cases.

Occasionally patients with chronic hepatitis have subsequently developed fulminant hepatitis associated with submassive necrosis resulting in graft failure (Figure 5).

Biliary disease

Histology

The usual features are those of low grade biliary obstruction, characterised by periportal fibrosis and marginal ductular proliferation (Figure 6). Cholestasis is generally mild or absent. Deposition of copper-associated protein is commonly observed in periportal hepatocytes, indicative of chronic cholestasis. Occasional cases have developed progressive portal fibrosis culminating in an early micronodular cirrhosis (Figure 7).

Aetiology

Ischaemia/technical problems

These account for most cases, resulting in strictures either at the biliary anastomosis or in the donor biliary tree. Factors implicated in

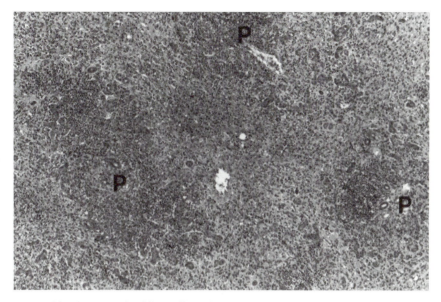

FIG 5—*Massive necrosis of liver allograft (?recurrent disease): section of hepatectomy specimen obtained 42 months following initial transplantation for fulminant non-A, non-B, non-C hepatitis. The liver was shrunken, weight 750 g. Histological examination shows severe hepatitis with panacinar necrosis. Surviving portal tracts (P) are surrounded by zones of ductular proliferation. Appearances are the same as those seen in the original hepatectomy specimen. (Haematoxylin and eosin; magnification × 75)*

the pathogenesis of biliary strictures include hepatic artery thrombosis, ABO incompatibility, prolonged cold ischaemia, and the obliterative arteriopathy that occurs in chronic rejection.[6] A higher incidence has been noted in paediatric patients, presumably due to the small sizes of vessels and ducts.

Recurrent primary biliary cirrhosis

Primary biliary cirrhosis (PBC) is also associated with features of biliary obstruction which develop as the disease progresses. Ductopenia and inflammatory (granulomatous) bile duct lesions, which are present in PBC, but not "pure" biliary obstruction, enable a diagnosis of recurrent PBC to be made.[3]

Recurrent primary sclerosing cholangitis

A higher incidence of biliary complications is present in patients receiving transplants for primary sclerosing cholangitis (PSC). This

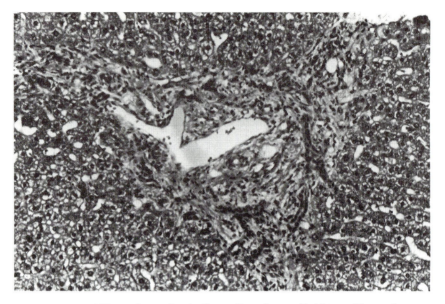

FIG 6—*Chronic biliary obstruction in liver allograft: needle biopsy, 13 months post-transplantation. Portal tract shows fibrous expansion with prominent marginal ductular proliferation. There is a light inflammatory infiltrate including several polymorphs. Small amounts of copper-associated protein were also deposited in periportal hepatocytes. A biliary problem was not suspected clinically at the time of biopsy, but was subsequently confirmed radiologically. (Haematoxylin and eosin; magnification × 120)*

may be related to the use of Roux anastomoses in these cases. In some cases periductal fibrosis and nodular scars have been observed – features typical of PSC[7] (Figure 8).

Clinical/biochemical changes

Many are asymptomatic at the time of biopsy. The "late" presentation and lack of clinical symptoms are probably manifestations of relatively mild disease. Cases with more severe biliary complications usually present within the first few months following transplantation. Most cases diagnosed histologically have cholestatic biochemistry (usually mild) and biliary problems are subsequently confirmed by radiology (ultrasonography with or without endoscopic retrograde cholangiopancreaticography). Occasional cases have become clinically jaundiced and some have developed signs of portal hypertension in association with progressive portal fibrosis. Corrective surgery may be required for cases in which biochemical and histological changes persist or progress.

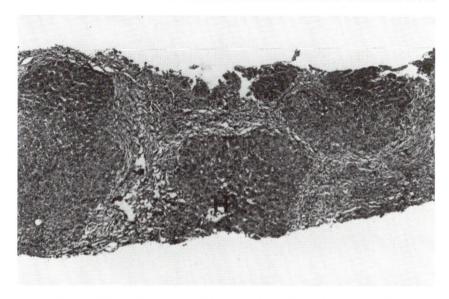

FIG 7—*Chronic biliary obstruction with early micronodular cirrhosis: needle biopsy, obtained 3 years post-transplantation during surgical reconstruction of biliary anastomosis. Histological examination shows periportal and bridging fibrosis with nodule formation. Occasional normally positioned hepatic venules (H) can still be seen. (Haematoxylin and eosin; magnification × 50)*

Recurrent primary biliary cirrhosis

Approximately 15% of PBC patients who are biopsied more than 12 months post-transplantation have histological features suggestive of recurrent disease.[3] Most have features of early disease and are clinically well with normal or mildly cholestatic biochemistry. The question of whether PBC recurs following liver transplantation remains controversial and is discussed further elsewhere in this book (see Chapter 13).

Rejection

Although rejection can occur any time after liver transplantation, it is an uncommon diagnosis more than 12 months post-transplantation, even in cases where immunosuppression is reduced. This may be a manifestation of "immune tolerance".[8]

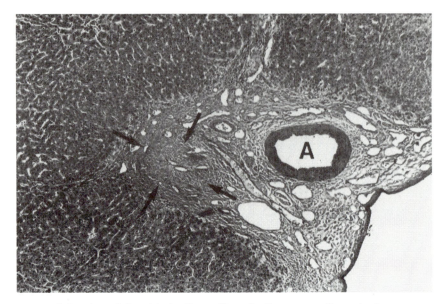

FIG 8—*Sclerosing cholangitis in liver allograft (?recurrent disease): hepatectomy specimen obtained at re-transplantation 44 months following initial transplantation for primary sclerosing cholangitis (PSC). Medium sized portal tract contains an artery (A) without an accompanying bile duct. In its place there is a nodular scar (outlines arrowed), typical of PSC. (Haematoxylin and eosin; magnification × 50)*

Two main patterns of rejection are recognised after the immediate postoperative period: "acute" and "chronic".[9] Both of these may occasionally be seen in "late" post-transplantation biopsies.

Acute ("cellular", "reversible") rejection

The classic triad of portal inflammation, bile duct damage, and venous endothelial inflammation is rarely seen more than a few weeks post-transplantation. Occasional cases have been observed more than 12 months post-transplantation, usually when immuno-suppression has been reduced as a result of, for instance, non-compliance or intercurrent disease.

Distinction from other causes of portal infiltrates (especially chronic hepatitis) may be difficult. Features favouring a diagnosis of

302

TABLE III—*Histological features distinguishing "acute" rejection from chronic hepatitis in biopsies taken late post-transplantation*

Feature	Acute cellular rejection	Chronic hepatitis
Portal tracts		
Inflammation	Mixed (lymphocytes, polymorphs, eosinophils, monocytes)	Mainly mononuclear (lymphocytes, plasma cells)
	Little spillover	Variable spillover ± piecemeal necrosis
Duct damage	Conspicuous	Usually mild
	Polymorphs + +	Mainly lymphocytes
Endothelial inflammation	Prominent	Absent or mild
Fibrosis	Absent	Variable, generally mild
Parenchyma		
Cholestasis	Usual	Unusual
	Can be marked	Mild
Inflammation	Absent or mild	Common (may be associated with confluent or bridging necrosis)

acute rejection versus chronic hepatitis are summarised in Table III.

Chronic ("ductopenic", "vascular", "irreversible") rejection

The two main diagnostic features of chronic rejection are progressive loss of intrahepatic bile ducts ("vanishing bile duct syndrome") and an obliterative vasculopathy affecting large and medium-sized arteries.[10] Secondary parenchymal changes of perivenular cholestasis and hepatocyte dropout are also present.

In the programme at Birmingham, changes of chronic rejection have very rarely occurred as a de novo phenomenon more than 12 months post-transplantation. Other centres, particularly in the USA, report "late" chronic rejection as a more common occurrence. Problems with the diagnosis of "late" chronic ductopenic rejection include a more insidious presentation and a tendency to coexist with other "late" patterns of graft damage, especially chronic hepatitis. In some cases, chronic hepatitis may evolve into chronic rejection.

Recurrent hepatitis B

This is discussed briefly in the section on chronic hepatitis above and is also considered separately in Chapter 13 in the section on recurrent disease.

Miscellaneous other findings

Many biopsies have other histological abnormalities, usually minor. These usually coexist with one of the main patterns described above, but may occasionally occur in isolation. A detailed description is not appropriate here but some of the minor changes seen are summarised below.

Unexplained ductopenia

A small number of long term post-transplantation biopsies have shown a paucity of bile ducts, sometimes as an isolated finding without any accompanying abnormalities. Some of these have been present in patients who previously had other histological and biochemical features of chronic (ductopenic) rejection, but in whom these other changes have subsequently resolved.[11]

Granulomata

Portal granulomata have only been observed in patients undergoing transplantation for PBC and are regarded as a manifestation of recurrent disease. Parenchymal granulomata, microgranulomata, have been observed in PBC patients, but also in other cases where their significance is uncertain.

Cholestasis, fatty change, siderosis

Minor degrees of cholestasis (usually perivenular), fatty change (usually macrovesicular), and siderosis are commonly observed in post-transplantation biopsies. The aetiology of these late changes is often uncertain.

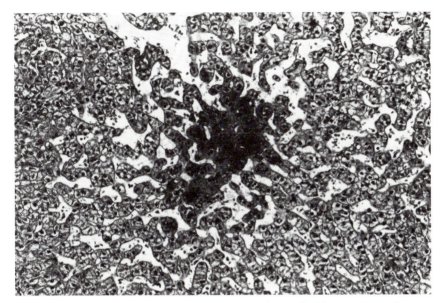

FIG 9—*Venous outflow obstruction in liver allograft: needle biopsy, 12 months post-transplantation from an asymptomatic patient. Perivenular area shows sinusoidal dilatation and congestion with closely packed erythrocytes present within liver cell plates. Phlebography subsequently demonstrated a narrowing at the caval anastomosis. (Haematoxylin and eosin; magnification × 120)*

Venous outflow obstruction

Occasionally, patients have had biopsies showing histological features of venous outflow obstruction (Figure 9). Although asymptomatic at the time, subsequent radiological investigations showed obstructive lesions in the vena cava, or hepatic veins. Features of veno-occlusive disease, possibly related to azathioprine, occur rarely and can resolve spontaneously.[12]

Conclusion

In summary, the great majority of liver allografts biopsied more than 12 months post-transplantation show histological abnormalities. The underlying aetiology is frequently uncertain. In some cases histological investigations may identify important causes of graft dysfunction (such as biliary or venous outflow obstruction) before these have become clinically evident. In other cases, minor

305

abnormalities progress, over a period of years, to life threatening complications such as cirrhosis or submassive necrosis. Some of these may result in regrafting. However, in most cases, histological changes are present in patients who are clinically well with normal or near normal biochemistry, and do not appear to have an adverse effect on graft survival. Most of the patients who have been monitored in this manner are still less than five years post-transplantation and it will clearly be important to determine the natural history of the predominantly minor changes documented so far.

References

1 Nakhleh RE, Schwarzenberg SJ, Bloomer J, Payne W, Snover DC. The pathology of liver allografts surviving longer than one year. *Hepatology* 1990; **11**: 465–70.
2 Hubscher SG. Chronic hepatitis in liver allografts. *Hepatology* 1990; **12**: 1257–58.
3 Hubscher SG, Elias E, Buckels JAC, Mayer AD, McMaster P, Neuberger JM. Primary biliary cirrhosis: histological evidence for disease recurrence after liver transplantation. *J Hepatol* 1993; **18**: 173–84.
4 Scheuer PJ. Classification of chronic viral hepatitis: a need for re-assessment. *J Hepatol* 1991; **13**: 372–4.
5 Harrison RF, Davies M, Goldin RD, Hubscher SG. Recurrent hepatitis B in liver allografts: a distinctive form of rapidly developing cirrhosis. *Histopathology* 1993; in press.
6 Sanchez-Urdazapal L, Gores GJ, Ward EM, *et al.* Ischaemic-type biliary complications after orthotopic liver transplantation. *Hepatology* 1992; **16**: 49–53.
7 Harrison RF, Hubscher SG. Sclerosing cholangitis in liver allografts: a histological perspective. *J Pathol* 1992; **167**: 150A.
8 Starzl TE, Demetris AJ, Murase N, Ildstad S, Ricordi C, Trucco M. Cell migration, chimerism and graft acceptance. *Lancet* 1992; **339**: 1579–82.
9 Hubscher SG. Histological findings in liver allograft rejection – new insights into the pathogenesis of hepatocellular damage in liver allografts. *Histopathology* 1991; **18**: 377–83.
10 Hubscher SG, Neuberger JM. Chronic rejection. In: Neuberger JM, Adams DH eds. *Immunology of Liver Allograft Rejection*. London: Edward Arnold, 1993: 216–29.
11 Hubscher SG, Buckels JAC, Elias E. McMaster P, Neuberger JM. Vanishing bile duct syndrome after liver transplantation: is it reversible? *Transplantation* 1991; **51**: 1004–10.
12 Gare E, Ranage J, Poitmann B, Williams R. Nodular regenerative hyperplasia of the liver following liver transplantation. *Gut* 1993; **34**: 544.

16: Incidental problems in management of liver transplant recipients

KIMBERLY ANN BROWN, JOHN R LOWES,
DAVID MAYER

Reproductive health

Contraception

As long term survival improves, issues over quality of life after transplantation become increasingly important. In the USA from 1988 to 1990, women accounted for 47% of liver transplant recipients, among whom 68% were of potential child bearing age.[1] These young women will be faced with issues surrounding menstruation and pregnancy. Specific questions that need to be explored are the return of menses post-transplantation, the potential for fertility, the risk to the transplant of pregnancy, and vice versa, and finally the teratogenic risk of immunosuppression.

It is clear that many women awaiting transplantation have alterations in menstrual patterns. Cundy *et al.* reviewed 44 women undergoing liver transplantation because of end stage liver disease, acute liver failure, or malignancy.[2] Forty-eight per cent of premenopausal women without a history of hysterectomy were amenorrhoeic for longer than one year prior to transplantation. Menses resumed in all premenopausal women with secondary amenorrhea within 10 months of the transplant. DeKoning *et al.* described 31 women who had received a liver transplant.[3] In 17 patients who were premenopausal prior to transplantation, six had normal menses, five had irregular menses and six were amenorrhoeic. Post-transplantation, 13 of 17 regained a normal pattern of menses within 1–28 months (median 8 weeks). Two patients continued with irregular menses and two with secondary amenorrhoea. It is evident from these two studies that menstruation resumes in the majority of premenopausal women following liver transplantation, and that early resumption of menses is not unusual. Therefore, it is advisable that women begin using contraception as soon as sexual activity resumes if pregnancy is not desired. Given the increased risk of infection with immunosuppressive therapy, it is recommended that intrauterine devices are avoided in these patients. Oestrogens may induce cholestasis and views on the use of oral contraceptives vary. Some centres advise use of physical barriers such as condoms, contraceptive sponges, or diaphragms. If these are not acceptable, then the use of an oral contraceptive is justified and the woman is made aware of the theoretical potential complications of inducing cholestasis or vascular thromboses. Many centres do allow use of an oral contraceptive if liver tests are normal, except in those grafted for Budd–Chiari syndrome.

Pregnancy

Perhaps the most important of these issues facing young women following liver transplantation is that of pregnancy. Can these patients become pregnant and, if so, what are the additional risks the pregnancy poses to the transplant recipient? Seventeen patients in one series by Scantlebury et al.[4,5] and 20 additional patients have been reported in the world literature as having successful pregnancies after liver transplantation. The information in all cases is incomplete, but the overall conclusion is that, in general, patients did fairly well. Of 33 pregnancies reported, 17 of 33 underwent caesarean section, a rate higher than the 24% national average in the USA. Only one intrauterine death was reported. Complications included toxaemia, hypertension, anaemia, and intrauterine growth retardation. In the largest series by Scantlebury and colleagues, 6 of 17 patients developed hypertension requiring treatment during their pregnancy. Four of these had associated toxaemia requiring caesarean section. Six of 17 developed anaemia with two requiring transfusion. Of the published cases where data are available, 17 of 35 births were pre-term and 12 of 34 reported intrauterine growth retardation.

Intrauterine growth retardation has been associated with cyclosporin A (cyclosporine) use in renal transplant recipients and probably contributes to the increased incidence of hypertension observed in these patients. Despite the increased rate of pre-term births, only one infant in the Scantlebury series required mechanical ventilation. In addition, although the use of prednisone and azathioprine is associated with increased risk of infection, this was not observed in the published reports.

Patients transplanted for Budd–Chiari syndrome deserve special comment. These patients remain on anticoagulants post-transplantation. Because pregnancy may be thrombogenic, the team at Birmingham generally advise against pregnancy in this group.

In summary, liver transplant recipients appear to have somewhat higher risk pregnancies than otherwise normal women. It would be recommended that these patients are monitored closely with particular attention to hypertension, development of toxaemia, and anaemia. If cyclosporin A is part of their regimen, the lowest possible dose should be used with frequent ultrasonography to monitor intrauterine growth. Obviously, these reports are far from adequate to predict how any one individual would proceed with pregnancy following liver transplantation. They do, however, suggest that pregnancy and the successful delivery of a normal child are possible, and provide hope for those wishing to conceive.

The potential for fatherhood of male liver transplant recipients deserves mention, because such recipients may be concerned about the effects of long term immunosuppressive therapy on fertility and fetal outcome. However, there have been no reports on male liver transplant recipients fathering children, making extrapolation from data on male renal transplant recipients necessary – for example, Penn et al. reported on 60 live births born to 50 fathers who were renal graft recipients.[6] Two infants had congenital defects. The fertility of these renal patients on long term immunosuppression was not commented upon.

Little has been written about the risk that pregnancy offers to the graft itself. Scantlebury described alterations in liver function tests during 19 pregnancies after orthotopic liver transplantation. In the period ante partum, 7 of 19 had mild to moderate elevations in liver tests. One patient had acute rejection and one had chronic rejection documented by biopsy.[7] Post partum, 10 of 19 had moderate elevations in liver tests with three resolving spontaneously. Four were treated with corticosteroids. Of these, only one of the four responded promptly suggesting that the enzyme abnormalities may not have been due to rejection. All tests eventually resolved with the exception of one patient with chronic hepatitis B and one patient with chronic rejection. Based on this report, it appears that pregnancy placed no undue risk on the transplanted liver itself.

What is the risk of chronic immunosuppression to the fetus? Cyclosporin A is highly lipid soluble and extensively distributed in the body. Venkataramanan et al. measured cyclosporin A and its metabolites in cord blood, the placenta, and umbilical cord of a pregnant woman after liver transplantation.[7] Relatively high concentrations of cyclosporin A and some of the metabolites were found in cord blood, umbilical cord, and especially in the placenta. It appears that the fetus is exposed not only to cyclosporin A but also to its metabolites. There is little evidence to suggest that cyclosporin A is mutagenic in the Ames test and does not produce any chromosomal abnormalities in animals. Although controlled studies do not exist, cyclosporin A, azathioprine and prednisone have all been associated with intrauterine growth retardation. Reports of pregnancies following kidney and liver transplantation suggest that most of these infants exposed to immunosuppressive drugs in utero are normal. Experience with FK506 is limited and, at present, its use is not recommended in pregnancy or in those wishing to become pregnant. However, long term studies are necessary to evaluate potential long term side effects on the offspring, including progress and development as well as fertility. Nevertheless, patients should at a minimum undergo frequent examination of ultrasonography to monitor fetal growth and, if possible, an obstetrician with expertise in high risk delivery should be available for consultation.

Parenthood

Finally, transplant recipients contemplating parenthood must face the reality that their survival is likely to be shorter than for other parents their age. With a three year survival of 69%,[1] many potential parents must face the prospect of leaving children for their spouse to raise. With this in mind, it does appear that patients considering parenthood can be reassured that pregnancy and the successful birth of a healthy baby are very possible.

Summary

Females	
Menstruation	Returns in > 90% of premenopausal women
	Median time 2–3 months
Pregnancy	
Effects on graft	Little evidence of significant deterioration
	Mild to moderate increased liver function tests common
	Documented rejection uncommon
Risks to mother	Hypertension, toxaemia, anaemia increased
	Increased rate of caesarean section
Risks to fetus	Intrauterine growth retardation common
Males	No data on fertility
	Unclear risk of fetal abnormalities due to chronic immunosuppressive therapy

Immunisation

One of the most serious complications following liver transplantation is infection. Because these patients are immunosuppressed, otherwise routine illnesses can become life threatening. Therefore, it seems reasonable that, where possible, infection should be prevented through the use of available vaccines. Many factors influence patient's access to, receipt of, and response to, immunisation. Often, as a result of the severity of illness before transplantation, immunisation is felt to be dangerous. In other cases, physicians worry that the immune response may not be adequate due either to the severity of the underlying illness or to the immunosuppressive medications that the patient may be receiving. As such, too often these patients are neglected when it comes to immunisation. The following summary will attempt to provide some guidelines as to the timing and appropriateness of various vaccines in both adults and children awaiting and undergoing liver transplantation.

It might be anticipated that patients most likely to benefit from

311

immunisation would be those patients in whom the consequences of illness may be most dramatic. Usually, mild viral illnesses in the immunosuppressed host are devastating. Many patients coming to liver transplantation, especially children, have been inadequately immunised against the usual childhood viral and bacterial pathogens. Ginsberg et al.[8] assessed the immunisation status of all children with chronic liver disease referred over a two year period for transplantation to the Children's Medical Center in Dallas. One hundred children aged from 4 months to 16 years (median 34 months) were evaluated. Of these, 44 patients (44%) were inadequately immunised at the time of evaluation. Half had never received diphtheria, pertussis, tetanus, or oral polio virus vaccine. Only one of 21 children aged 15 months or older had received mumps, measles, and rubella (MMR) immunisation. None of the 14 patients who were eligible to receive immunisation against *Haemophilus influenzae* Pittman type b had been immunised. Infants had the highest rate of inadequate immunisation with only 22% aged less than six months being completely immunised as compared with 100% of those over 40 months. All these patients had received almost constant medical surveillance before referral; indeed, 22% of the children had never received any form of immunisation. Reasons for this included physicians telling parents that the child was too ill to be immunised, and fear that the potential febrile response may be difficult to distinguish from injection. None of these concerns warrants exclusion of these patients from adequate immunisation. Nevertheless, certain vaccines, in particular live virus vaccines, are contraindicated in patients receiving immunosuppressive medications. As such, patients requiring transplantation should be identified early and aggressively immunised so as not to miss the opportunity to protect patients from such infections both before and after transplantation. The following describes the safety and efficacy of various vaccines and guidelines for their use are provided in some tables.

Killed vaccines

In general, patients on immunosuppressive agents can safely be given denatured protein, carbohydrate, and killed virus vaccines. These include diphtheria, pertussis, tetanus (DPT), inactivated polio virus (IPV), and *Haemophilus influenzae* Pittman type b (Hib) (Table I). Patients on immunosuppressive therapy, before or after liver

TABLE I—*Childhood immunisation*

Vaccine	Type	Comments/Schedule
Diphtheria ⎱⎰ (DPT)	Toxoid	Safe before or after transplantation
Pertussis	Inactivated bacteria	Schedule: 2 months, 4 months, 6 months
Tetanus	Toxoid	18 months, 4–6 years
Haemophilus influenzae Pittman type b (Hib)	Bacterial polysaccharide conjugated to protein	Safe before or after transplantation Schedule: 2 months, 4 months, 6 months, 15 months
Oral polio vaccine (OPV)	Live virus	Unsafe post-transplantation and in patient siblings and contacts
Inactivated polio vaccine (IPV)	Inactivated virus	Safe before or after transplantation Schedule: 2 months, 4 months, 15 months, 4–6 years
Measles, mumps, rubella (MMR)	Live	Unsafe post-transplantation. Safe in siblings and contacts. If possible, give at age 15 months at least one month prior to transplantation
Heptavax	Recombinant	Safe Schedule: birth, 2 months, 9 months

Schedules are taken from Rudolph[10] and based on US Public Health Service recommendations.
For patients starting immunisation after infancy schedules are included in Rudolph.[10]

transplantation, should not be given live viral or bacterial vaccines; these include oral polio vaccine (OPV), measles, mumps, and rubella (MMR), yellow fever, or Bacillus Calmette–Guérin (BCG) because they are at risk of developing clinical disease from the attenuated bacterium or virus. As such, the American Academy of Pediatrics recommended that patients older than 12 months should have their serological titres against measles, mumps, and rubella measured. Those with negative titres should be given MMR vaccine, preferably

TABLE II—*Immunisation*

Vaccine	Comment
Pneumococcal	Safe
	Should be given after age 24 months
	May require re-immunisation
Influenza	Should be given on a yearly basis to patients
	before or after transplantation
Varicella-zoster	Live virus
	Cannot be given post-transplantation
	Not currently licensed for use in the USA
Cytomegalovirus	Live virus
	Investigational
Heptavax	Should be given to adults in a series of three
	injections one month apart

one month or more before transplantation.[9] Only inactivated polio vaccine (IPV) should be given to transplant recipients. Immunologically normal siblings and household contacts of patients receiving liver transplants should not receive live oral polio vaccine (OPV) because of the potential for shedding the virus and transmission to immunosuppressed siblings. However, siblings and household contacts may receive MMR vaccine and IPV because transmission of these viral vaccines does not occur.[10] Many patients presenting at older ages will have been inadequately immunised. Immunisation schedules for the general population should be followed, avoiding live viral vaccines after transplantation.[10]

Pneumococcal infection

Pneumococcal infections may present a serious threat both to paediatric and to adult transplant recipients. In general, patients either with chronic liver disease or after liver transplantation should receive the polyvalent vaccines if aged 24 months or older (Table II). Although patients with chronic liver disease have not been studied with regard to this vaccine, it is possible to derive several points from data concerning its use in renal transplant recipients. Linneman and colleagues studied 104 renal transplant recipients receiving long term prednisone and azathioprine, and 33 patients on haemodialysis.[11] All were given Pneumovax (a pneumococcal vaccine) and a positive response was defined as a 40% rise in serum antibody concentration.

Based on this definition, 91% of transplant recipients and 88% of dialysis patients were considered to be responders. Antibody levels after immunisation were lowest in patients immunised in the first six months following transplantation. Follow up of these patients over two years revealed a threefold decrease in antibody levels during this period, with greater decreases seen in the dialysis patients. More importantly, patients who were re-immunised had no serious reactions, and overall the rate of pneumococcal infections fell as they had after the original immunisation programme.[12] These data suggest that chronically ill patients and patients on immunosuppressive medications can and do respond to pneumococcal immunisation with a resultant decrease in serious infection. Antibody titres may fall more rapidly than in normal patients and re-immunisation may be required. At present, however, the exact timing is not well defined. Even so, it is recommended in many centres that all patients awaiting liver transplantation and those post-transplantation should receive Pneumovax as part of their medical care.

Influenza

Similarly, influenza infection in patients with end stage liver disease and in liver transplant recipients may cause significant morbidity and mortality. In these patients, routine annual influenza immunisation should be considered. Most reports in the literature have found impaired immunological responsiveness especially in renal allograft recipients given influenza vaccine. In some, this appeared to be related to poor graft function. None of the studies found any relation between impaired serum antibody responses to immunisation and the dose or duration of immunosuppressive therapy although one author suggested that cyclosporin A may impair antibody response more than azathioprine.[13] This author evaluated 59 renal transplant recipients, 28 patients on dialysis, and 29 healthy volunteers. All were given influenza vaccine on day 0 with most patients receiving a booster on day 30. No serious side effects from immunisation were noted. Mean titres were significantly lower in the cyclosporin A treated patients as compared to either patients receiving azathioprine or controls, and no difference was observed in the azathioprine treated patients as compared to controls. Booster immunisation appeared beneficial only in the haemodialysis group. Despite the fact that the vast majority of patients receiving liver transplants are on cyclosporin A, and given the few data available and the potential serious consequences of influenza in this population, yearly immunisation with influenza vaccine is recommended.

Hepatitis B

Hepatitis B is yet another virus that may pose a threat to certain transplant recipients, in particular those with sexual exposure or health care workers. Clearance of hepatitis B is very poor in the liver transplant. Active immunisation with hepatitis B is highly effective in most normal individuals. The ability of active immunisation to elicit an antibody response in patients with chronic liver disease and to protect against hepatitis B has been studied. Van Thiel et al. evaluated 144 patients awaiting liver transplantation[14] who received Heptavax once a month for a total of three injections. Antibody response in these patients was significantly lower than in controls (44–53% compared with 93%). No difference was found between patients completing their immunisation course either before or after transplantation. Sokal found a higher response in 30 children with extrahepatic atresia before and after transplantation.[15] Protection against hepatitis B was observed in 73% of children before transplantation. This was 55% in children immunised after transplantation. Carey found that only 20% of adults awaiting liver transplantation mounted a significant antibody response to Heptavax.[16] In addition, rechallenging non-responders with three injections of double dose vaccine provided no additional benefit. Unfortunately, a cost–benefit ratio for the use of Heptavax in this population cannot be derived from these data. Given the potentially devastating effects of hepatitis B infection in liver transplant recipients, this group should receive the vaccine until more data are available.

Varicella-zoster

Varicella-zoster vaccine is a live attentuated virus vaccine. Its safety and efficacy in normal children have been established, and it is now generally used in Japan and Korea and used for immunocompromised patients in other countries. Broyer and Boudailliez established the efficacy of the vaccine in uraemic children awaiting renal transplantation in France.[17] Twenty of 23 seronegative uraemic children were able to seroconvert after receiving vaccine. Although antibody titres were low, the frequency of varicella-zoster and herpes zoster infections decreased dramatically in patients following the introduction of systemic varicella-zoster immunisation. As it is a live virus vaccine, its use post-transplantation is contraindicated. At present, the vaccine is not licensed for use in the USA.

Cytomegalovirus

Cytomegalovirus is often a devastating problem in patients post-transplantation and many agents have been used in an attempt to prevent or treat cytomegalovirus associated infection. Although immunisation with the vaccine has been shown to produce seroconversion in healthy subjects, and in most renal transplant recipients, clinical trials have not proved its benefit. At present, this vaccine should be considered investigational and patients should receive it only in the context of controlled trials.

In summary, infection is one of the most serious threats to patients following liver transplantation due primarily to depressed cell mediated immunity with immunosuppressive agents. Childhood viral illness, pneumococci, influenza, and hepatitis B all represent potentially avoidable threats through the use of immunisation. The most important point to make is the need for careful attention to these patients. Live virus vaccines should be given at appropriate ages prior to transplantation if possible, and all patients with end stage liver disease and post-transplantation should be immunised against these common pathogens. Other vaccines are documented in Box A.

Drug treatment of intercurrent disease

The treatment of intercurrent disease in a patient who had undergone liver transplantation needs to be considered carefully. The main problems relate to:

- Interactions with immunosuppressive agents
- The treatment of patients who are immunosuppressed
- The avoidance of hypotension.

Problems may also be encountered in the pharmacodynamics and pharmacokinetics of some drugs if patients either are temporarily

BOX A   Vaccines

Live attenuated vaccines

BCG	Poliomyelitis (OPV)
Measles	Typhoid (oral)
Mumps	Varicella-zoster
Rubella	Yellow fever

Inactivated vaccines, capsular antigens, toxoids

Anthrax	Japanese encephalitis
Cholera	Meningococcus
Diphtheria	Poliomyelitis (inactivated, IA)
Haemophilus influenzae	Pneumococci
Pittman type b (Hib)	Rabies
Hepatitis B	Tick borne encephalitis
Hepatitis A	Typhoid
Influenza	Whooping cough

undergoing external biliary drainage or are cholestatic as a result of the marked alteration in levels of drugs that are handled by the liver.

Many drugs alter the levels of cyclosporin A (cyclosporine) and FK506 by inducing or inhibiting metabolising enzymes, so dose monitoring of drug levels is required.

This section will consider the treatment of a range of common conditions affecting patients with liver allografts.

Headaches

Headaches are a side effect of cyclosporin A or FK506 therapy. If headaches occur with therapeutic cyclosporin A levels, then simple analgesics such as paracetamol (acetaminophen) up to 1 g six hourly may be given.

Migraine

Conventional anti-migraine therapy is rarely of value in treating migraine. There is little experience with the use of 5-hydroxytrypt-amine-1 agonists – for example, sumatriptan. Nifedipine or pro-

---

BOX B   Non-steroidal anti-inflammatory drugs

Non-steroidal anti-inflammatory drugs with lower incidence of side effects
 Ibuprofen
 Naproxen
 Diclofenac

Non-steroidal anti-inflammatory drugs to be avoided in liver transplant recipients
 Indomethacin
 Phenylbutazone

---

pranolol may be of value. In disabling cases it may be necessary to reduce the cyclosporin A dose which could result in sub-therapeutic levels. In this instance, alternative long term immunosuppression with corticosteroid therapy or other therapy must be introduced before cyclosporin A levels fall.

Hypertension

Hypertension may be primary or be a side effect of cyclosporin A or corticosteroid therapy. Sustained diastolic pressure of over 90–100 mm Hg should be treated depending on age. Nifedipine, nicardepine, and isradipine are employed as first line treatments. If these or other calcium channel antagonists are ineffective, then β-blockade with a cardioselective agent such as atenolol or metoprolol should be used.

Analgesia

Paracetamol can be used in standard doses following liver transplantation. The use of opiate analgesics, dihydrocodeine, buprenorphine, pethidine, or morphine, when indicated, need not be restricted in those with good liver function. Non-steroidal anti-inflammatory drugs should be used with caution and preferably for short duration. A list of suitable and unsuitable agents is given in Box B.

319

Infections

Bacterial infections

Chest infections Penicillin derivatives such as co-amoxiclav (amoxycillin + clavulanic acid) or cephalosporins are well tolerated in non-allergic individuals. In penicillin sensitive subjects, ciprofloxacin can be given although renal function should be monitored. Erythromycin will increase cyclosporin A levels. Intravenous co-trimoxazole (sulphamethoxazole + trimethoprim) may markedly reduce blood levels of cyclosporin A, but this has not been reported with oral administration.

Urinary tract infections Oral trimethoprim, co-trimoxazole, amoxycillin, or a cephalosporin may be usd for a community acquired urinary tract infection.

Urinary tract infections acquired in hospital are more likely to be caused by *Pseudomonas aeruginosa* and other multi-resistant organisms; antibiotic sensitivites are available to guide treatments. Gentamicin and other aminoglycosides should be avoided because of their nephrotoxicity.

Boils Staphylococcal skin infections should be treated with flucloxacillin. In penicillin sensitive individuals, erythromycin may have to be used, but cyclosporin A levels should be carefully monitored.

Infectious diarrhoea In addition to supportive treatment with oral (or intravenous) fluids, as clinically required, specific antibiotic treatment should be given to immunosuppressed patients who develop infectious diarrhoea. Stool cultures should be obtained in patients with bloody or chronic diarrhoea, diarrhoea associated with fever or systemic symptoms. Evidence of infection with *Clostridium difficile* and toxin production should be sought. If positive, then treatment with oral vancomycin should be given (500 mg daily for 7–10 days). Other specific infections should be treated according to the sensitivities of the organism concerned. Ciprofloxacin is effective against many pathogenic coliforms, and co-trimoxazole is effective in salmonellosis and shigellosis. Symptomatic campylobacter enteritis requires treatment with erythromycin, and, as indicated above, care with cyclosporin A levels is required.

Tuberculosis In many centres, patients of Asian or Afro-Caribbean origin, or those grafted for alcoholic liver disease, may receive anti-tuberculous prophylaxis while receiving immunosuppressive therapy. This therapy ceases 6–12 months after transplantation. Active tuber-culous infection in patients receiving immunosuppression carries a poor prognosis.

Prophylactic antibiotics

The use of prophylactic antibiotics for invasive procedures, such as dental surgery, varies between centres. At Birmingham, the practice is to use guidelines developed for some cardiac patients, advised by the British Society for Antimicrobial Chemotherapy. Thus, for adults, the advice at Birmingham is to give amoxycillin 3 g as a single oral dose 1 hour before the procedure (children 5–10 years, 1·5 g; children less than 5 years, 0·75 g). For patients who are sensitive to penicillin, clindamycin 600 mg is given orally 1 hour before and 6 hours after the procedure. An alternative of erythromycin stearate 1·5 g orally 1–2 hours before and 0·5 g 6 hours after the procedure can be used, but erythromycin can interact with cyclosporin A and FK506 metabolism.

For patients undergoing general anaesthesia who may require antibiotic prophylaxis, amoxycillin 1 g intramuscularly in 2·5 ml 1% lignocaine (lidocaine) should be given before induction, followed by 0·5 g amoxycillin orally 6 hours later. For patients who are penicillin sensitive, vancomycin 1 g by slow intravenous infusion (over 30 minutes), followed by intravenous gentamicin 120 mg, is suggested.

Liver biopsy

In the allograft, liver biopsy is a safe procedure, although in those with intrahepatic sepsis, or those with a Roux loop, liver biopsy may induce sepsis. For such patients, antibiotic prophylaxis is recommended.

Viral infections

Herpes simplex Herpes simplex infections of the mouth should be treated with acyclovir cream five times daily. Treatment should be started as soon as there is clinical suspicion of herpes simplex infection.

Herpes simplex keratitis should be treated with acyclovir ophthalmic ointment.

Herpes simplex encephalitis   Intravenous acyclovir should be administered if there is a clinical suspicion of herpes simplex encephalitis in a dose of 10 mg/kg every 8 hours for 10 days.

Varicella-zoster   This potentially lethal infection in immunocompromised individuals should be treated as soon as possible with intravenous acyclovir 10 mg/kg every 8 hours.

Infections caused by opportunist organisms

Pneumocystis carinii pneumonia   Infection with *Pneumocystis carinii* pneumonia (PCP) is rare unless high doses of immunosuppressive agents are employed and/or co-trimoxazole prophylaxis is omitted. Co-trimoxazole and pentamidine isethionate are effective. Specialist assistance should be sought in the management of this complication which should initially involve a significant reduction in immunosuppressive therapy.

Diabetes mellitus

Patients may have impaired glucose tolerance as a result of a variety of causes. Diabetes should be managed in a conventional manner with diet, oral hypoglycaemic agents (where available), or insulin if required.

Depression

A depressive illness is not uncommon after transplantation. Most patients recover spontaneously and may be helped by postoperative counselling. This is discussed elsewhere. A small number of patients require pharmacological intervention. In general, tricyclic antidepressants are safe to use, but mianserin is probably best avoided as it has been associated with bone marrow suppression.

Hormone replacement therapy

Menopausal symptoms should be treated with hormone replacement therapy (HRT) if required, and this can be either a combination of oestrogen and a progestogen or an oestrogen alone in those patients who have previously undergone hysterectomy. Progestogens may inhibit cyclosporin A metabolism leading to higher levels, but dosage adjustment is rarely required to cyclosporin A after the introduction of cyclical HRT.

Osteoporosis

This is difficult but not uncommon after transplantation, particularly in those women who received a transplant for chronic cholestatic liver disease. Cortiscosteroid therapy should be withdrawn as soon as is practicable and according to local protocols.

Established osteoporosis remains a difficult condition to reverse. Oral calcium, either alone or in conjunction with diphosphonates, may be beneficial, but there is little evidence of therapeutic benefit.

The use of drugs to treat specific intercurrent illnesses are discussed below in systems. The classification of the *British National Formulary* has been used.

Gastrointestinal drugs

Antacids

Antacids may be used for the symptomatic treatment of acid related disorders. Only if ascites is still a problem in the first few months after transplantation should low sodium compounds be used. Sodium bicarbonate tablets may be helpful in treating hyperkalaemia associated with cyclosporin A induced metabolic alkalosis.

Ulcer healing drugs

After liver transplantation, suppression of acid secretion is routinely employed for the first three months. Cimetidine may lead to a rise in cyclosporin A levels. Ranitidine, famotidine, nizatidine, and omeprazole do not affect cyclosporin A levels to any significant extent, and may be used to treat peptic ulceration and other acid related disorders as required. Sucralfate and tripotassium dicitratobismuthate may also be used. Omeprazole is particularly useful in treating reflux oesophagitis, but in view of its profound acid inhibitory properties it may predispose to oesophageal candidiasis. Colloidal bismuth should be avoided if there is nephrotoxicity.

Drugs used to treat inflammatory bowel disease

There are no specific contraindications to the use of standard drugs – aminosalicylates and corticosteroids – in the treatment of Crohn's disease and ulcerative colitis. Infective agents, especially *Clostridium difficile*, must be excluded as the cause of any relapse.

Additional systemic corticosteroids may be required to control inflammatory bowel disease.

Bile salts and chelating agents

Ursodeoxycholic acid may be used as a cholorrhetic agent in patients with biliary sludge or cholestasis post-transplantation but is of unproven value. Cyclosporin A levels may increase.

Cholestyramine may be used to treat pruritus. However, its use may reduce absorption of cyclosporin A.

Cardiovascular drugs

Diuretics

Ascites may take some time to resolve after transplantation. Diuretics may be employed but care should be taken to avoid hypovolaemia. Potassium sparing diuretics such as spironolactone, amiloride, and triamterene may compound hyperkalaemia secondary to cyclosporin A therapy. Careful monitoring of renal function and serum potassium is required. Thiazide diuretics may increase cyclosporin A levels.

Anti-arryhthmics and other cardiac drugs

Some cardiac drugs may affect cyclosporin A and FK506 levels as outlined in Box C and in Chapter 11.

BOX C Cardiac drugs that increase blood levels of cyclosporin A or FK506

Drug	Increases levels of:
Amiodarone	Cyclosporin A
Diltiazem	Cyclosporin A
Nicardipine	Cyclosporin A
	FK506
Verapamil	FK506

Cyclosporin A may increase the plasma concentration of nifedipine. Digoxin may be used to control atrial fibrillation although care should be used in dosage in the presence of renal impairment. β-Adrenoreceptor blockers may be used, but if possible cardioselective agents, such as atenolol or metoprolol, should be employed in order to minimise reduction of hepatic blood flow. These drugs may be used to control supraventricular tachyarrhythmias and angina, but dosage levels and blood pressure should be monitored carefully to avoid hypotension that may predispose to hypoperfusion of the transplanted liver and hepatic artery thrombosis.

Anti-hypertensive therapy

Hypertension is common in patients receiving cyclosporin A. Calcium channel antagonists that cause vasodilation such as nifedipine, isradipine, and nicardipine are used as first line treatments, although β-adrenoceptor blockade may be used. Thiazide diuretic therapy may increase cyclosporin A levels and exacerbate renal impairment, and is not routinely employed. Angiotensin converting enzyme inhibitors should be avoided if possible, as they may exacerbate hyperkalaemia, and sudden episodes of hypotension may prejudice hepatic blood supply.

Anticoagulants

Oral anticoagulants   In patients with no evidence of cholestasis there is no contraindication to the use of warfarin (coumadin) if clinically indicated. Patients grafted for Budd–Chiari syndrome are normally anticoagulated after surgery.

Heparin   Heparin may also be used. Thrombocytopenia may occur in patients who also are taking myelotoxic drugs such as azathioprine.

Anti-platelet agents   In the absence of other contraindications, aspirin may be used as an anti-platelet agent if required, although it may exacerbate renal dysfunction.

Respiratory system drugs

Bronchodilators

There are no contraindications to the use of β_2-adrenoceptor stimulants or anti-muscarinic bronchodilators.

Theophylline may increase cyclosporin A levels, and patients may also readily acquire toxic levels of theophylline, consequently, careful monitoring of the levels of both drugs is required if they are required in combination.

Corticosteroids

Systemic corticosteroids should be given as usual in severe asthmatic attacks. Systemic corticosteroids may reduce plasma FK506 levels (but not cyclosporin A levels).

Cortiscosteroids can be used but particular attention to inhaler technique should be made, with the use of 'spacer devices' where possible to reduce the incidence of oropharyngeal candidiasis.

Central nervous system drugs

Hypnotics and anxiolytics

The usual care should be employed when initiating therapy with benzodiazepines, but no specific precautions are required.

Drugs used to treat psychoses

Phenothiazines may be used to treat organic or functional psychoses. The dosages should be carefully titrated to avoid hypotension. Chlorpromazine may cause neutropenia and caution should be taken when used together with azathioprine. Haloperidol may be better tolerated than chlorpromazine as it is less prone to induce hypotension.

Antidepressant drugs

Tricyclic antidepressants should be used where necessary to treat depressive illness. Amitriptyline is commonly employed and is well tolerated. Mianserin should be avoided as it has been associated with myelotoxic side effects.

Analgesics

Headaches Paracetamol should be employed initially. If this is unhelpful, prophylaxis with nifedipine, verapamil, or pizotifen should be tried. Treatment of acute attacks of migraine is difficult. Ergotamine containing compounds cause arterial vasoconstriction, and this may predispose to problems with hepatic arterial blood flow and so should be avoided. Severe symptoms may necessitate reconsideration of the immunosuppressive regimen. Some patients have been treated with the new 5-hydroxytryptamine-1 agonist, sumatriptan, orally or by subcutaneous injection. This drug may also cause coronary artery spasm and should be employed with caution.

Non-steroidal anti-inflammatory drugs There is an increased risk of nephrotoxicity with non-steroidal anti-inflammatory drugs and cyclosporin A and these drugs should be used with caution (see Box B).

Opiate analgesics There are no specific problems with opiate analgesics and these should not be withheld if symptoms dictate.

Anti-epileptics

Cyclosporin A may induce convulsions and many patients with spike activity on electroencephalograms after transplantation may require anticonvulsant therapy, particularly while receiving intravenous therapy. Anti-epileptic treatment will reduce cyclosporin A and FK506 levels (Box D).

Drugs used in the treatment of infections

Anti-bacterial drugs

Before initiating any anti-bacterial therapy it is important that cultures of blood, urine, sputum, and, where appropriate, ascites and bile are taken. In life threatening sepsis, however, initiation of therapy

---

BOX D   Anti-epileptic drugs which decrease cyclosporin A and FK506 levels

Phenytoin
Carbamazepine
Phenobarbitone (phenobarbital)

BOX E   Anti-bacterial drugs

Anti-bacterials that increase cyclosporin A and FK506 levels
  Erythromycin
  Doxycycline
  Troleandomycin (FK506 only)

Anti-bacterials that decrease cyclosporin A levels
  Intravenous co-trimoxazole

Anti-bacterial agents that should be avoided where possible because of additive nephrotoxicity
  Aminoglycosides
  Sulphonamides
  Vancomycin
  4-Quinolones

Anti-bacterial agents that should be avoided where possible because of additive neurotoxicity with FK506
  Ciprofloxacin and the other 4-quinolones
  Norfloxacin
  Imipenem

---

should not await the results of such cultures, but may be subsequently modified according to the organism(s) isolated and their antibiotic sensitivities. In patients not allergic to penicillin, with presumed septicaemia, a combination of co-amoxiclav and an anti-pseudomonal cephalosporin such as ceftazidime may be employed. In penicillin allergic individuals a combination of ciprofloxacin and metronidazole may be employed.

A number of antibacterial agents have important interactions with cyclosporin A and FK506. These are outlined in Box E.

TABLE III—*Suggested intravenous amphotericin dosage regimen for adult patient with life threatening fungal or yeast infection*

Dose (mg)	Volume of 5% dextrose (ml)	Day	Duration of infusion (hours)
1	250	1	2
24	1000	1	6
25	1000	1	6
50	1000	2 *et seq.*	6

Slower incremental rates may be employed in individuals with less life threatening infections.

Anti-tuberculous drugs

This has been discussed previously (p 320).

Anti-fungal drugs

Prophylactic anti-fungal therapy is usually required when patients are taking high doses of corticosteroids in addition to other immuno-suppressive agents. This therapy is aimed at preventing oropharyn-geal candidiasis; oral nystatin suspension and amphotericin lozenges are effective.

Systemic fungal infection in the presence of immunosuppressive agents carries a poor prognosis. In the presence of systemic fungal infection, the immunosuppressive regimen should be reduced or even stopped temporarily, but only after discussion with the transplant centre. Systemic anti-fungal agents can be employed and prolonged treatment is required.

Systemic amphotericin may be given, but side effects are common and nephrotoxicity is a major problem. Immediate side effects may be reduced by gradually increasing the dose. A suggested regimen for adult patients is outline in Table III. Liposomal amphotericin may reduce some side effects but is costly.

There is a reluctance to employ flucytosine in the treatment of systemic infection because the side effects of myelotoxicity and nephrotoxicity render it particularly hazardous in patients after transplantation.

Ketoconazole is significantly better absorbed than the other imida-zole anti-fungal agents, but is metabolised by the liver and will increase cyclosporin A levels. Fluconazole and itraconazole may be of benefit in treating extensive mucocutaneous candidiasis, and may have a role in the treatment of systemic candidiasis. These triazole anti-fungals may increase cyclosporin A levels.

Antiviral therapy

Herpetic lesions related to mucous membranes should be treated with topical acyclovir early. Systemic herpetic lesions, varicella-zoster, and herpes simplex encephalitis should be treated on clinical suspicion with systemic acyclovir.

Ganciclovir should be reserved for the treatment of cytomegalovirus disease (not seroconversion). Severe cases may also require hyper-immune γ-globulin.

Drugs used in disorders of the endocrine system

Diabetes mellitus

Iatrogenic diabetes is not uncommon following transplantation. Conventional approaches should be used.

Thyroid drugs

In general the treatment of thyroid disorders is unaffected by liver transplantation, but caution should be taken when using carbimazole and azathioprine. Hyperthyroidism should be controlled with either radioactive iodine treatment, surgery, or β-adrenoceptor blockade.

Steroids

Corticosteroids may decrease FK506 levels, but otherwise should be administered as dictated by the underlying clinical condition.

If possible the use of danazol (danazole) in the treatment of endometriosis should be avoided; its combination of side effects, especially neutropenia and thrombocytopenia, and its ability to increase cyclosporin A levels make it a difficult drug to handle in transplant recipients.

Conclusions

If there is any doubt about the advisability of introducing further therapeutic agents, the transplant centre concerned should be contacted for advice.

Surgery after liver transplantation

Patients who have undergone liver transplantation may subsequently require surgical procedures for conditions that may not necessarily be associated with their liver transplant. The underlying liver disease may be associated with diseases of other organs – for example, ulcerative colitis in patients with primary sclerosing cholangitis. As with other abdominal operations, liver transplantation may result in adhesions within the peritoneal cavity, and this, in turn, results in intestinal obstruction. Steroids predispose to peptic ulceration and chronic immunosuppression is associated with an increased incidence of tumours, in particular skin cancers and lymphomas. Although operations on the liver graft, such as biliary reconstruction, should be undertaken by the transplant surgeon, other procedures will be performed by an appropriate specialist.

The surgical team should be aware of the special problems that can occur in the liver transplant recipient during the perioperative period. Coagulation may be defective if the liver is not functioning perfectly. In addition, many patients with chronic liver disease have an enlarged spleen and continue to exhibit hypersplenism with a low platelet count for many months post-transplantation. The enlarged spleen is also in danger of surgical trauma. Upper abdominal structures, such as the stomach and duodenum, are often intimately adherent to the liver and to structures at the porta hepatis following liver transplantation. Moreover, vascular and biliary reconstruction at the time of transplantation may have disturbed the normal anatomy in the region of the porta hepatis and may have involved construction of a Roux loop of jejunum or occasionally an aortic conduit from the infrarenal aorta. The abdominal surgeon therefore needs to know the technical details of the transplant operation before performing a laparotomy.

Except in the septic patient, in whom immunosuppression may have to be reduced to control infection, immunosuppression should not be stopped during the perioperative period. For patients on oral steroids doses of equivalent intravenous steroids should be

331

substituted. Azathioprine should be given at the same dose intravenously as was prescribed orally. If cyclosporin A cannot be taken orally, it should be given as an intravenous infusion at one-fifth of the oral dose. Cyclosporin A, particularly if given intravenously, is nephrotoxic. Urine output should be monitored carefully with daily measurement of blood creatinine and urea, and the patient should be kept well hydrated. Other potentially nephrotoxic drugs, in particular aminoglycosides, should be avoided. A number of drugs affect cyclosporin A metabolism and blood levels of cyclosporin A should be monitored daily. Because immunosuppressed patients are at high risk from infection, prophylactic antibiotics appropriate to organisms likely to be liberated from the site of surgery should be administered. In those with a Roux loop, antibiotic prophylaxis is suggested before liver biopsy.

References

1 Belle SH, Beringer KC, Murphy JB, *et al*. Liver transplantation in the United States: 1988 to 1990. In: Terasaki, P, ed. *Clinical Transplants* 1991: 13–28.

2 Cundy TF, O'Grady JG, Williams R. Recovery of menstruation and pregnancy after liver transplantation. *Gut* 1990; **31**: 337–8.

3 deKoning ND, Haagsma EB. Normalization of menstrual pattern after liver transplantation: consequences for contraception. *Digestion* 1990; **46**: 239–41.

4 Scantlebury V, Gordon R, Tzakis A, *et al*. Childbearing after liver transplantation. *Transplantation* 1990; **49**: 317–21.

5 Laifer SA, Darby MJ, Scantlebury VP, *et al*. Pregnancy and liver transplantation. *Obstet Gynecol* 1990; **76**: 1083–8.

6 Penn I, Makowski EL, Harris P. Parenthood following renal and hepatic transplantation. *Transplantation* 1980; **30**: 397–400.

7 Venkataramanan R, Koneru B, Wang CCP, *et al*. Cyclosporine and its metabolites in mother and baby. *Transplantation* 1988; **46**: 468–9.

8 Ginsburg CM, Andrews W. Orthotopic hepatic transplantation for unimmunised children: A paradox of contemporary medical care. *Pediatr Infect Dis J* 1987; **6**: 764–5.

9 Committee on Infectious Diseases American Academy of Pediatrics. Immunodeficient and immunosuppressed children. In: Peter G, Lepow ML, McCracken GH, Phillips CF, eds. *Report of the Committee on Infectious Diseases*, 22nd ed, 1991; 47–51.

10 Rudolph AM, ed. *Rudolph's Pediatrics*, 19th Ed. Prentice Hall: Appleton and Lang, 1991: 34–7.

11 Linnemann CC, First MR, Schiffman G. Response to pneumococcal vaccine in renal transplant and hemodialysis patients. *Arch Intern Med* 1981; **141**: 1637–40.

12 Linnemann CC, First MR, Schiffman G. Revaccination of renal transplant and hemodialysis recipients with pneumococcal vaccine. *Arch Intern Med* 1986; **146**: 1554–6.

13 Versluis DJ, Beyer WEP, Masurel N, *et al*. Impairment of the immune response to influenza vaccination in renal transplant recipients by cyclosporine, but not azathioprine. *Transplantation* 1986; **42**: 376–9.

14 Van Thiel DH, El-Ashmawy L, Love K, *et al*. Response to hepatitis B vaccination by liver transplant candidates. *Dig Dis Sci* 1992; **37**: 1245–9.

15 Sokal EM, Ulla L, Otte JB. Hepatitis B vaccine response before and after transplantation in 55 extrahepatic biliary atresia children. *Dig Dis Sci* 1992; **37**: 1250–2.

16 Carey W, Pimental R, Westveer MK, *et al*. Failure of hepatitis B immunization in liver transplant recipients: Results of a prospective trial. *Am J Gastroenterol* 1990; **85**: 1590–2.
17 Broyer M, Boudailliez B. Varicella vaccine in children with chronic renal insufficiency. *Postgrad Med J* 1985; **61**: 103–6.

17: Management of children after liver transplantation

MICHAEL J NOWICKI,
SUSAN PEDERSEN RYCKMAN, MARY BETH BECHT,
FREDERICK C RYCKMAN, WILLIAM F BALISTRERI

Coupled with the increasing experience in the perioperative care of children following liver transplantation has been the acquisition of broad based knowledge regarding their postoperative care. The end result is a high survival rate and quality of life. In this chapter, the focus is specifically on the following issues:

- Quality of life
- Growth and nutrition
- Infections
- Immune suppression.

Quality of life

Liver transplantation has proved to benefit children with end stage liver disease through improved survival. However, live transplantation is not without significant potential morbidity. Rather than curing the underlying liver disease, the operation replaces it with another form of "chronic illness" which is easier to manage. Therefore the following question must be addressed: Does the child undergoing liver transplantation have an improved quality of life? The answer depends upon the criteria used to assess quality of life:

- Life expectancy
- Return to normal functioning in school or the work force

- Decreased time spent in the hospital
- Improvement in growth and development
- Subjective feeling of well-being.

There are few studies which directly assess these issues; therefore, surrogate markers must be used in the context of the premorbid and/ or pre-transplantation condition of the child.

The child with end stage liver disease has not only a chronic illness, but a life threatening condition. Therefore, it is not surprising that significant dysfunction in intrafamilial interactions may occur. Commonly, there is a strong parental need to shelter the affected child, often manifested as isolation of the family and overprotection of the child.[1] The child is often characterised as being dependent, demanding, and difficult to comfort.[1] These characteristics are similar to those seen in families in other transplantation groups. Although there may be a sense of relief, and even euphoria, following a successful transplantation, it is often short lived.[2] Families may become disillusioned when they realise that liver transplantation is a disease unto itself, with many complications. Children may become anxious or overtly depressed, whereas parents often develop a sense of hopelessness.[1] Children who are well adjusted before liver transplantation tend to progress in a healthy manner psychologically, whereas children with difficulties pre-transplantation tend to show increased dependency.[3]

Variables in families that correlate with a "positive" post-transplantation course include intact marriages, minimal financial stress (including, in North America, private insurance) and higher intellectual/developmental functioning of the child at the time of transplantation.[4]

Emotional adaptation of children who have received a liver transplant is not significantly different from that of children with another chronic illness, diabetes mellitus. Windsorová et al. compared paediatric liver transplant recipients to children with insulin-dependent diabetes mellitus and found no differences in depressive symptoms, level of anxiety, or self-concept.[5] Compared with healthy children, self-assessment tests reveal that liver transplant recipients score in the normative range for depression, anxiety, and self-esteem; however, when objective testing is being used, children who have survived liver transplantation have higher levels of depression and anxiety, and lower self-esteem compared with healthy children.[5]

335

Follow up studies have shown that over three-quarters of children were in age appropriate grade levels following liver transplantation.[6] Any school delay was most commonly attributed to chronic illness *before* transplantaion and/or emotional immaturity. Objective testing has documented recovery of gross motor skills, behavioural scores, and interactive functions one year after transplantation.[6]

Long term neurological dysfunction has been noted in both adults and children following liver transplantation. Neuropsychological testing of adults with chronic liver disease reveals that they frequently exhibit deficits limited to visuospatial and perceptual–motor skills; verbal testing and global measures of intellectual functioning are equivalent to controls.[7] In contrast to patients with adult onset liver disease, children with chronic liver disease show defects on global intellectual measures, as well as specific neuropychological measures; these deficits persist following liver transplantation.[8] In comparing children who have undergone liver transplantation with those who have another chronic illness, cystic fibrosis, the liver transplant recipients had significantly lower scores on non-verbal intelligence tests, lower academic achievement, and lower scores in areas of abstraction and conception formation, visuospatial function, and motor function. No differences were seen on tests of verbal intelligence, or in areas of alertness or concentration, perceptual–motor skills, and sensory–perception.[8] Two factors that have been associated with poor neurological outcome are early onset of liver disease and significant growth retardation.[9, 10] It has been suggested that the reason for the differences seen between adults and children with chronic liver disease relates to the developing brain being more vulnerable to the possible cerebrotoxic effects of liver disease.[8] Many of these findings are also seen in children with end stage renal disease and poor nutritional status.

Neuropsychological abnormalities are supported by pathological findings on postmortem examination of brain tissue taken from children who died after liver transplantation. However it is unclear what degree of contribution comes from morbidity pre-transplantation or other factors (prolonged intensive care, etc.). Hall and Martinez studied brains from 35 paediatric liver transplant recipients who had died following transplantation; neuropathological lesions were found in all of them.[11] Vascular lesions, the most common finding (86%), included infarction, ischaemia, thrombosis, and haemorrhage. Alzheimer type II astrocytes, a characteristic feature of chronic liver disease, were found in 69% of the children; infection with fungi was detected in 29%.[11] Compared to adults, children tended to have a higher incidence of intracranial haemorrhage (27% vs 20%), cerebral ischaemic lesions (32% vs 18%), and global brain ischaemia (49% vs 20%).[12]

Injury leading to central nervous system (CNS) lesions can occur at any time during the transplantation experience. In the pre-transplantation period significant malnutrition, growth failure, vitamin E deficiency, and chronic liver failure all contribute to neurological dysfunction. During the operative phase, neurological injury may occur due to shifts in electrolytes, hypotension, and decreased cerebral perfusion pressure (CPP). Potter et al. studied CPP in patients undergoing liver transplantation for fulminant liver failure.[13] During induction of anaesthesia, the CPP was in an acceptable range; however, during the pre-clamp phase there was an increase in intracranial pressure (ICP) and a resultant decrease in CPP. Slight improvement was seen in the CPP during the anhepatic phase. However, with reperfusion of the new liver, a marked increase in ICP was documented with a concomitant decrease in CPP.[13] The increased ICP lasted for up to 10 hours following transplantation, implying that careful attention to ICP must be continued until resolution has been documented. The risk for neurological injury remains in the post-transplantation patient, occurring both directly and indirectly to immunosuppression. Cyclosporin A (cyclosporine) has been shown to cause white matter changes, detectable on computed tomography.[14] Immunosuppression increases the risk of infections including meningoencephalitis (with resultant CNS damage) and sepsis (with hypotension leading to ischaemic damage).

Regarding quality of life, a major justification for liver transplantation in children is that recipients will require fewer hospitalisations than patients with chronic liver disease. Thus, a true measure of quality of life is time spent at home. Following liver transplantation, children experience significantly fewer hospital admissions and fewer days in the hospital, and receive less medication.[15, 16]

Growth and nutrition

Nutritional deficiencies associated with growth failure are common in children with end stage liver disease; these problems often continue following successful liver transplantation. Growth retardation, a common complication of immune suppression with the widespread use of cyclosporin A, contributed to the poor quality of life. Recent efforts, which have focused on the recognition and management of nutritional deficiencies in both the pre- and the postoperative periods, along with a decreased reliance on steroids, have decreased the incidence of growth retardation.

Malnutrition is prevelant among children awaiting liver transplantation; 60% of children with end stage liver disease had depleted fat stores and 20% had evidence of more chronic malnutrition.[17, 18] Major contributing factors to malnutrition include: anorexia, early satiety secondary to ascites and organomegaly, and fat malabsorption due to decreased bile flow.[19, 20] Additional factors in protein–energy malnutrition include abnormalities in amino acid metabolism, deficiency of fat soluble vitamins, and increased energy requirements.[21, 22]

Correction of protein–calorie malnutrition before transplantation can increase the probability of a suggestive outcome of liver transplantation. At Cincinnati the preferred route of nutrition is enteral. Often the need to provide increased calories requires concentration of the feed (which also decreases the fluid load) or the addition of glucose polymers and/or medium-chain triglycerides to bolster the caloric density. If voluntary oral intake is not sufficient to ensure adequate caloric intake for growth, nasogastric routes are used.

Aggressive nutritional support in the immediate postoperative period can help achieve a positive nitrogen balance, facilitate weaning from ventilatory support, and shorten the stay in the intensive care unit.[23] The approach used at Cincinnati to the nutritional management of the child who has undergone liver transplantation is shown in Box A.

It is often difficult to ensure adequate nutrition following liver transplantation. Children often develop oral defensiveness following prolonged intubation, thus limiting oral intake. Infants who required exclusive nasogastric feeds before transplantation may lose their ability to feed orally. Feeding disorders are also seen in the infant with developmental delay due to chronic liver disease. Often the medications given present another confounding factor which leads to persistence of poor nutrition; immunosuppressant medication may have common side effects of diarrhoea, constipation, vomiting, and anorexia (Table I).

BOX A Nutritional management following orthotopic liver transplantation in the paediatric patient*

1 Supply adequate calories: 100–130 cal/kg per day. (May vary dependent upon needs for catch-up growth and increased metabolic rate)
2 Increase caloric density of formulae via:
   – glucose polymers
   – concentrated infant formulae or adult nutritional products
3 Supply adequate protein: 2·5–3·0 g/kg per day
4 Increase calcium intake to offset catabolism and osteoporosis
5 Calorie counts and daily weight to assess adequacy of intake
6 Fluid and/or sodium restriction as appropriate
7 Enteral feedings if:
   – inadequate caloric intake
   – weight loss with oral intake (nocturnal nasogastric feedings preferred)

* Modified from Becht et al.[23]

Nutritional rehabilitation following liver transplantation is dependent upon:[24, 25]

- Improved hepatic synthetic function with normal levels of visceral proteins
- Enhanced bile flow, and thus adequate absorption of fat and fat soluble vitamins
- Better appetite.

Catch up growth can be seen when the caloric intake is between 100 and 130 cal/kg per day with a minimum of 2·5–3·0 g protein/kg per day.[23] In a study by Stewart et al., significant improvement in weight, head circumference, and anthropometric measurements, was found within one year of transplantation.[26] Linear growth did not improve appreciably and increments in length varied inversely with steroid dosage.[26] Other studies have documented improved linear growth with increased growth velocities despite corticosteroid use. Vicente et al. reported accelerated growth in 76% of children undergoing liver transplantation; however, they comment that catch up growth occurred during chronic steroid therapy if a "low dose" was used.[27] Moukarzel et al.[28] found the following results in their liver transplant population: 13%, improvement in height percentiles

TABLE I—*"Nutrition-related" side effects of immunosuppressive medications used post-transplantation*

Immunosuppressive agent	Nutritional side effects
Cyclosporin A	Hyperkalaemia Hypomagnesaemia Hyperlipidaemia Hyperglycaemia Gingival hyperplasia
Prednisone	Fluid/sodium retention Hyperglycaemia Increased appetite Gastrointestinal ulceration Mood swings Osteoporosis
Azathioprine	Nausea/vomiting Oesophagitis Altered taste acuity
OKT3	Nausea/vomiting Diarrhoea Loss of appetite Fluid retention
FK506	Nausea/vomiting Abdominal pain

Modified from Becht MB *et al.*[23]

into the normal range; 43%, maintenance of height in the normal range; 31%, maintenance of height below the fifth percentile; and 11%, height falling below the fifth percentile. Linear growth velocity improved in 38%, remained unchanged in 23%, and decreased in 39%.[28] When growth velocity was compared to steroid dose, a significant difference in catch up growth was noted between those receiving less than 5 mg prednisone/day (55%) and those receiving more than 5 mg prednisone (22%).[28] Thus it appears that chronic use of high dose steroids is associated with impaired linear growth, similar to the experience seen in the renal transplant population.[29] It has also been found at Cincinnati that linear growth can be improved by the use of low dose or alternate day steroids, or the use of "steroid sparing" immunosuppressants alone when feasible (Figure 1).

Other factors that contribute to poor linear growth following liver

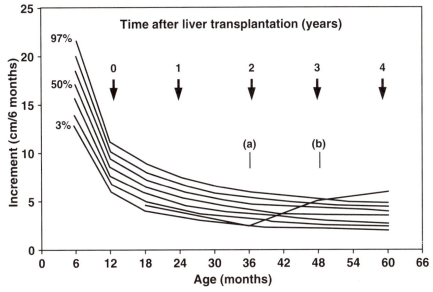

FIG 1—*Diagrammatic height–velocity chart of a five-year-old patient four years following liver transplantation. Note the increasing growth velocity which occurred following the decrease of the oral prednisone dose to 0·1 mg/kg on alternate days, and subsequent withdrawal. (a) Every other day dosing predicted; (b) discontinuation predicted. (Reproduced, with permission, from Becht et al[23])*

transplantation include: poor graft function, the need for multiple operations, chronic rejection, and the vanishing bile duct syndrome.[28, 30] Continued improvements in nutritional support, surgical technique, and immunosuppression that spares the use of corticosteroids, perhaps combined with the selective use of recombinant human growth hormone,[31] will allow improved linear growth following liver transplantation to become the norm for paediatric patients.

Infection

One of the most significant causes of morbidity and mortality following liver transplantation in children is infection. Overall, the incidence of infectious complications following transplantation is 80%; infection is the major contributing factor in at least 20–40% of morbidities after transplantation.[32–35] In a study by Kusne *et al.*, infection was associated with 89% of deaths in their liver transplant

341

population.[36] Of the infections following liver transplantation, bacteria are the causative agent in 60% of the cases, viruses in 35–60%, and fungi in approximately 40%, with multiple infections ocurring in some patients.[32] George et al. studied the patterns of infection in paediatric liver transplant recipients.[37] At least one infection was documented in 72% of the patients; more infections occurred when prophylactic anti-lymphocyte antibodies were used than when they were not given (2·9 vs 1·0 infection per transplantation).[37] Bacteria were the most common pathogens isolated during all periods except the third and fourth weeks post-transplantation when viruses were the most common cause of infection.[37] The highest percentage of infections (44%) occurred in the first two weeks following transplantation, when bacteria and fungi accounted for virtually all infections. There was a steady decline in the number of infections seen after the first two weeks. Most viral infections occurred in the third and fourth weeks following liver transplantation.[37]

Bacterial infections

Bacterial infections, as stated above, occur most commonly in the immediate post-transplantation period. The most common pathogens isolated are Gram-negative enteric organisms, enterococci and staphylococci. The most common sites infected are the blood stream and the abdomen (intra-abdominal abscesses and infected seromas); other less common sites are the surgical wound and the lungs.[37] The risk of early postoperative infection is increased by poor nutrition, immunosuppression, and indwelling catheters. The prolonged use of prophylactic antibiotics may select for resistant organisms or lead to Clostridium difficile enterocolitis.

Fungal infections

Fungi may also cause a significant problem in the immediate post-transplantation period. The most common isolated fungal pathogen is Candida spp., followed by Aspergillus sp.[36] The use of bowel decontamination in the period before transplantation has been shown to be efficacious in eliminating Candida spp. from the gastrointestinal tract of adults.[38, 39] This therapy is less practical in the paediatric population because of the poor palatability of the medication and because of the long period that children spend waiting for transplantation. An alternative method for children is to culture the gastrointestinal tract at the time of transplantation, and then to treat selectively those patients in whom *Candida* sp. is isolated. Using this strategy, the incidence of fungal infections in children following liver transplantation can be decreased.[39] Another potential means of decreasing the incidence of fungal infection may be the use of fluconazole as prophylaxis. In a retrospective study, Torre-Cisneros *et al.* reported that the incidence of aspergillosis was significantly less (0·2%) in patients who received FK506 than in those who received cyclosporin A (2·4%); the mortality rate was also less in those receiving FK506 against those on cyclosporin A (50% vs 94%).[40]

Viral infections

The peak incidence of viral infections occurs later than the peak for bacterial and fungal infections. Most early and severe viral infections are caused by herpes viruses, including cytomegalovirus, Epstein–Barr virus, and herpes simplex virus. The high incidence of infection with these viruses may be related to: their ability to remain latent in the host, and to reactivate following induction of immuno-suppression; and the high prevalence of these viruses in the general population. In a study of opportunist viral hepatitis following liver transplantation, cytomegalovirus was most commonly the causative agent, being found in 82% of the patients; Epstein–Barr virus (10%) and herpes simplex virus (5%) were found less frequently.[41]

Cytomegalovirus

The likelihood of developing cytomegalovirus infection is influenced by the preoperative status of the donor and recipient. The highest risk occurs when a seronegative recipient receives an organ from a seropositive donor; the second highest risk occurs when an organ from a seropositive donor is placed in a seropositive patient.[42] This poses a significant problem in the paediatric popula-tion where the seroprevalence of cytomegalovirus neutralising anti-bodies is low. Breinig *et al.*[43] prospectively studied the incidence of viral infection in 51 consecutive paediatric patients who had received liver transplants. The incidence of seropositivity for cytomegalovirus in this pre-transplantation population was 19%, compared to 79% in adults; primary cytomegalovirus infection developed in 17% of patients who were initially seronegative, and reactivation occurred in 88% of patients with a history of previous cytomegalovirus infection.[41] The overall prevalence of cytomegalovirus infection in children undergoing liver transplantation (30%) is significantly less than that for adults (77%).[43] The incidence of symptomatic cytomegalovirus infection can be decreased by the combination of passive immunisation (with intravenous immune globulin or hyperimmune anti-cytomegalovirus immune globulin) and antiviral therapy (ganciclovir and acyclovir). However, seroconversion is almost universal in seronegative patients who receive an organ from a seropositive donor. Unlike the case for fungal infections, FK506 does not appear to be beneficial in decreasing the incidence of cytomegalovirus infections following liver transplantation when compared to cyclosporin A.[44] Cytomegalovirus infection is suggested by the development of fever, leucopenia, maculopapular rash, sore throat, and lymphadenopathy. Other possible presenting features include hepatocellular abnormalities, respiratory insufficiency, and gastrointestinal haemorrhage. Diagnosis can be established by direct assays or culture of cytomegalovirus from urine or tissue biopsies (liver or gastrointestinal tract), by immunohistochemical identification on biopsy, by detection of viral genome in tissue biopsy using in situ hybridisation, or by identification of antibodies to cytomegalovirus in the blood. Treatment should be initiated while awaiting the results of diagnostic tests, to allow the best chance for success.

Epstein–Barr virus

Epstein–Barr virus can either cause a primary infection or reactivation following initiation of immunosuppression. The seroprevalence of Epstein–Barr virus in the paediatric pre-transplantation population is 50%, significantly less than the prevalence seen in adults (92%). Primary Epstein–Barr virus infection is seen in 67% of seronegative children receiving a liver transplant; reactivation occurs in 48% of children with previous Epstein–Barr virus infection.[43] The overall prevalence of Epstein–Barr virus infection in the paediatric liver transplant population (57%) is higher than that seen in adults (36%).[43] Epstein–Barr virus infection following liver transplantation has a wide spectrum of presentation; it may occur as a mononucleosis-like syndrome, hepatitis simulating rejection, and post-transplantation lymphoproliferative disease (PTLD). PTLD is a potentially fatal abnormal proliferation of B lymphocytes which can occur in any situation where there is immunosuppression; it occurs in 4% of paediatric solid organ transplant recipients.[45] There are several recognisable clinical syndromes (Table II). Both primary infection, and reactivation of latent infection, with Epstein–Barr virus can precede the development of PTLD, but primary infection is more common.[37] Active Epstein–Barr infection causes B cell proliferation; with the use of immunosuppressant agents cytotoxic T cell activity is inhibited and Epstein–Barr virus proliferation goes unchecked. The incidence of PTLD correlates with the level of immunosuppression, being highest in those receiving high levels of immunosuppressants.[47] Treatment of PTLD consists of decreasing the level of immunosuppression and initiating antiviral chemo-therapy with either ganciclovir or acyclovir.[48]

Other viruses

The prevalence of adenoviral infection following liver trans-plantation is much less than that of the herpes viruses; however, it is still a significant problem. Adenoviral hepatitis is seen in 3·2% of liver transplant recipients of all ages and in 2·5% of paediatric recipients.[41,49] Diagnosis can be made by characteristic features on liver biopsy and immunohistochemistry; the virus can also be identified in hepatic tissue by electron microscopy. Mortality rate from hepatitis caused by adenovirus approaches 30%; no effective therapy exists, although lowering the amount of immunosuppres-sion may be beneficial.[49]

Varicella-zoster, although a relatively benign disease in healthy children, is a serious, potentially life threatening disease in immuno-compromised hosts. The child receiving immunosuppression fol-lowing a liver transplantation is at risk for severe varicella-zoster infection. McGregor et al. studied 47 children following liver transplantation who were susceptible to varicella-zoster.[50] Fifteen were not exposed to varicella-zoster during the study period. Twenty-five children who were exposed to varicella-zoster received immunoprophylaxis with varicella-zoster immune globulin (VZIG) within 72 hours of exposure; 28% developed clinical varicella-zoster. One patient who received VZIG 94 hours following exposure

TABLE II—*Clinical syndromes: lymphoproliferative disease*

Subtype	Clinical	Histology	Immunological cell typing	Cytogenetics	IgG gene rearrangements	Therapy
Benign polyclonal lymphoproliferation	Infectious mononucleosis-like syndrome	Polymorphic diffuse B cell hyperplasia	Polyclonal B cell proliferation	Normal	Normal	Acyclovir
Early malignant transformation	Infectious mononucleosis-like syndrome	Polymorphic B cell lymphoma	Polyclonal B cell proliferation	Clonal cytogenetic abnormalities	Present	Acyclovir + ↓immunosuppression
Malignant monoclonal lymphoma	Localised solid tumour masses	Polymorphic B cell lymphoma	Polyclonal B cell proliferation	Clonal cytogenetic abnormalities	Present	Discontinue Immunosuppression Chemotherapy Radiotherapy Surgical resection

Modified from Hanto.[46]

TABLE III—*Late post-transplantation or outpatient immunosuppression protocol*

Time after transplantation (months)	Prednisone dose (mg/kg)	Cyclosporin A level (μg/l) (whole blood monoclonal radio-immunoassay)	Azathioprine
1	0·7	350 ± 50	Discontinue
2	0·6	300–350	between
3	0·6	300 ± 50	1 and 3
6	0·2	250 ± 50	months
12	0·1	200	after
18–24	0·1*	150–200	operation
30–36	Discontinue	150 ± 50	

* Alternate-day dosing. Monitoring through frequent protocol measurement of liver enzymes and serum interleukin-2 receptor levels.
Modified from Becht et al.[23]

also developed clinical varicella-zoster. All the patients who did not receive immunoprophylaxis following exposure developed varicella-zoster infection. Overall, 61% of children exposed to varicella-zoster following liver transplantation developed clinical disease, irrespective of VZIG use. Of the 14 patients who developed varicella-zoster, 13 were hospitalised and received intravenous acyclovir; 11 patients recovered and 2 died as a result of disseminated varicella-zoster. Both deaths occurred in children receiving a higher than normal dose of immunosuppressant agents at the time of infection. Based on their experience, McGregor et al. suggest that susceptible liver transplant recipients should receive immunoprophylaxis within 72 hours of exposure to varicella-zoster; if clinical varicella-zoster infection develops, intravenous acyclovir should be initiated within 24 hours of eruption of cutaneous lesions.[50]

Immunosuppression

Current maintenance therapy consists of cyclosporin A, prednisone, and occasionally azathioprine. The protocol used at Cincinnati is shown in Table III. Episodes of acute rejection unresponsive to steroid recycling may require the use of monoclonal (OKT3) or polyclonal anti-lymphocyte antibody preparations. Recently,

TABLE IV—*Adverse side effects associated with cyclosporin A and FK506*

	Cyclosporin A	FK506
Central nervous system	Tremors, paraesthesiae, seizures	Tremors, hyperaesthesiae, photophobia, seizures, confusion, dysarthria, insomnia
Renal	Decreased glomerular filtration rate, decreased creatinine, increased serum creatinine, hypertension, hypercalcaemia, hyperuricaemia	Decreased glomerular filtration rate increased serum creatinine, hyperkalaemia, hypertension
Gastrointestinal	Diarrhoea, constipation, nausea, vomiting, abdominal pain, pancreatitis	Not specified
Hepatic	Hepatotoxicity (increased alanine transaminase, aspartate transaminase, bilirubin, alkaline, phosphatase) Cholelithiasis	Not specified
Infectious diseases	Increased incidence of bacterial, fungal, and viral infections	Increased incidence of bacterial, fungal, and viral infections
Cosmetic	Hypertrichosis, gingival hyperplasia, facial dysmorphisms	Not specified
Immune	Anaphylactoid reactions, rashes	Not specified
Endocrine	Insulin-dependent diabetes mellitus	Insulin-dependent diabetes mellitus
Drug interactions	Co-trimoxazole Ketoconazole, erythromycin, rifamycin (induction of cytochrome P450)	Not specified
Miscellaneous	Post-transplantation lymphoproliferative disease	Post-transplantation lymphoproliferative disease

FK506, an immunosuppressive agent derived from *Streptomyces tsukubaensis*, has been evaluated in children. In a study comparing FK506 to cyclosporin A, Tzakis *et al.*[51] showed a trend favouring improved patient and graft survival in the FK506 group. The number of rejection episodes was similar in the two groups, but rejection episodes were easier to manage in the FK506 group. Increasing the dose was enough to reverse rejection 1·5-fold more frequently in the FK506 group compared to cyclosporin A; conversely, OKT3 was used 2·5-fold and steroid recycling 4·4-fold more frequently in the cyclosporin A group. There was a lower requirement for steroid use, with less than 10% of FK506 patients requiring chronic steroids, against an almost universal requirement in patients treated with cyclosporin A. Hypertension was significantly less common in the FK506 group, and infections were less common and less severe in patients receiving FK506.[52]

Despite the beneficial effect of inhibiting rejection, both FK506 and cyclosporin A have significant adverse side effects (Table IV). Improved methods of immunosuppression may therefore be associated with less adverse effects, reliable control of rejection, and improved patient survival.

Conclusion

Liver transplantation has greatly improved both the duration and the quality of life of children with end stage liver disease. This has offered them the opportunity to reach their full potential for growth and development. Further refinements in immunosuppression, nutritional support, infection control, and psychosocial support should increase the odds.

References

1 Bradford R. Children's psychological health status – the impact of liver transplantation: a review. *J R Soc Med* 1991; **84**: 550–3.
2 Serrano J, Verougstraete C, Ghislain T. Psychological evaluation and support of pediatric patients and their parents. *Transplant Proc* 1987; **19**: 3358–62.
3 Penn I, Bunch D, Olenik D, *et al.* Psychiatric experience with patients receiving renal and hepatic transplants. *Semin Psychiatr* 1971; **3**: 54–65.
4 Kennard BD, Petrik K, Stewart SM, *et al.* Identifying factors in post-operative successful adaptation to pediatric liver transplantation. *Social Work in Health Care* 1990; **15**: 19–33.
5 Windsorová D, Stewart SM, Lovitt R, *et al.* Emotional adaptation in childen after liver transplantation. *J Pediatr* 1991; **119**: 880–7.
6 Zitelli BJ, Gartner JC, Malatack JJ, *et al.* Liver transplantation. In: Balistreri WF, and Stocker JT, eds. *Pediatric Hepatology*. New York: Hemisphere Publishing Corporation, 1990: 363–76.
7 Bernthal P, Hays A, Tarter RE, *et al.* Cerebral CT scan abnormalities in cholestatic and hepatocellular disease and their relationship to neuropsychological test performance. *Hepatology* 1987; 7: 107–14.

8 Stewart SM, Hiltbeitel C, Nici J, et al. Emotional adaptation in children after liver transplantation. Pediatrics 1991; **87**: 367–76.

9 Stewart SM, Uauy R, Waller DA, Kennard BD. Mental and motor development correlates in patients with end-stage biliary atresia awaiting liver transplantation. Pediatrics 1987; **79**: 882–8.

10 Stewart SM, Uauy R, Kennard BD, et al. Mental development and growth in children with chronic liver disease of early and late onset. Pediatrics 1988; **82**: 167–72.

11 Hall WA, Martinez AJ. Neuropathology of pediatric liver transplantation. Pediatr Neurosci 1989; **15**: 269–75.

12 Martinez AJ, Ahdab-Barmada M. The neuropathology of liver transplantation: comparison of main complications in children and adults. Mod Pathol 1993; **6**: 25–32.

13 Potter KD, O'Grady J, Peachey T, et al. Intracranial and cerebral perfusion pressure changes before, during, and immediately after orthotopic liver transplantation for fulminant hepatic failure. Q J Med 1991; **79**: 425–33.

14 deGroen PC, Aksamit AJ, Rakela J, et al. Central nervous system toxicity after liver transplantation. The role of cyclosporin and cholesterol. N Engl J Med 1987; **317**: 861–6.

15 Zitelli B, Gartner C, Malatack A, et al. Pediatric liver transplantation: patient evaluation and selection, infectious complications, and life-cycle after transplantation. Transplant Proc 1987; **19**: 3309–16.

16 Zitelli B, Miller J, Gartner C, et al. Evaluation of the pediatric patient for liver transplantation. Pediatrics 1988; **82**: 173–80.

17 Kaufman SS, Murray ND, Wood RP, et al. Nutritional support for the infant with extrahepatic biliary atresia. J Pediatr 1987; **110**: 679–86.

18 Kaufman SS, Scrivner DJ, Guest JE. Preoperative evaluation, preparation and timing of orthotopic liver transplantation in the child. Semin Liver Dis 1989; **9**: 176–83.

19 Andrews W, Fyock B, Gray S, et al. Pediatric liver transplantation: the Dallas experience. Transplant Proc 1987; **19**: 3267–76.

20 Snover DC, Sibley RK, Freese DK, et al. Orthotopic liver transplantation: a pathological study of 63 serial biopsies from 17 patients with special reference to the diagnostic features and natural history of rejection. Hepatology 1984; **4**: 1212–22.

21 Busuttil RW, Sou P, Millis JM, et al. Liver transplantation in children. Ann Surg 1991; **213**: 48–57.

22 Malatack JJ, Schaid DJ, Urbach AH, et al. Choosing a pediatric recipient for orthotopic liver transplantation. J Pediatr 1987; **111**: 479–89.

23 Becht MB, Pedersen SH, Ryckman FC, Balistreri WF. Growth and nutritional management of pediatric patients after orthotopic liver transplantation. Gastroenterol Clin North Am 1993; **22**: 367–80.

24 Silverman A, Roy CC. Pediatric Clinical Gastroenterology, 3rd Ed. St Louis: CV Mosby, 1983.

25 Hehir DJ, Jenkins RL, Bistrain BR, Blackburn GL. Nutrition in patients undergoing orthotopic liver transplantation. Journal of Parenteral and Enteral Nutrition 1985; **9**: 695–700.

26 Stewart SM, Uauy R, Waller DA, et al. Mental and motor development, social competence, and growth one year after successful pediatric liver transplantation. J Pediatr 1989; **114**: 574–81.

27 Vicente J, Spolindoro N, Berquist WE, et al. Growth acceleration in children after orthotopic liver transplantation. J Pediatr 1988; **112**: 41–4.

28 Moukarzel AA, Najm I, Vargas J, et al. Effect of nutritional status on outcome of orthotopic liver transplantation in pediatric patients. Transplant Proc 1990; **22**: 1558–91.

29 Pennisi AJ, Costin G, Phillips LS, et al. Linear growth in long-term renal allograft recipients. Clin Nephrol 1977; **8**: 415–21.

30 Snover DC, Freese DK, Sharp HL, et al. Liver allograft rejection: an analysis of the use of biopsy in determining outcome of rejection. Am J Surg Pathol 1987; **11**: 1–10.

31 Benfield MR, Parker KL, Waldo B, et al. Treatment of growth failure in children after renal transplant. Transplantation 1993; **55**: 305–8.

32 Andrews WS, Wanek E, Fyock B, et al. Pediatric liver transplantation: a 3-year experience. J Pediatr Surg 1989, **24**: 70–6.

33 Busuttil RW, Colonna JO, Hiatt JR, *et al*. The first 100 liver transplants at UCLA. *Ann Surg* 1987; **206**: 387–99.

34 Krom RAF, Wiesner RH, Rettke SR, *et al*. The first 100 liver transplantations at the Mayo Clinic. *Mayo Clin Proc* 1988; **64**: 84–94.

35 Iwatsuki S, Starzl TB, Gordon RD, *et al*. Experience in 1000 liver transplants under cyclosporin-steroid therapy: a survival report. *Transplant Proc* 1988; **20**: 498–504.

36 Kusne S, Dummer JS, Singh N, *et al*. Infections after liver transplantation: an analysis of 101 consecutive cases. *Medicine* 1988; **67**: 132–43.

37 George DL, Arnow PM, Fox A, *et al*. Patterns of infection after pediatric liver transplantation. *Am J Dis Child* 1992; **146**: 924–9.

38 Wiesner R, Hermans PE, Rakela J, *et al*. Selective bowel decontamination to decrease gram negative aerobic bacterial and candida colonization and prevent infection after orthotopic liver transplantation. *Transplantation* 1988; **45**: 570–4.

39 Andrews W, Siegel J, Renaro T, *et al*. Prevention and treatment of selected fungal and viral infections in pediatric liver transplant recipients. *Clin Transplantation* 1991; **5**: 204–7.

40 Torres-Cisneros J, Manes R, Kusne S, *et al*. The spectrum of aspergillosis in liver transplant patients: comparison of FK506 and Cyclosporin immunosuppression. *Transplant Proc* 1991; **23**: 3040–1.

41 Markin RS, Langnas AN, Donovan JP, *et al*. Opportunistic viral hepatitis in liver transplant recipients. *Transplant Proc* 1991; **23**: 1520–1.

42 Millis JM, McDiarmid SV, Hiatt JR, *et al*. Randomized prospective trial of OKT3 for early prophylaxis of rejection after liver transplantation. *Transplantation* 1989; **47**: 82–8.

43 Breinig MK, Zitelli B, Starzl TE, Ho M. Epstein–Barr virus, cytomegalovirus, and other viral infections in children after liver transplantation. *J Infect Dis* 1987; **156**: 273–9.

44 Alessiani M, Kusne S, Fung JJ, *et al*. CMV infection in liver transplantation under cyclosporin of FK506 immunosuppression. *Transplant Proc* 1991; **23**: 3035–7.

45 Ho M, Jaffe R, Miller G, *et al*. The frequency of Epstein–Barr virus infection and associated lymphoproliferative syndrome after transplantation and its manifestations in children. *Transplantation* 1988; **45**: 719–27.

46 Hanto DW. Association of lymphoma and viral disease. *Roundtable Report*. Raintan, NJ: Ortho Biotech, 1992: 13–16.

47 Schroeder TJ, Gramse DA, Mansour ME, *et al*. Monoclonal antibody therapy in pediatric transplantation. *Transplant Proc* 1992; 24(Suppl 1): 2–10.

48 Stephanian E, Gruber SA, Dunn DL, *et al*. Post-transplant lymphoproliferative disorders. *Transplant Review* 1991; **5**: 120–9.

49 Konaru B, Atchinson R, Jaffe R, *et al*. Serological studies of adenoviral hepatitis following pediatric liver transplantation. *Transplant Proc* 1990; **22**: 1547–8.

50 McGregor RS, Zitelli BJ, Urbach AH, *et al*. Varicella in pediatric orthotopic liver transplant recipients. *Pediatrics* 1989; **83**: 256–61.

51 Tzakis AG, Fung JJ, Demetris AJ, *et al*. Use of FK506 in pediatric patients. *Transplant Proc* 1991; **23**: 924–7.

52 Fung JJ, Todo S, Tzakis AG, *et al*. Conversion of liver allograft recipients from cyclosporin to FK506-based immunosuppression: benefits and pitfalls. *Transplant Proc* 1991; **23**: 14–21.

53 Tzakis AG, Rayes J, Todo S, *et al*. FK506 versus cyslosporin in pediatric liver transplantation. *Transplant Proc* 1991; **23**: 3010–15.

VI: Public health issues

18: Ethical issues in liver transplantation

MARTIN BENJAMIN

Introduction

Since the introduction of transplantation into clinical practice, there has been an increasing awareness of ethical problems associated with the procedure. Areas of concern range from whether the procedure should be performed at all to the impact of transplantation on resources that are already limited. The development of newer techniques such as living related organ donation and the use of financial incentives to donate organs have given additional areas of concern. Ethical problems relate in part to the different methods of health care delivery. In North America, the area of ethical issues is being addressed in depth and, therefore, this chapter will concentrate on those ethical issues with particular relevance to North America. Clearly, not all these considerations will apply to other countries but to cover all aspects of the ethical issues involved in transplantation would be beyond the scope of this book.

Ethical issues in liver transplantation, as in transplantation more generally, may be divided into three main categories: (1) procurement; (2) allocation; and (3) payment. The first deals with proposals for increasing the supply of transplantable organs; the second deals with methods and principles for distributing a limited number of organs to a larger number of patients who can benefit from them; and the third deals with determining how (or whether) to pay for these expensive procedures. The three categories are interrelated. Success (or failure) in one will often affect the others.

Procurement

As the science and technology of transplantation continue to improve, the demand for organs places increased strain on a limited supply. Yet proposals to increase the supply of organs raise complex ethical issues.

Ethical issues often require choice between two or more actions or policies, each of which can be supported by a well grounded rule or principle. In organ procurement, ethical considerations seem to pull in opposing directions. On the one hand, the importance of extending life and improving its quality for those suffering from end stage organ failure requires that we do everything in our power to increase the supply of transplantable organs. On the other hand, respect for such values as individual autonomy and altruism, as well as the sensibilities of the bereaved and the fact that transplantation depends on the good will of the public without whose dollars and donated organs the procedure would be impossible, appear to constrain what we may do to increase the supply. The one set of values, in this instance, seems to conflict with the other, and there is no obvious set of higher-order values that will resolve the matter. What follows is a brief review of major issues.

"Encouraged voluntarism"

At its inception both in the USA, and in many other countries, transplantation relied on the voluntary donation of organs. Concern about negative public reaction to the idea of transplantation, together with a respect for a deeply entrenched legal and cultural emphasis on personal autonomy, led to a procurement system in which organs could not be removed for transplantation without the fully informed consent of the donor or his or her family.[1] Dubbed "encouraged voluntarism" by Arthur Caplan, the system encourages individuals to donate organs after their death, and to indicate their willingness to do so by filling out individual donor cards or driver's licences.[2] Those devising the system, according to Virnig and Caplan:[3] "hoped this approach to organ donation, grounded in voluntarism, would result in procurement of sufficient organs while promoting altruism and protecting patient self-determination" (p. 2155). Yet the system has not yielded as many organs as we would like. Each year the list of those awaiting transplantation grows longer, whereas a large portion of the public, though aware of the need for donor organs, remains reluctant to fill out donor cards or to consent to donation from relatives. There is, moreover, some reason to believe that many health professionals are reluctant to raise the possibility of organ donation with the families of patients pronounced dead by brain criteria.[4,5] The result is a number of transplantable organs going to the grave while patients with organ failure languish and die on waiting lists. In 1990, for example, 2206 patients died while awaiting organs.[6]

Against this background, a number of proposals have been made for changing the procurement system so as to increase the supply of transplantable organs. These range from more or less modest reforms of the system of encouraged voluntarism to more radical proposals for replacing this system with, for example, a system in which consent to organ donation is presumed rather than explicitly obtained.

Required request

Noting that health professionals are often reluctant to raise the possibility of transplantation with the families of potential cadaveric donors, Arthur Caplan proposed that hospitals be required to make and document such requests.[7] If hospitals were required to make such requests, making it a routine procedure might both reduce the psychological stress associated with infrequent asking, and lead to the appointment and training of individuals best suited to the task. Called "required request", the first such law was passed in Oregon in 1985, with 42 states and the District of Columbia following suit within four years. The effect of such laws on the overall rate of organ procurement is, at this point, not entirely clear.[3]

Required request laws constitute no significant departure from the values underlying encouraged voluntarism. They provide a mechanism for increasing the number of donors while preserving both altruism, and the right of individuals and families to refuse or consent to donation. Two other proposals – presumed consent and providing some form of financial compensation, incentive, or reward for donation – call for more radical change.

Presumed consent

Encouraged voluntarism is sometimes characterised in terms of "opting-in" – that is, the presumption that an individual is *not* an organ donor unless and until that individual (or his or her next of kin) goes out of his or her way to donate. One must, in other words, "opt-in" to being a donor. Proposals for establishing a system of "presumed consent" are, by contrast, characterised in terms of "opting-out". In a system of presumed consent an individual is presumed to be a donor unless and until that individual (or his or her family) takes explicit steps to opt-out of the system. Arguments for replacing encouraged voluntarism (a system in which one must go out of one's way to opt-in) with presumed consent (in which one must go out of one's way to opt-out) turn not only on the possibility of increasing the supply of transplantable organs, but also on opinion polls indicating a widespread willingness among the public to donate organs upon death. Indeed, it has been argued that, absent evidence to the contrary, one is more likely to respect the autonomy of possible organ donors by presuming their consent to donation than not.[8] Moreover, a number of European countries, such as Austria, Belgium, France, Portugal, Finland, and Norway, have already passed some form of presumed consent law governing transplantation.[9]

The issues are, however, complex. There is, for example, little compelling evidence that the existence of presumed consent laws has yielded a significant increase in organ procurement in those countries that have adopted them. Land and Cohen conclude a recent review of European transplant laws by observing that: "Only in one country, Austria, and in a few regions are the developments promising and encouraging. There is no obvious correlation between high postmortem organ removal rates and the existence of presumed consent laws" (p. 2167). Moreover, the practical difficulties of implementing a system of presumed consent (and a practical, reliable mechanism for opting-out) in a country as culturally heterogeneous and litigious as the USA are formidable.[10] Although expressing an important ideal and a goal towards which societies aspiring to social solidarity ought to strive, a fair, workable system of presumed consent is still something that must, at this time, be argued for rather than implemented. Only when explicitly understood and endorsed by a large majority of a nation's population will this system of procurement significantly increase the supply of organs while respecting the rights and autonomy of potential donors.

Market approaches

In most other contexts shortages of valuable commodities are relieved by increased financial incentives for those producing them or making them available. Many believe similar economic considerations should be applied to organ procurement. The best way to increase the supply of organs while respecting people's autonomy is to provide financial incentives or rewards for those making them available. It is important, in this connection, to distinguish cadaveric from living sources of organs. Given differences in risk, it is much easier to justify market based approaches to obtaining organs from cadavers than from living "donors". The following discussion will therefore be limited to market based proposals involving cadaveric organs. Unless and until such proposals can be justified, there is little point in addressing the more complex and controversial question of financial inducements for living "donors".[11]

If people are unwilling to donate their (or their relatives') (cadaver) organs, perhaps they would be willing to sell them if the price were right. And, the argument goes, what could possibly be wrong with this? People are allowed to sell their labour in a wide variety of risky jobs – all of which involve greater potential harm than the removal of organs from a cadaver. Moreover, in many states market considerations already govern the transfer of blood and blood products. If, therefore, providing some sort of financial incentive or outright payment for cadaveric organs is likely to increase the overall supply, it is not only permissible but perhaps also mandatory to implement such a system.

Specific proposals for economically driven systems of organ procurement range from the simple provision of burial expenses or a US$1000 cash benefit to families who consent to cadaver donation[12] to elaborate schemes for future delivery markets.[13-15] Yet the very idea of payment for organs engenders ethical opposition.[16] Some question the presumption that human organs are, like other goods to which market considerations can be applied, rightly conceived of as commodities. Human body parts, it might be argued, are, rightly, different from other things that can be bought and sold – they are not property. Yet the arguments for and against conceiving the body as property are extraordinarily complex and far reaching, requiring more detailed analysis and assessment than can be provided here.[17-19] Other objections to market governed approaches include:

- Possible detrimental effects on an already limited sense of altruism and social solidarity
- The prospect that they will be ineffective in increasing the supply of organs.

The system of encouraged voluntarism provides a refreshing and unusual outlet for altruistic behaviour in a society whose members are, for the most part, motivated by economic self-interest. Ours would be a better society, it could be plausibly argued, if the sense of social solidarity and altruistic motivation characteristic of organ donation were extended to other spheres. Yet replacing, or even supplementing, the current system of encouraged voluntarism with one or another market based approach may, some believe, further undermine social solidarity and altruism.[20] Whether this is true is, however, a matter of dispute.[17-19] As to whether market based approaches will actually increase the supply of organs, Childress[17] contends that: "the fears and attitudes that [presently] reduce the effectiveness of a system based on voluntary donations can reasonably be expected to destroy a system based on sales. If, for example, someone is reluctant now to sign a donor card for fear that proper care may not be received in the hospital, it is easy to imagine that person's fears about accepting money (even in the form of health insurance reductions) for delivery of organs upon death" (p. 2146). It is not so much the particular system as the fear of a premature declaration of death, Childress suggests, that stands in the way of increasing the supply of organs.

Whether to adopt or experiment with one or another market based approach to organ procurement remains an open question. Those in favour of such approaches have been developing more refined proposals that avoid criticisms levelled at the prospect of exploitative bidding wars,[13, 15] whereas those opposed to them point to promising reforms and refinements in the system of encouraged voluntarism.[17, 20, 21]

New sources of organs

Problems of procurement might be eased – or conceivably eliminated – by the development of new sources of organs, including:

- Anencephalic infants and patients in persistent vegetative state (PVS)

- Living non-renal donors
- Non-traditional donors
- Xenografts
- Artificial organs.

Anencephaly and PVS

Anencephalic infants and those in PVS are totally and permanently unconscious, but they are not, under current conceptions, regarded as dead. Death, as presently conceived, requires permanent cessation of all brain activity, including that of the brain stem. Anencephalic infants and those in PVS have permanent cessation of neocortical function but have functioning brain stems. An anencephalic infant's heart might, for example, be transplanted into an infant with hypoplastic left heart syndrome and parents of an anencephalic infant often wish to donate their infant's organs for transplantation. Despite strenuous efforts by some parents and medical centres to effect use of such organs for transplants, a number of legal, ethical, and medical questions have, at least for the present, forced a moratorium on the practice.[22]

Whether those in PVS should be considered dead, and hence potentially part of the donor pool, is also a matter of controversy. Some ethicists argue that total and permanent loss of consciousness (that is, PVS) is tantamount to death. One, John Fletcher of the University of Virginia, has gone so far as to include a clause in his living will indicating that if he lapses into PVS he wants his organs donated at that time for transplantation.[23] Fletcher acknowledges that this is largely an effort at consciousness raising, but he and a number of other ethicists believe that the identification of PVS with death is an idea whose time has come. It is usually estimated that, in the USA, there are about 10 000 individuals in PVS. If those in PVS were to be pronounced dead, there would be a significant increase in the pool of potential organ donors.

Living non-renal donors

Recent developments in transplantation of parts of the small intestine, lung, pancreas, and liver from living donors raise both promise and problems. The promise is that of a larger pool of transplantable organs. The problems centre on ethics, as illustrated

361

by liver transplantation with living donors. Before implementing a protocol for transplanting a liver lobe from a parent to a non-critically ill infant with advanced liver disease, a group of transplant surgeons and clinical ethicists at the University of Chicago "convened a yearlong series of seminars and discussions that were open to the entire University community".[24] The group examined a variety of issues involving balance of risks and benefits, selection of donor and recipient, and informed consent. The procedure has proved medically feasible as well as ethically justifiable, and should provide some increase in the supply of transplantable livers, as well as other benefits.[25]

Non-traditional donors

One way to expand the supply of organs is the use of more high risk or marginal donors – for example, older donors or those with conditions such as diabetes, hypertension, hypotension, treatable infections, non-heart-beating donors, and those with abnormal organ function, high risk of viral infection, and past history of malignancy. "This approach", as Alexander puts it, "has the distinct disadvantage that the success rate might not be as high as with the use of optimal donors, and certain legal risks exist for the transplant team. On the other hand, the use of non-traditional donors could make transplantation available to a substantially larger number of patients with an overall improvement in survival from end-stage organ failure".[6] A central ethical issue is whether at least some of the 2206 patients who died while awaiting an organ in 1990 would have been better off if they had received an organ from a non-traditional donor (assuming these were the only alternatives).

Xenografts

Scientific progress in successfully transplanting the organs of non-primate animals into humans would do much to alleviate the organ shortage.[26] Primates, though perhaps posing fewer scientific problems, raise special ethical problems – due to their higher mental capacities – and practical problems – due to their limited numbers. Ethical problems will also arise in using non-primate donors. If however, livers from pigs could be transplanted into those with end stage liver disease with something like the same success currently experienced with human livers, it would be difficult for a society that routinely dines on pork and bacon to object. Indeed, given the nutritional adequacy of an informed vegetarian diet, regretfully taking the life of a pig for purposes of transplantation seems more justifiable than taking its life in order to please the palate.[27]

Artificial organs

The development of, say, an effective, practical artificial (or manufacturable) liver would, of course, yield as many transplantable livers as money could buy. But that is the hitch. How expensive would such organs be? And would we, as individuals and as a society, be willing and able to pay for them, especially as the percentage of the gross domestic product spent on health care continues to rise? Answers to this question require considering procurement issues alongside those of payment, which is done below.

Allocation

So long as supply falls short of demand, we shall have to devise methods and principles for allocating transplantable organs. Determining such methods and principles is not a purely scientific or value neutral undertaking. It is inescapably a matter of ethics – involving conflicts between such values as loyalty to particular patients, maximising overall medical utility (saving the greatest number of person-years of life or quality adjusted life years (QALYs)), justice or equity, and respect for autonomy.[28]

Selecting patient selection criteria

Any proposed system of allocation must ultimately be conveyed to, and directly or indirectly ratified by, the public, without whose money and donated organs transplantation would be impossible. A guiding thought, therefore, as we consider arguments for or against various proposals should be whether we can reasonably expect that a particular proposal would be ratified by the public, especially by those patients in need of a transplant who will not meet the proposed selection criteria.

The philosopher Thomas Scanlon suggests that an act can be justified if it follows from a system of rules which, on reflection, cannot reasonably be rejected by anyone seeking informed, unforced, general agreement about the matter in question.[29] Extended to organ allocation, this suggestion implies that our aim should be a set of patient selection criteria which, given scarcity and the need for general agreement, cannot reasonably be rejected by anyone seeking a fair, efficient, and workable system for allocating organs. Foremost in our minds should be medically eligible patients who will not receive organs under the chosen policy. Given the facts and the need for agreement on a uniform policy, can we reasonably expect them to endorse the criteria we have employed?

That a patient who could benefit from a new organ does not receive one is always unfortunate, but it need not be unfair.[30] There is little we can do in the immediate future to eliminate the scarcity of organs and the corresponding need to select some patients for transplantation over others. We can, however, try to ensure that the criteria guiding these unfortunate decisions could be acknowledged as the best available by all to whom they apply.

General principles

The Ethics Committee of the United Network for Organ Sharing (UNOS)* recently developed a statement of general principles to be employed in organ allocation.[31] The Committee identified three principles for providing an adequate framework for most allocation decisions:

- Utility (interpreted as net medical benefit)
- Justice (requiring fair or equitable treatment to all awaiting organs)
- Autonomy (respecting informed self-directing patient choice, even if this may not in certain instances maximise utility or promote equitable distribution).

*Annual Report of the US Scientific Registry for Organ Transplantation and the Organ Procurement and Transplantation Network 1990, UNOS, Richmond, Virginia and the Division of Organ Transplantation, Health Resources and Services Administration, Bethesda, Maryland.

The Committee acknowledged the possibility of conflicts between these principles and addressed means of resolving them.

One strategy is to establish a fixed ranking of the principles – to prioritise or lexically to order them in some way – and always to follow this ranking. This was however, rejected as overly rigid. Whatever ranking one establishes ahead of time, it is always possible to imagine a situation in which adhering to it would be absurd. A second strategy is to address conflicts as they arise by appeal to one's intuitions. The problem here is that people's intuitions differ widely on these matters, resulting in deadlock or a lack of uniformity from one transplant centre to another.

A third strategy, which the Committee endorsed, is to acknowledge the complexity of the situation and the impossibility of fully eliminating conflict among the three principles. With regard to conflicts between utility and justice, for example, the Committee states:[31]

> While members of the Committee hold diverging positions regarding the ethically correct relations between utility and justice, a consensus has been reached for purposes of policy relative to organ and tissue allocation: utility ... and justice (or fairness in distribution) should be given equal status. This means that it is unacceptable for an allocation policy to single-mindedly strive to maximize aggregate medical good without any consideration of justice in distribution or for a policy to be single-minded about promoting justice at the expense of the overall (medical) good.   (page 2229)

The general idea is that in cases of conflict justice and utility require equal consideration. The Committee reasoned as follows:

> We make this proposal fully realizing that it may not square with the personal morality of many people. Some would insist on higher priority for utility; others for equity. In fact, whole classes of people might be so inclined invariably to favor one of these principles or the other. The fact that one group would give very heavy weight to one or the other of the principles cannot, for public policy purposes, settle the matter. Inasmuch as: (1) neither side can provide conclusive arguments for its position; (2) each side can provide plausible arguments for its position; and (3) ours is a pluralistic society in which individual views cover the entire spectrum from pure utilitarianism to extreme egalitarianism, we believe that giving equal consideration to each is a fair and workable compromise.
> (page 2230)

This general position seems to underlie the computerised UNOS point system for allocating livers. Candidates for particular livers in the USA are awarded a certain number of points for such facts as *blood type* (recipients with the same ABO type as the donor are awarded 10 points, those with compatible but not identical types are given 5 points, and those with incompatible types receive no points), *time on the waiting list* (10 points for those waiting longest with fewer points for those with shorter tenure), and *degree of medical urgency* (ranging from 24 points for the most urgent to no points for the least urgent). Taking account of blood type seems to reflect utilitarian considerations, considering time on the waiting list reflects considerations of justice, and awarding points for degree of medical urgency some combination of both.

Some variation or refinement of the UNOS Ethics Committee's statement of general principles in organ allocation may be as close as we can come to one that could not be reasonably rejected by anyone seeking informed, unforced, general agreement. Policies that are true to the complexity of the issues and of ourselves often require trade-offs among a number of important principles, none of which, on reflection, we, as a society, are prepared to relinquish. Well grounded compromises that mirror our ambivalence while acknowledging all of the things we value may, in some situations, be the best we can do.[28]

Alcoholism and liver transplantation

An issue special to liver transplantation is whether carefully selected, abstinent alcoholics who meet the conventional criteria should be allowed to compete equally with non-alcoholics for livers available for transplantation. There are three main positions. The first argues that patients whose end stage liver disease is attributable to alcohol consumption are personally responsible for their organ failure in a way that other patients are not and they should, accordingly, always have a lower priority for receiving a new liver than patients whose liver failure is attributable to other factors.[32] The second position maintains that carefully selected, alcoholic patients meeting the criteria should, as a matter of justice, be allowed to compete equally with non-alcoholic patients.[33] A third position is a compromise between the two. The fact that alcohol consumption is likely to have contributed to a carefully selected transplant candidate's end stage liver disease should, on this view, be given some weight in allocation decisions, but not so much that such candidates invariably have a lower priority than others. A recent analysis of these views concludes that there is little practical difference between the second and third and that each is preferable, from an ethical point of view, to the first.[34]

Payment

Transplantation is very expensive. Proposals in the late 1980s to cut medical costs or to ration health care often recommended dropping public payment for transplantation in favour of more cost effective forms of care.[35, 36] Improvements in the success rates of transplantation have since altered such recommendations.[37, 38] Although the earliest versions of the State of Oregon's proposal to ration health care for Medicaid recipients eliminated payment for all non-renal transplantation, the most recent version includes payment for all transplantation except for alcohol related liver failure. Questions remain, however, about whether ability to pay should ever be a condition for being placed on a waiting list for a new organ.

There is a compelling argument, based on the special nature of transplantation, for making access to transplantation available to all who can benefit, regardless of ability to pay. The argument assumes a nationwide procurement system based on either encouraged voluntarism (with or without required request) or presumed consent. Prospective donors in such systems are urged to provide organs for the good of the public or community as a whole, not only for the good of those who can afford to pay for the operations and the follow up care. Moreover, individuals or their families are asked to donate organs regardless of their financial status. If one's income or insurance coverage is irrelevant to one's status as a donor, the argument maintains, it should be similarly irrelevant to one's status as a recipient. The injustice of urging those who cannot themselves afford to be recipients to become donors is compounded when one considers that transplantation is heavily dependent (for research, training, the organ sharing system) on public funds to which all, poor and rich, must be presumed to contribute. Under such circumstances it is *unfair*, and not simply unfortunate, that one might qualify as a donor but not, because of one's limited income, as a recipient.

This argument is grounded not on an absolute right to access to an organ, but rather on fairness and the special nature of transplantation. *If* the transplantation system depends on public funding and is

367

designed for the welfare of the community as a whole, access to new organs ought to be available to all who can benefit, regardless of personal ability to pay. The argument does, however, have limitations. It will not apply as strongly to xenografts or the implantation of artificial organs – for these do not require personal donation. (It may be useful, in this connection, to distinguish the *trans*plantation of human organs from the *im*plantation of animal or artificial organs.) Still, to the extent that the research, development, and training necessary for successful employment of xenografts and artificial organs are publicly funded, there is a case for access to all who can benefit, regardless of ability to pay.

Interrelationships

Although distinguished here for analytical purposes, issues of procurement, access, and payment are closely interrelated.[39] Success in organ procurement, for example, depends on public donation. If the public perceives what it regards as significant injustices in either allocation or payment, support for organ donation is likely to suffer. A reduction in support for donation will, in turn, further increase the gap between supply and demand for organs and, as a result, intensify dilemmas of allocation.

Another relationship involves procurement and payment. The overall cost of transplantation is currently limited by the correspondingly limited supply of organs. The development of successful xenografting or artificial organs is, however, likely to result in a significant change. If the supply of organs, like that of dialysis machines, is limited only by our willingness or ability to pay for them, a new series of issues will emerge about access to transplantation and its cost effectiveness compared to other demands on the limited health care monies.

No other area of medicine is at this time so directly dependent on public support as organ transplantation. And no other area raises as many different, but interrelated, ethical issues. Insensitivity to some of these issues, Caplan suggests, has provided "important reasons to worry that the public trust requisite for both the provision of organs and the money to pay for them is eroding".[39] The trust of the public, both now and in the future, depends as much on attention to ethical issues as it does on success in the laboratory and in the operating room.

References

1 Caplan AL. Requests, gifts, and obligations: the ethics of organ procurement. *Transplant Proc* 1986; **18** (Suppl 2): 49–56.
2 Caplan AL. Organ transplants: the costs of success. *Hastings Center Report* 1983; **13**: 23–32.
3 Virnig BA, Caplan AL. Required request: what difference has it made? *Transplant Proc* 1992; **24**: 2155–8.
4 Youngner SL, Allen M, Bartlett ET, *et al.* Psychosocial and ethical implications of organ retrieval. *N Engl J Med* 1985; **313**: 321–4.
5 Youngner SL. Psychological impediments to procurement. *Transplant Proc* 1992; **24**: 2159–61.
6 Alexander JW. High-risk donors: diabetics, the elderly, and others. *Transplant Proc* 1992; **24**: 221–2.
7 Caplan AL. Ethical and policy issues in the procurement of cadaver organs for transplantation. *N Engl J Med* 1984; **311**: 981–3.
8 Cohen C. The case for presumed consent to transplant human organs after death. *Transplant Proc* 1992; **24**: 2168–72.
9 Land W, Cohen B. Postmortem and living organ donation in Europe: transplant laws and activities. *Tranplant Proc* 1992; **24**: 2165–7.
10 Sadler BL. Presumed consent to organ transplantation: a different perspective. *Transplant Proc* 1992; **24**: 2173–4.
11 Daar AS. Rewarded gifting. *Transplant Proc* 1992; **24**: 2207–11.
12 Peters TG. Life or death: the issue of payment in cadaveric organ donation. *JAMA* 1991; **265**: 1302–5.
13 Schwindt R, Vining AR. Proposal for a future delivery market for transplant organs. *J Health Polit Policy Law* 1986; **11**: 483–500.
14 Cohen LR. Increasing the supply of transplant organs: the virtues of a futures market. *George Washington University Law Review* 1989; **58**: xx.
15 Blumstein, JF. The case for commerce in transplantation. *Transplant Proc* 1992; **24**: 2190–7.
16 Pellegrino ED. Families' self-interest and the cadaver's organs: what price consent? *JAMA* 1991; **265**: 1305–6.
17 Childress JF. The body as property: some philosophical reflections. *Transplant Proc* 1992; **24**: 2143–8.
18 Andrews LB. The body as property: some philosophical reflections – a response to J. F. Childress. *Transplant Proc* 1992; **24**: 2149–51.
19 Tomlinson T. Inducements for donation: benign incentives or risky business. *Transplant Proc* 1992; **24**: 2204–6.
20 Sells RA. The case against buying organs and a futures market in transplants. *Transplant Proc* 1992; **24**: 2198–202.
21 Evans RW. Need, demand, and supply in organ transplantation. *Transplant Proc* 1992; **24**: 2152–4.
22 Cranford RE. Anencephalic infants as organ donors. *Transplant Proc* 1989; **24**: 2218–20.
23 Kolata G. Ethicists debating a new definition of death. *New York Times*, 21 April 1992.
24 Singer, Peter A, *et al.* (1989). Ethics of liver transplantation with living donors. *N Engl J Med* **321**: 620–2.
25 Siegler M. Liver transplantation using living donors. *Transplant Proc* 1992; **24**: 2223–4.
26 Reemstra K. Xenografts. *Transplant Proc* 1992; **24**: 2225.
27 Benjamin M. Ethics and animal consciousness. In: Mappes, TA, Zembaty JS, eds. *Social Ethics: Morality and Social Policy*, 3rd Ed. New York: McGraw-Hill, 1987: 476–84.

369

28 Benjamin M. Value conflicts in organ allocation. *Transplant Proc* 1989; **21**: 3378–80.
29 Scanlon TM. Contractualism and utilitarianism. In: Sen A, Williams B, eds. *Utilitarianism and Beyond*. Cambridge: Cambridge University Press, 1982: 103–28.
30 Engelhardt HT. Allocating scarce medical resources and the availability of organ transplantation. *N Engl J Med* 1984; **311**: 66–71.
31 Ethics Committee United Network for Organ Sharing. General principles for allocating human organs and tissues. *Transplant Proc* 1992; **24**: 2227–37.
32 Moss AH, Siegler M. Should alcoholics compete equally for liver transplantation? *JAMA* 1991; **265**: 1295–8.
33 Cohen C, Benjamin M, *et al*. Alcoholics and liver transplantation. *JAMA* 1991; **265**: 1299–301.
34 Benjamin M, Turcotte JG. Ethics, alcoholism, and liver transplantation. In: Lucey, MR, Merion R, Beresford TP, eds. *Liver Transplantation and the Alcoholic Patient*. Cambridge: Cambridge University Press, 1993; in press.
35 Welch HG, Larson EB. Dealing with limited resources: the Oregon decision to curtail funding for organ transplantation. *N Engl J Med* 1988; **319**: 171–3.
36 Callahan D. *What Kind of Life: The Limits of Medical Progress*. New York: Simon and Schuster, 1990.
37 Evans RW. *Executive Summary: The National Cooperative Transplantation Study*, BHARC-100-91. Seattle: Battelle–Seattle Research Center, 1991.
38 Turcotte JG. Supply, demand, and the ethics of organ procurement: the medical perspective. *Transplant Proc* 1992; **24**: 2140–2.
39 Caplan AL. Problems in the policies and criteria used to allocate organs for transplantation in the United States. *Transplant Proc* 1989; **21**: 3381–7.

19: The costs and benefits of liver transplantation

STIRLING BRYAN, MARTIN J BUXTON

Introduction

Within appropriate equity constraints, priority in funding for health care programmes or procedures should be given to those activities that generate the most health gain for every pound or dollar of resources that is devoted to them. Liver transplantation should be no exception. Considerable resources are already being devoted to liver transplantation and as it develops further the potential is for the demand for resources to increase considerably. It is therefore most important that future funding decisions be based on good information about both benefits and costs. Transplantation of other solid organs, particularly kidneys and hearts, has been subject to a number of rigorous evaluations, and hence decisions about these can be made on a relatively firm basis of good information on what is achieved and at what cost. There is, as a result, widespread agreement that renal transplantation is a relatively attractive technology to fund in terms of its cost effectiveness ratio, and several studies of heart transplantation show that, although it is less cost effective than kidney transplantation, it is more cost effective than many other well established and routinely funded procedures. Liver transplantation has not been evaluated to the same degree. Although there is little doubt that liver transplantation has become increasingly successful in extending the lives of some specific categories of patients with end stage liver disease, there appears to be a very high cost associated with this complex intervention.

The starting point, from an economist's perspective, in making decisions about any health care technology is the concept of resource scarcity. Society will always be unable to produce all desired outputs and thus choices between health care technologies will have to be made. Economic evaluation can be defined as "the comparative analysis of alternative courses of action in terms of both their costs and consequences".

It addresses the question of whether a particular health care technology, such as liver transplantation, should be funded when compared with the other activities, such as other solid organ transplantation, that could be provided with equivalent resources. The cost of a technology should be calculated to reflect all the resources devoted to it regardless of their source, and so should include patients' own resources as well as those of the health care sector. An assessment of the consequences of deploying a technology should include the impact it has on the patient's expected survival and the quality of that survival. The results of economic evaluations are commonly expressed as a ratio of cost to effect – for example, net cost per additional year of survival gained or net cost per quality adjusted year of survival (QALY) gained. The latter requires a weighting to be attached to the years of survival to reflect the associated quality of life.[1] The "cost per QALY" approach to the assessment of the cost effectiveness of health care interventions has been applied extensively in North America and is increasing in popularity in the UK and the rest of Europe.

This form of analysis can then be used to establish priorities on the basis of efficiency: technologies with a lower cost per unit of effect should be given funding ahead of those with a higher cost per unit of effect. Liver transplantation will have several different cost effectiveness ratios because the benefits and costs of the procedure almost certainly differ according to the nature of the underlying disease instigating the need for transplantation. Thus, the cost effectiveness ratio for liver transplantation for patients with primary biliary cirrhosis is likely to differ from the ratio for patients with carcinoma of the liver.

This chapter will review our current level of knowledge on the benefits and costs of liver transplantation and, in the process, will identify key parameters on which information has to be generated if the cost effectiveness ratios relating to the procedures are to be established.

Costs

In assessing the cost of a transplant procedure, several distinct components should be considered: evaluation and screening;

candidacy and organ procurement; transplantation; and post-trans-plantation. Evaluation and screening costs are those associated with "working up" a patient to determine if he or she is a suitable candidate for a transplant. Candidacy and organ procurement costs are incurred immediately following the acceptance of a patient as a transplant recipient through to the period immediately before the transplantation. Transplantation costs are accumulated during the surgical procedure itself, and postoperative costs are any costs arising subsequently, including the costs of long term immunosup-pression and monitoring.

Very few studies to date have included a comprehensive analysis of the costs of liver transplantation; most focus on the costs of the transplantation episode itself. The study reported by Kankaanpaa[2] of a small ($n = 32$) heterogeneous group of US liver transplant recipients details an average hospital stay of 64 days. All studies to date have measured accumulated charges which are subject to local pricing variance. A formal prospective assessment of charges, which have been captured and weighted appropriately, has not been conducted. The National Health Services and Practice Patterns Survey[3] of liver transplant operating costs undertaken across many hospitals in the USA provides similar results for the levels of resource use as those already indicated. They report an average hospital length of stay of 67 days with an average stay in intensive care of 19 days. Their survey also investigated operating time and found the average surgical time to be 19 hours. A more recent UK study[4] suggests that, as with the transplantation of other organs, experience and improved immunosuppression have reduced length of inpatient stay post-transplantation. For a small ($n = 23$) hetero-geneous group of UK liver transplant recipients, Burroughs et al.[4] describe in detail the nature of the resources devoted to the care of patients. The median stay in intensive care post-transplantation was four days and the median total hospital stay, excluding readmission due to complications, was 43 days. The total health service cost in the first six months post-transplantation was estimated to be £16 000 (1991 US$25 000)*. This price is considerably less than that reported from the USA – for example, Evans estimated that the median accumulated charges for the liver transplant procedure in the USA was US$145 795 (£97 200).[5]

*All cost figures have been converted to 1991 US dollar equivalents using the OECD GDP purchasing power parity index and the gross domestic product (GDP) price index.

The importance in cost terms of the choice of appropriate drug therapy is demonstrated in the USA by Staschak et al.[6] who showed that total hospital charges for a liver transplant recipient could be significantly reduced by switching from one type of immunosuppression (cyclosporin A or cyclosporine) to another (FK506). The reduction in hospital charges per patient were estimated to be in excess of US$100 000 (1991 US$108 600) which largely reflected reduced hospital inpatient stay from an average of 36 days with cyclosporin A to only 16 days with FK506, and a reduced number of postoperative problems. Although there can be little doubt that the need to provide an extended period of hospital inpatient care contributes greatly to the cost of a liver transplant, Bonsel et al.[7] show that the requirement for intensive pharmaceutical provision is also a significant factor in determining overall cost. They estimate that in the Netherlands drugs account for about 12% of the total cost in the first year post-transplantation. Liver transplant recipients will receive drug regimens that include immunosuppression, treatment of acute cellular rejection, and treatments for viral and bacterial infections when required.

A problem with many of the existing cost analyses of liver transplantation is that they tend not be explicit with regard to the resource parameters included in the analysis. However, even when studies are explicit in this respect it is evident that their coverage of resources is incomplete. This makes cost comparisons across studies particularly difficult. The most comprehensive analysis of the costs of liver transplantation and the cost of the alternative of non-transplant care has been undertaken as part of the evaluation of the Dutch liver transplant programme which calculated the net cost of a liver transplant, including postoperative costs for up to five years, to be Dfl190 000 (1991 US$96 000). This estimate of cost is probably the most accurate that currently exists but may be very specific to the patients in that study, the practices of the single transplant centre involved, and the Dutch health care setting. Although this study provides an excellent example of the rigorous evaluation work that is required, additional studies are needed elsewhere to determine whether the cost effectiveness results obtained are generalisable.

To determine the true net cost of a transplant procedure requires that some form of alternative care be costed for the patient. This would consist of whatever care the patient would have received had the transplant not been offered. Attempts to calculate such alternative costs have (in the absence of a formal comparative study) resulted in estimates that vary greatly. However, in terms of the costs of the procedure itself, there is general agreement that the high degree of complexity associated with a liver transplant makes it one of the most costly of all solid organ transplant procedures. Set against this is the fact that caring for a patient who, in the absence of a liver transplant, will progressively deteriorate and die is itself a costly option and must be considered as part of any assessment of the additional resource requirements of a liver transplant.

Benefits

Survival

Information on survival after liver transplantation is widely reported in the literature, but it too tends to relate to results from specific centres with the problem that the number of patients considered then tends to be relatively small. The exceptions to this are the reports that are based on the liver transplant registries, notably the United Network for Organ Sharing Scientific Liver Transplant Registry at the University of Pittsburg (PITT-UNOS LTR),[8] which gives a broader picture of the survival paths, based on larger numbers of transplantations. A general pattern which is clearly evident is that the survival rates have improved markedly over time. As McMaster and Dousset[9] show, liver transplantation in Europe prior to 1984 had a one year survival rate of only 33%, but the 1635 patients grafted in 1990 had a 74·6% survival rate at one year. In the USA, one year patient survival for patients undergoing transplantation between October 1987 and September 1988 was 72%, and one year graft survival was 64%.[8] Several authors report significant differences in patient survival for patients in different diagnostic categories. The PITT-UNOS LTR data show the worst outcome to be for patients with either fulminant liver failure or malignancies (one year survival of 58% and 57% respectively) and better outcomes for patients with cholestatic cirrhosis or "other" cirrhosis (one year survival of 76% and 77% respectively). Results of the European Liver Transplant Registry reported by Bismuth[10] for all liver transplantations between 1968 and 1986 indicate that, in terms of three year survival, better results have been achieved in patients with post-hepatic cirrhosis (68·5%) and primary biliary cirrhosis (65·5%), and less favourable outcomes for patients with hepatocellular carcinoma (41%). Direct comparison of the results from the two registries is inappropriate because of differences in the time periods covered by the two registries, differences in the length of survival considered, and possible differences in the case-mix of patients transplanted.

Focusing specifically on liver transplantations in children, a recent paper by Salt et al.[11] described the survival experience of 100 children receiving transplants in the UK between 1983 and 1990. Most underwent transplantation because they suffered from biliary atresia. The survival rate at one year was 71%, falling to 64% at just over two years. This is generally consistent with the sort of survival figures being quoted by the European and US registries, and stresses the apparently favourable survival picture being provided by paediatric liver transplantation for biliary atresia.

As with costs, the more difficult question to assess is what would have happened without transplantation. The reported survival rates discussed above beg the question of the survival patients would have achieved in the absence of transplantation but with the best alternative therapy. This issue has never been addressed in the context of a randomised clinical trial but has been considered in other ways, mainly for patients with primary biliary cirrhosis (PBC). Neuberger et al.[12] detailed the survival experience of 29 PBC patients receiving transplants before April 1984 and is one of the first studies also to have estimated survival in the absence of transplantation. The latter was estimated using a statistical model derived from historical data collected on PBC patients who did not receive a transplant. The poor results reported actual survival with transplantation exceeding expected survival without transplantation in only 11 out of 29 cases. This, in part, is a reflection on the early stage of development of the technology. Bonsel et al.[13] also report survival estimates for PBC patients without liver transplantation. They conclude that, for PBC patients with Child–Pugh classes B and C, transplantation significantly improves long term survival. Other studies have consistently reported one year survival for PBC patients to be in excess of 65% and up to 82%.

The general picture that emerges from studies of liver transplantation in patients with PBC is that most deaths in transplant recipients occur in the first two or three months post-surgery, and, thus, the survival rate in transplant recipients is similar to the expected survival without transplantation (generated using statistical models) over this initial period. Beyond the first few months, however, the observed and expected survival rates differ significantly in all studies of PBC patients, and thus liver transplantation does appear to improve long term survival for PBC patients. One caveat is that the models used to predict survival without transplantation have all been based on historical PBC patients, and therefore may have tended towards overestimating the benefits of transplantation if the results of non-transplant therapy have improved, or if it is the case that the more severe PBC patients are not referred for transplantation but such patients are included in the control population.

The general improvement in survival post-transplantation seen in the late 1980s and early 1990s has not resulted from the selection of more straightforward cases, according to McMaster and Dousset,[9] but may in part be explained by a change in the patient categories selected for grafting. In Europe, as a proportion of all liver transplantations, fewer are being undertaken in patients with tumours, and more children and adolescents are undergoing transplantations.

Quality of life

As the evidence on the effectiveness of liver transplantation to improve survival becomes more convincing, it is appropriate to ask questions about the quality of that extended survival. A very interesting sociological investigation into the "impact" of a liver transplant programme has been undertaken in the Netherlands.[14] Most of the patients in the study had previously been suffering from a prolonged illness and some, once they had received a new liver, experienced difficulties in adjusting psychologically to their changed situation. It is clear that liver transplantation was successful in most cases with many patients being happy with their physical condition post-transplantation. However, there were unavoidable difficulties related to the requirements for both prolonged after care post-transplantation and prolonged medication. Varying degrees of immunosuppressive, drug-related side effects were experienced, such as changes in appearance, which patients found unpleasant and annoying but seldom complained about. The older patients, those over 50 years, were positive about liver transplantation despite its problems because, for example, they could now "enjoy watching their grandchildren grow up". The younger patients too viewed the procedure positively, although there is the suggestion that the need for long term medication, with its associated adverse side effects, has the potential to upset their newly found "mental balance" especially if this is viewed as a constraint on their career or social ambitions. Overall, the authors conclude that, for many, liver transplantation provides great improvement in various aspects of functioning, and only for a minority is there little or no benefit. Although liver transplant recipients appear in this study to have, on average, more physical, social, and emotional problems than might be expected for a comparable group of "normal" individuals, they nevertheless tend to view the situation with satisfaction and hope.

The problem with such detailed qualitative analysis, however, is that it does not lend itself to comparative analysis of the health related quality of life benefits from different procedures. The most commonly used quantitative generic indicator of quality of life in studies of liver transplantation in adults has been the Sickness Impact Profile (SIP), developed in the USA, which quantifies the impact of disease on everyday functioning in terms of physical, cognitive, and behavioural limitations. The studies that have used the SIP show that adult liver transplant recipients improve on virtually all SIP scales post-transplantation but show some impairment compared to "normal" scores for parameters relating to sleeping, eating, working, and recreation. Two evaluative studies have assessed quality of life using the Nottingham Health Profile (NHP), a similar but shorter generic quality of life measurement instrument developed in the UK which examines an individual's physical, social, and emotional functioning. Liver transplant recipients tended to show general improvements on the NHP scales compared to their scores pre-transplantation, and in comparison with community "norm" scores showed fewer problems related to emotional reactions but greater problems related to physical mobility.

A small number of studies have assessed, in the context of paediatric liver transplant recipients, a range of parameters that may broadly be included under the heading quality of life for paediatric patients. Generally, it appears that liver transplantation is associated with accelerated patient growth, improved patient behaviour, improved patient activity tolerance, normal IQ, and placement in age appropriate school classes.

Comparing costs and benefits

In the USA, Evans[15] reported original estimates of the cost effectiveness of liver transplantation. He quoted a cost effectiveness ratio of US$38 000 (1991 US$47 500) per life year gained. It is difficult to comment on the accuracy or validity of this estimate because he gave virtually no detail on how the estimate was derived. Another USA based study is reported by Kankaanpaa[2] which, rather unhelpfully, analysed separately liver transplant recipients surviving less than one year (1991 US$291 700 per life year saved) and those surviving more than one year (1991 US$62 000 per life year saved). This distinction is unhelpful from a policy perspective. It is more important to know, given expected survival results, the average costs and benefits for the group of patients offered liver transplantation.

The medical technology assessment of liver transplantation in the Netherlands collected data on cost, survival, and patients' quality of life for non-alcoholic cirrhosis patients managed with and without transplantation.[7] They integrated the cost information with the benefit data to express their results as cost per life year gained and cost per quality adjusted life year (QALY) gained. The cost effectiveness ratios ranged from Dfl47 000 to Dfl133 000 (1991 US$23 800 to US$67 300) per life year gained, depending to a large extent on the severity of disease at the time of transplantation. When quality of life adjustments were made to the gained years of life, the cost effectiveness ratios were similar: Dfl51 000 to Dfl133 000 (1991 US$25 800 to US$67 300) per QALY gained. This reflects the finding that patients who survive a liver transplantation tend then to experience a relatively unimpaired life which they value highly. This is the only comprehensive economic evaluation of liver transplantation to have been undertaken in Europe.

Discussion

Should scarce health care resources be dedicated to the activity of liver transplantation and, if so, what level of resources is appropriate? There can be little doubt that for some indications – for example, PBC and biliary atresia – transplantation of the liver has a positive impact on both patient survival and quality of life. However, for some other indications – for example, tumours – the prognosis following transplantation is accepted as being poor. Common to all indications is the fact that liver transplantation is intensive in resource use and, thus, is associated with a high cost. Can the high cost be justified in terms of the benefits it achieves? At the present time we have to say that adequate evidence is not available. Uncertainty exists with regard to the net benefit and net cost associated with the procedure as a treatment for specific causes of liver failure and this is, in part, because it has never been the subject of a randomised controlled trial and because non-experimental methods of calculating net survival for liver transplantation are not particularly satisfactory.

In comparison with research on other solid organ transplant procedures, for example, the major evaluative studies of heart transplantation undertaken in the USA,[16] in the UK,[17] and in the Netherlands,[18] it is evident that relatively little evaluative research on liver transplantation has been funded. From the perspective of evaluation, there are clearly many differences between heart and liver transplantation, most notably the fact that unlike heart transplantation, liver transplantation is indicated for a large number of underlying diseases, and the profiles of benefits and costs differ markedly depending on the disease. Although the published evaluation work undertaken in the Netherlands provides some information on the value of liver transplantation for patients with non-alcoholic cirrhosis, questions remain regarding its value for other indications and the extent to which information on costs and benefits can be transferred from one country or continent to another. For each patient group considered for liver transplantation, defined in part by the nature of the liver disease, evidence is required on survival, quality of life, and costs both for transplant recipients and for similar patients who have not received a transplant. For some indications, it may be that the expected prognosis with liver transplantation is similar to that with the conventional alternative therapy. For such indications, controlled trials are called for to establish the net effectiveness and net costs of the technology. As this basic evaluative evidence is patchy, it should not be surprising to discover that other evaluation questions have not been addressed. Thorough analysis of the relationship between the activity level of a liver transplant centre or surgeon, and patient outcome and cost, has not been undertaken. Thus, there is only very limited evidence on which to base policy on the appropriate distribution and appropriate scale of liver transplant centres. The current proliferation of centres in Europe might then appropriately be questioned, especially given the evidence from other fields of surgery indicating a link between increased scale and improved results.

Even if funding is available, as the demand continues to grow transplant teams will increasingly be faced with the need to decide which patients should be given priority within the constraints of the supply of available donor organs. There may, therefore, have to be a reconsideration of whether it is appropriate to offer transplantation to patients with indications that have poor prognosis, such as the "hopeless transplantation in the final end stage cirrhosis".[9] An efficiency perspective would suggest that priority of claim for a compatible liver should be given to the patient who is expected to benefit most in terms of improvements in survival and quality of life, assuming the cost to be similar for different indications. Questions of equity then become very important: should patients with self-inflicted injuries be given priority over those with injuries that are apparently not self-inflicted? For example, consider the situation of a patient who has taken an overdose of paracetamol (acetaminophen) and who, for the sake of this example, is expected to have a better prognosis than and a similar resource requirement to another patient who, through no obvious fault of his or her own, also requires a liver transplant operation. It would be more efficient to use the available and compatible liver for the paracetamol overdose patient but it may be that the equity considerations of society dictate that patients with self-inflicted injuries should always be given a lower priority. If this were the case then a clear equity–efficiency trade-off exists.

In conclusion, the existing evidence indicates that liver transplantation is effective in improving survival and quality of life for specific indications. The extent of the benefit provided is uncertain because comprehensive information is lacking on the survival and quality of life of patients in the absence of transplantation. The true net cost of providing a transplant is also unclear; estimates vary widely and clearly differ from one country to another. What is certain is that the cost is high and this accentuates the need to establish that the benefits provided by liver transplantation are themselves sufficiently large to justify the cost. It is not clear that all the indications for which liver transplantation is currently provided represent a cost effective use of health care resources. If liver transplantation is to be more widely accepted as an appropriate technology for funding, then a responsibility lies with the community of liver transplant surgeons and physicians to be active in working to establish clearly the specific indications for which it is an effective technology and which have cost effectiveness ratios that are within a reasonable range. Until that is known, the onus must be on health care purchasers to ensure that liver transplantation is only purchased from centres actively involved in properly designed research which can assess the costs and benefits of this exciting but expensive technology.

References

1 Weinstein MC, Fineburg HV. *Clinical Decision Analysis*. Philadelphia: WB Saunders, 1980.
2 Kankaanpaa J. Cost-effectiveness of liver transplantation – how to apply the results in resource allocation. *Prevent Med* 1990; **19**: 700–4.
3 National Health Services and Practice Patterns Survey. *First Year Report on Adult Liver Transplantation Operating Costs, Medicare Payments and Utilisation Rates*. Washington: MTPPI Press, 1988.
4 Burroughs AK, Blake J, Thorne S, Else M, Rolles K. Comparative hospital costs of liver transplantation and the treatment of complications of cirrhosis: a prospective study. *Eur J Gastroenterol Hepatol* 1992; **4**: 123–8.
5 Evans RW. *The National Co-operative Transplantation Survey: Final Report*. Battelle, Seattle, Washington DC, 1991.
6 Staschak S, Wagner S, Block G, *et al*. A cost comparison of liver transplantation with FK506 or CyA as the primary immunosuppressive agent. *Transplant Proc* 1990; **22**: 47.
7 Bonsel GJ, Essink-Bot ML, de Charro FT, van der Maas PJ, Habbema JDF. Orthotopic liver transplantation in the Netherlands: the results of a medical technology assessment. *Health Policy* 1990; **16**: 147–61.
8 Detre KM, Belle SH, Beringer KC, Murphy JB, Vaughn WK. PITT–UNOS Liver Transplant Registry. In: Terasaki P, ed. *Clinical Transplants 1989*, Los Angeles, CA: ULCA Tissue Typing Laboratory, 1989.
9 McMaster P, Doussett B. The improved results of liver transplantation. *Transplant Int* 1992; **5**: 125–8.
10 Bismuth H, Castaing D, Aldridge MC. Hepatic transplantation in Europe: improved survival. *Eur J Gastroenterol Hepatol* 1989; **1**: 79–82.
11 Salt A, Noble-Jamieson G, Barnes ND, *et al*. Liver transplantation in 100 children: Cambridge and King's College Hospital Series. *BMJ* 1992; **304**: 416–21.
12 Neuberger J, Altman DJ, Christensen E, Tygstrup N, Williams R. Use of prognostic index in evaluation of liver transplantation for primary biliary cirrhosis. *Transplantation* 1986; **41**: 713–16.
13 Bonsel GJ, Kompmaker IJ, van't Veer F, Habbema JDF, Sloof MJH. Use of a prognostic model for assessment of value of liver transplantation in primary biliary cirrhosis. *Lancet* 1990; **335**: 493–7.
14 Tymstra TJ, Bucking J, Roorda J, van der Henvel WJA, Gips CH. The psychological impact of a liver transplant programme. *Liver* 1986; **6**: 302–9.

15 Evans RW. Cost-effectiveness analysis of transplantation. *Surg Clin North Am* 1986; **66**: 603–16.
16 Evans RW, Manninen DL, Overcast TD, *et al. The National Heart Transplantation Study: Final Report*. Battelle Human Affairs Research Centres, Seattle, Washington DC, 1984.
17 Buxton M, Acheson R, Caine N, Gibson S, O'Brien B. *Costs and Benefits of the Heart Transplant Programmes at Harefield and Papworth Hospitals: Final Report*. London: HMSO, 1985.
18 van Hout B, Bonsel G, Habbema D, van der Maas P, de Charro F. Heart transplantation in the Netherlands: costs, effects and scenarios. *J Health Econ* 1993; **12**, 73–93.

Index